A CULTURAL HISTORY
OF MEDICINE

VOLUME 4

A Cultural History of Medicine
General Editor: Roger Cooter

Volume 1
A Cultural History of Medicine in Antiquity
Edited by Laurence Totelin

Volume 2
A Cultural History of Medicine in the Middle Ages
Edited by Iona McCleery

Volume 3
A Cultural History of Medicine in the Renaissance
Edited by Elaine Leong and Claudia Stein

Volume 4
A Cultural History of Medicine in the Enlightenment
Edited by Lisa Wynne Smith

Volume 5
A Cultural History of Medicine in the Age of Empire
Edited by Jonathan Reinarz

Volume 6
A Cultural History of Medicine in the Modern Age
Edited by Todd Meyers

A CULTURAL HISTORY OF MEDICINE
IN THE ENLIGHTENMENT

Edited by Lisa Wynne Smith

BLOOMSBURY ACADEMIC
LONDON • NEW YORK • OXFORD • NEW DELHI • SYDNEY

BLOOMSBURY ACADEMIC
Bloomsbury Publishing Plc
50 Bedford Square, London, WC1B 3DP, UK
1385 Broadway, New York, NY 10018, USA
29 Earlsfort Terrace, Dublin 2, Ireland

BLOOMSBURY, BLOOMSBURY ACADEMIC and the Diana logo are trademarks
of Bloomsbury Publishing Plc

First published in Great Britain 2021
This paperback edition first published 2024

Copyright © Bloomsbury Publishing, 2021

Lisa Wynne Smith has asserted her right under the Copyright, Designs
and Patents Act, 1988, to be identified as Editor of this work.

Cover image: © Heritage Images / Getty Images

All rights reserved. No part of this publication may be reproduced or transmitted in any
form or by any means, electronic or mechanical, including photocopying, recording, or
any information storage or retrieval system, without prior permission in writing from
the publishers.

Bloomsbury Publishing Plc does not have any control over, or responsibility for, any third-party
websites referred to or in this book. All internet addresses given in this book were correct at
the time of going to press. The author and publisher regret any inconvenience caused if
addresses have changed or sites have ceased to exist, but can accept no responsibility
for any such changes.

A catalogue record for this book is available from the British Library.

Library of Congress Cataloging-in-Publication Data
Names: Cooter, Roger, editor.
Title: A cultural history of medicine / general editor, Roger Cooter.
Description: London ; New York : Bloomsbury Academic, 2021. |
Series: The cultural histories series | Includes bibliographical references and index. |
Identifiers: LCCN 2020051490 | ISBN 9781472569936 (hardback)
Subjects: LCSH: Medicine–History.
Classification: LCC R131 .C78 2021 | DDC 610.9—dc23
LC record available at https://lccn.loc.gov/2020051490

ISBN:	HB:	978-1-4725-6990-5
	Set:	978-1-4725-6987-5
	PB:	978-1-3504-5160-5
	Set:	978-1-3504-5164-3

Series: The Cultural Histories Series

Typeset by RefineCatch Limited, Bungay, Suffolk
Printed and bound in Great Britain

To find out more about our authors and books visit www.bloomsbury.com
and sign up for our newsletters.

CONTENTS

LIST OF ILLUSTRATIONS   vii
ACKNOWLEDGEMENTS   ix
GENERAL EDITOR'S PREFACE   x
    Roger Cooter

Introduction   1
    Lisa Wynne Smith, Claudia Stein and Roger Cooter

1   Environment   13
    Erin Spinney

2   Food   29
    E.C. Spary

3   Disease   51
    Lina Minou

4   Animals   73
    Monica Mattfeld

5   Objects   103
    Marieke M.A. Hendriksen

6   Experiences   125
    Micheline Louis-Courvoisier

7	Mind/Brain *Claudia Stein and Roger Cooter*	151
8	Authority *Angela Haas*	169
REFERENCES		193
NOTES ON CONTRIBUTORS		227
INDEX		229

ILLUSTRATIONS

INTRODUCTION

0.1	The Enlightenment Gallery at the British Museum.	2
0.2	Sir Hans Sloane, by J. Faber, Junior.	3
0.3	Trade card recommending 'Sir Hans Sloane's Milk Chocolate'.	4

CHAPTER 1

1.1	*The Torrid Zone, or, Blessings of Jamaica*.	14
1.2	The port of Marseille during the plague of 1720.	15
1.3	A physician wearing a seventeenth-century plague prevention costume.	16
1.4	Johnny New-Come in the island of Jamaica *c.* 1800.	23

CHAPTER 2

2.1	Diet in the classical repertoire.	32
2.2	A German view of the dangers of coffee drinking for health.	33
2.3	An early eighteenth-century Dutch posset pot with Chinese decoration.	34
2.4	Thea Bohea.	36
2.5	Sanctorius on his scales.	40
2.6	Jacob Powell, butcher, of Stebbing in Essex.	41
2.7	Quantifying breakfast.	44

CHAPTER 3

3.1	Eight heads depicting the human passions.	56
3.2	Jacques Callot, *Envy*.	58

3.3	Face showing peaceful joy.	63
3.4	Face showing anger.	66

CHAPTER 4

4.1	Woodcut of an elephant.	82
4.2	Handbill advertising the exhibition at 'Mr Becket's, Trunk Maker, No. 31, Hay Market'.	89
4.3	James Gillray, *Monstrous Craws*.	100
4.4	Thomas Rowlandson, *The Monstrous Craw; or a New Discovered Animal*.	101

CHAPTER 5

5.1	Opaque glass apothecary jar for preparation of the human skull.	107
5.2	Page from Hans Sloane's catalogue of fossils.	108
5.3	Wet preparation of the vertebrae of a six-month-old foetus.	114
5.4	Ercole Lelli, female skeleton.	118
5.5	The birthing phantom at Rijksmuseum Boerhaave.	120

CHAPTER 6

6.1	Astonishment with fright, compassion and violent movements.	126
6.2	Two figures showing the brain, spine and nerves.	128
6.3	The face of a man expressing simple bodily pain.	136
6.4	A man suffering acute pain.	138
6.5	Abatement.	145

CHAPTER 7

7.1	The pathway of burning pain.	153
7.2	A woman breastfeeding her child.	159
7.3	Franz Joseph Gall leading a discussion on phrenology with five colleagues, by Thomas Rowlandson.	167

CHAPTER 8

8.1	The tomb of M. de Pâris.	176
8.2	*Le bacquet de Mr. Mesmer*.	187
8.3	*Le Mesmerisme a tous les diables*.	189

ACKNOWLEDGEMENTS

Thank you to the contributors; you have been a pleasure to work with and I have learned a lot from your scholarship. Thank you to Claudia Stein, Elaine Leong, Laurence Totelin and Jonathan Reinarz – editors of other volumes – for their advice and support. And thank you, above all, to series editor Roger Cooter and Bloomsbury editors Laura Reeves and Rhodri Mogford for their encouragement and patience throughout the project, and their assistance during difficult times.

GENERAL EDITOR'S PREFACE

ROGER COOTER

The cultural history of medicine is all-embracing. Virtually nothing can be excluded from it – the body in all its literary and other representations over time, ideas of civilisation and humankind, and the sociology, anthropology and epistemology of health and welfare, not to mention the existential experiences of pain, disease, suffering and death and the way professionals have endeavoured to deal with them. To contain much of this vastness, the volumes in this series focus on eight categories, all of contemporary relevance: environment, food, disease, animals, objects, experience, mind/brain, and authority. From the ancient through to the postmodern world these themes are pursued with critical breadth, depth and novelty by dedicated experts. Transnational perspectives are widely entertained. Above all, these volumes attend to and illuminate what exactly is a *cultural* history of medicine, a category of investigation and an epistemological concept that has its emergence in the 1980s.

Introduction

LISA WYNNE SMITH, CLAUDIA STEIN AND ROGER COOTER

In celebration of its 250th anniversary in 2003, the British Museum opened a new permanent exhibition: the Enlightenment Gallery. Housed in its restored King's Library, built in 1823, thousands of objects from the Museum's collection were put on display, diverse objects from all over the globe. The aim was to show how Europeans and Americans understood their world in the Age of Enlightenment – a period roughly between 1680 and 1820. The emphasis was and is on the Enlightenment's passion for collecting, cataloguing and classifying everything: objects natural and human-made – fossils, botanical and animal specimens, precious stones, Greek and Roman vases, Chinese porcelain, ancient scripts, coins and technical instruments. The exhibition dazzles in order to inspire the visitor and perhaps to rekindle their scientific curiosity to unlock today's mysteries of the universe. Material things and their journeys, along with the ordering of knowledge, stand at the core of this indeed wondrous presentation.

Much of what is on display is the legacy of one man: Sir Hans Sloane (1660–1753), one of Britain's most famous Enlightenment physicians. By the time of his death, aged ninety-three, Sloane had amassed a formidable collection of 50,000 books and manuscripts, 12,000 botanical specimens, 10,000 animal specimens, 32,000 coins and much more. Valued at over £80,000 at the time, this was the stuff that actually constituted the foundation of the British Museum in 1753. It also supplied the material for several other world-famous institutions, among them the British Library and Natural History Museum in London.

In 1727 Sloane succeeded Sir Isaac Newton to become the president of the Royal Society – or, as per its full name as of 1663, which revealed proto-Enlightenment aspirations, the Royal Society of London for Improving Natural Knowledge. Sloane had been the Royal Society's secretary from 1693 to 1713

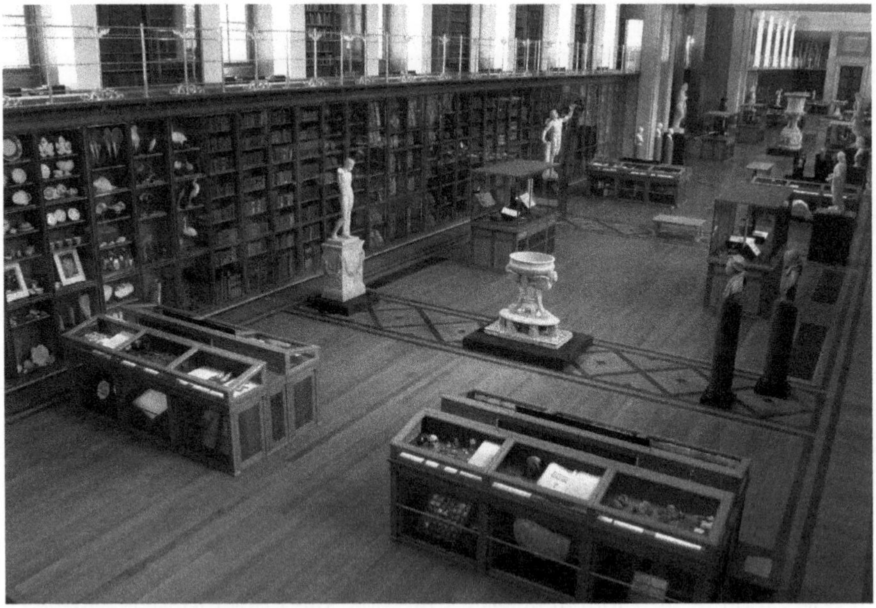

FIGURE 0.1: The Enlightenment Gallery at the British Museum. Credit: The Trustees of the British Museum, London.

and was, as such, responsible for publishing one of the world's most prestigious scientific journals of the Enlightenment: the Royal Society's *Philosophical Transactions*. But Sloane was no Newton; he was neither a great thinker nor in any way a philosopher or theoretician. He was, rather, a great mediator of knowledge systems and practices, in this respect not unlike his successor as president of the Royal Society, the naturalist Sir Joseph Banks. Like Banks, Sloane was remarkably good at networking, collaborating and using polite sociability (Smith 2019). His epistolary network covered the globe; every significant natural philosopher of the eighteenth century was known to him either personally or through letters. Sloane's correspondence enables us to see what the Enlightenment was in terms of ideas and expectations. The surviving thousands of letters are a rich source of information on scientific discourse, collections of antiquities, curiosities and books. As well, they provide rich pickings on patients' illnesses, medical treatments and family history; patients' experiences of embodiment; popular and medical understandings of *materia medica*; and physicians' constructions of disease. Sloane's medical practice was not, however, separate from his collecting, although this has long been obscured by attention being focused only on his collecting and networking. There is a story to be told about the intimacy of his medical practice in relation to his collecting, not to mention about the construction of his identity as a physician

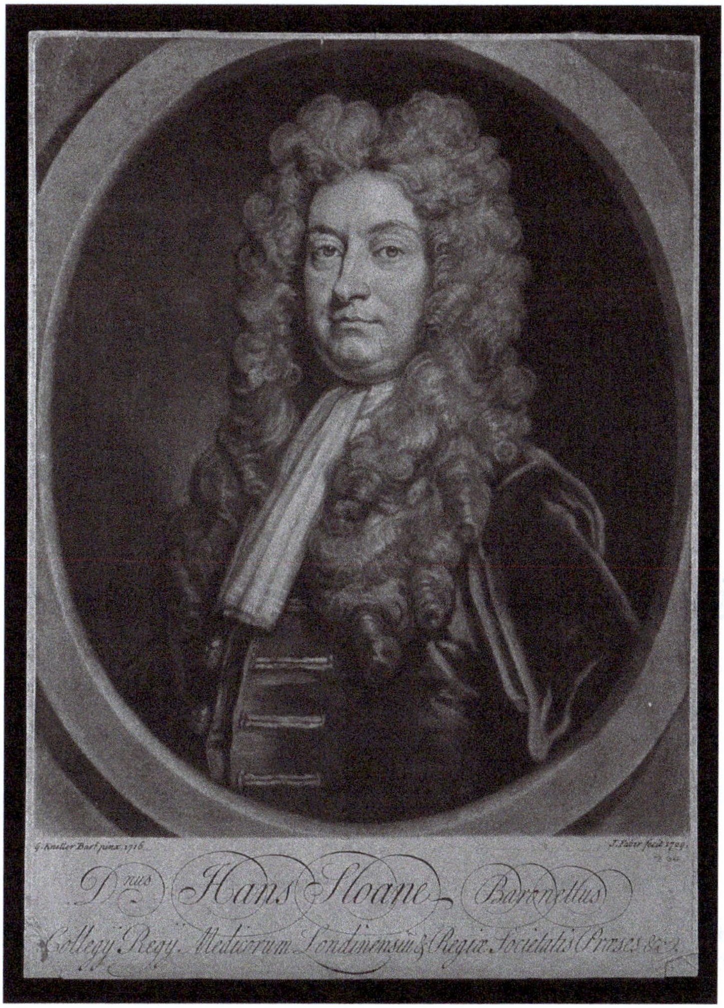

FIGURE 0.2: Sir Hans Sloane, by J. Faber, Junior, 1729 (after Sir G. Kneller, 1716). Credit: Wellcome Collection, London/Public Domain.

(Smith 2019). But that is not the intention here; rather, with Sloane in mind, we wish to draw attention to the question of the Enlightenment itself in its relation to the presentation and representation of the history of medicine.

The British Museum's Enlightenment Gallery is all about representations, too. Significantly, although Sloane is present in busts and such-like, the exhibition does not celebrate Sloane – the man after whom countless London streets and squares have been named, as well as a chocolate bar and hot chocolate, and even some peoples' identity ('Sloane Rangers' in the 1980s). Sloane was at once everywhere in the Enlightenment Gallery (through his

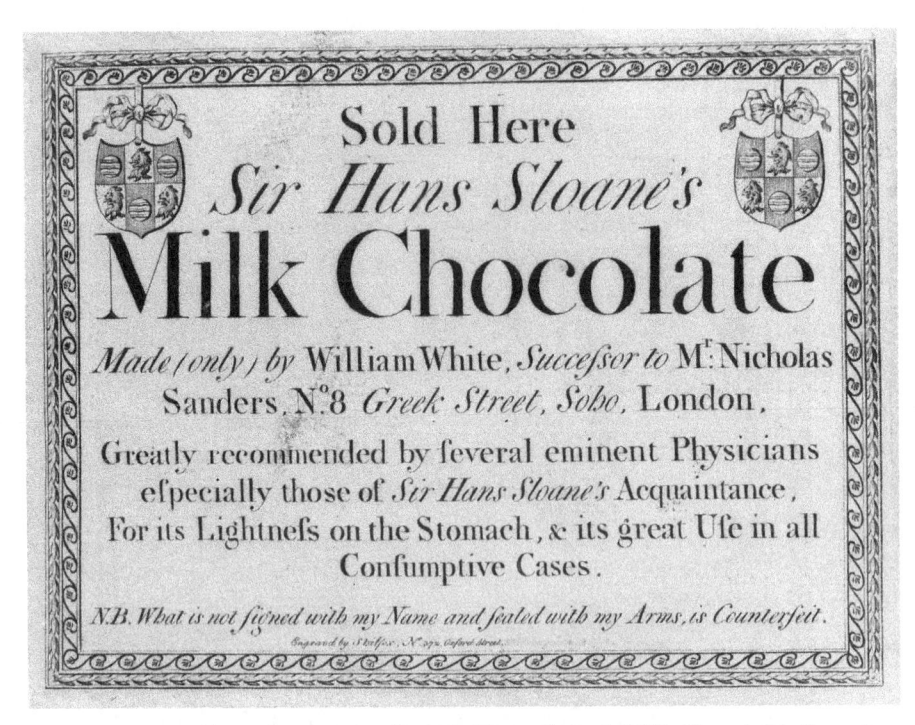

> Sold Here
> Sir Hans Sloane's
> # Milk Chocolate
> Made (only) by William White, Successor to Mr Nicholas Sanders, N.º 8 Greek Street, Soho, London,
> Greatly recommended by several eminent Physicians especially those of Sir Hans Sloane's Acquaintance, For its Lightness on the Stomach, & its great Use in all Consumptive Cases.
> N.B. What is not signed with my Name and sealed with my Arms, is Counterfeit.

FIGURE 0.3: Trade card recommending 'Sir Hans Sloane's Milk Chocolate'. Sloane's association with milk chocolate is long-standing, if largely a myth to promote sales (as per Delbourgo 2017: 199–200). Credit: Wellcome Collection, London/Public Domain.

collection) and nowhere (his easily missed bust was on a plinth in the corner). He has, however, long been the subject of popular biography and is a familiar figure among scholars in the history of science (Brooks 1954; De Beer 1953; Delbourgo 2012, 2017; MacGregor 1994; Walker et al. 2012). It is noteworthy that the British Museum's exhibition did not play him up or make much of the many other contemporaries – some women, but mostly men – who contributed to the variety of materials on display. Like Sloane, they were all well-to-do explorers, diplomats, or natural philosophers and medical men.

The reason for not celebrating Sloane in the exhibition is twofold. First, these collectors, and especially Sloane, have been tarnished by our remodelled views of justice and equality. By any standard, their gains were ill-gotten. In Sloane's case they were made on the back of slavery. The extent of his collecting could never have been reached if it had not been for his marriage in 1695 to a wealthy heiress of one of the largest sugar plantations in Jamaica, then the British Empire's hot spot for sugar production and slavery. While his successful medical practice among the English elite brought him a handsome income, it was from the slave labour on his wife's Jamaican sugar plantation that he bankrolled his voracious appetite for collecting.

The other reason for the exhibition's playing down the individual lives and ambitions of Enlightenment men and women while playing up a material-focused narrative is that of a general shift in historical understanding, particularly of the Enlightenment, and of slavery not least.[1] The whole conception and execution of the British Museum's exhibition is testimony to the success and popularization of a new way of looking at, and writing about, the Enlightenment. This historiographical shift first became noticeable in the humanities and social sciences in France in the 1970s, especially among French linguists and philosophers. It was then taken up wholeheartedly by Anglo-American scholars in the 1980s and 1990s. One outcome was the 'new' cultural history to which historians of science and medicine of the eighteenth century were major contributors. In fact, their contribution has been central to a rewriting of history aimed at 'demystifying' the older narrative of the Enlightenment – the meta-narrative that the British Museum's new exhibition sought to bury for good.

The older historiography of the Enlightenment was essentially intellectualist, concentrating on analysis of the written text. History wasn't history if it was not in written culture, it was claimed – a distinction that separated it from anthropology. There was some appreciation that the Enlightenment as an intellectual movement had regional variations and that England was always a little different. (Anglophones had a peculiar desire to identify a single Enlightenment, whereas scholars of Europe were always more comfortable with the idea of its manifold forms; Spary 2011: 93; Edelstein 2010.) The movement was celebrated overall for its the triumph of reason and rationality over superstition, and scientific method (empiricism) over magic and witchcraft. The making of the modern world, the narrative claimed (including the rise of equality and democracy), was largely the result of scientific societal 'progress', the success of rationally thinking brains fearlessly searching for the 'laws' of nature, both human and natural. In truth, this was the seventeenth century's empirical method applied to the study of man. At its core was the notion of the perfectibility of human nature: trust in the abilities of humans to raise themselves through education and knowledge. It was through this that humans were alleged to have moved from states of savagery to civilization. The proper study of mankind is man, Alexander Pope famously declared – a thoroughly human-centric view in which 'man' was the white European virtuoso or intellectual.

The Enlightenment 'project', with its enthusiasm for scientific progress and human betterment, has attracted the attention of historians of medicine ever since the discipline was invented around the turn of the nineteenth century. What interested early medical historians was the written testament of important Enlightenment physicians, their theories and 'scientific breakthroughs'. There was much to write about, much written evidence to work through. Although the empirical method and practices such as experimentation were not 'invented' in the Enlightenment, their widespread medical application and institutionalization can be readily observed in the period. Key medical and scientific theories, such as inoculation and electricity, were then first developed and put into practice. An international scientific 'republic of letters' emerged (in which Sloane was a key figure), which debated, tested, and approved or discarded these new ideas and practices. Modern scientific medicine was identified as transpiring in the Enlightenment, and medical historians – who were often doctors themselves – busied themselves writing retrospective histories of such medical progress.

In the 1930s a new focus emerged, inspired largely by socialist ideals. The rise of state public health became a central focus. Here too the Enlightenment had much to offer, for it was during the eighteenth century that states began seriously to appreciate the importance of healthy citizens for work and war. Governments began to set up health authorities (developed from civic health boards and royal medical commissions during the Renaissance). Their target was the productivity of nations. Women and their reproductive bodies, as well as the fight against epidemic disease, became central to administrators who began to think in terms of populations as a whole. New institutions such as maternity hospitals, epidemic wards in hospitals and institutions for those who did not fit the agenda of reason and rationality (such as the 'mad') emerged all over Europe. New mathematical achievements such as probability theory and statistics allowed doctors to trace and check the rise and fall of populations, with the rise becoming a matter of pride and economic success among individual states. Historians of medicine, inspired by sociological methods, became themselves obsessed with numbers, hoping to identify medical, scientific and societal progress through elaborate collections of archival statistics and numbers.

But in the 1970s this narrative of progress and enlightened achievement began to come unstuck. The civil rights movements shone a light on the inherent contradictions of a story that left out the masses of the poor and uneducated, women, and Indigenous populations that had in fact been oppressed by white European imperialists. The authority of medicine and the sciences also came under scrutiny. It became all too clear that the narrative of Enlightenment as a striving for equality and happiness for all looked good only on paper. Civil rights activists and left-liberal-leaning academics – including, increasingly, historians of medicine – began to argue that modern society's shortcomings and evils were actually part and parcel of the keeping alive of the old narrative. To heal modernity's ills the narrative needed to change; the 'myth' of the Enlightenment needed to be demystified.

The social history of medicine that emerged in the 1970s contributed to this project. Written within a sociological paradigm mainly by left-leaning academics trained in history departments rather than in medical schools, it turned its back on the story of medical progress. The figure of the doctor as representative of the state and of its institutions began to be eyed with suspicion. Instead, 'the patient's view', as popularized by the sociologist Nicholas Jewson and later by the medical historian Roy Porter, shifted to centre-stage (Jewson 1976; Porter 1985). Jewson, supposing that modern hospital patients had been rendered passive in medical interactions (a supposition not unsupported at the time), argued that patients actually played an active role in shaping medical theory in the eighteenth century, or at least those patients who were well-off patrons for physicians. Agency was thus restored to patients in history-writing, a circumstance well instanced historically in Sloane's medical correspondence. Later, in the 1980s and 1990s, Anglo-American scholarship built on Jewson's work, depicting an eighteenth-century marketplace in which patients had extensive choice from a wide array of practitioners. Accordingly, physicians were required to develop a good bedside manner, to market themselves as celebrities, to make themselves useful or to develop expertise in natural philosophy and new remedies (Porter and Porter 1989; Cook 1994). The patient's view is an approach that in recent years has flourished, drawing attention to illness experiences as shaped by gender, age or family life (Stolberg 2011; Churchill 2012b; Withey 2011; Newton 2012). Olivia Weisser (2015) and Sasha Handley (2016). The recent work shows how the patient's point of view easily slips into cultural history. Weisser, for example, primarily looks at physical and emotional experiences of illness, while Handley looks at the cultural construction of sleep and how the intersection of culture, materiality and biology shapes people's experiences. Again we can see Sloane featuring here, his medical correspondence providing extensive insight into patient experience and medical decision-making and the patient–practitioner relationship (Smith 2003, 2006; Churchill 2012b) at the same time as informing on the construction of illness and the experience of the body (Smith 2008, 2011).

But this emphasis, this take-up of Jewson's article, only came later. In the 1970s–1980s, in the hey-day of the social history of medicine, the 'patient's view' that was stressed was the alleged voice of the dispossessed. It was attention to the poor, to women, to children, to the 'mad', to people of ethnic and racial exclusion, and so on, that then provided an inspiring counter-narrative to the Enlightenment progress narrative. It was only in the 1980s that these kinds of interests morphed into the cultural history of medicine. In truth, this was more a 'socio'-cultural history, for the change was not clear-cut and the interests of the old left-liberal social historians lingered on; it was social historians, after all (people like Roy Porter), who did much to open up the new spaces of cultural history. Ultimately, however, the cultural history of medicine came to focus more on the middling sorts rather than on the poor and dispossessed, on networks rather than class, on global connections, markets, consumers, the production of knowledge (historical epistemology) and knowledge systems.[2] More or less, these interests were connected, directly or indirectly, to the other major force that undermined the old Enlightenment story: poststructuralism, or more generally, postmodernism. (For a fuller version of this historiography, see

Stein's introduction to the forthcoming Renaissance volume in this Cultural History of Medicine series, and Cooter and Stein 2013.)

Poststructuralism was very much the child of French linguistic theorists, all of whom targeted the Enlightenment as the key period in which the 'meta-narratives' of modernity were fabricated: progress, celebrations of reason and rationality, and such. These were increasingly seen as 'myths' that had to be understood as historical constructions specific to time and place. The Enlightenment itself was now to be cast for the first time as a 'meta-narrative'. Although it was registered as an important historical development, the Enlightenment was now considered to be a historically specific 'project'.

For the history of medicine and science, no one did a better job at 'demystification' than the French philosopher Michel Foucault. Indeed, it can be argued that it was due to him that the discipline of the history of medicine was catapulted to the academic front lines. This is not to say that Foucault's books on the history of madness, the rise of the modern clinic and sexuality did not disturb; after all, they revealed how even the most intimate body experience expressed in the past had to be treated with suspicion. For Foucault, there was to be no transhistorical 'experience' of disease, of pain or of sexual pleasure; any knowledge, especially scientific and medical knowledge commonly thought to be 'neutral', was always inextricably linked to strategies and practices of power. The target of these technologies of power was the human body. Thus emerged the 'history of the body' in the 1980s and 1990s, which focused on discursive formations (for examples, see Schiebinger 1993; Laqueur 1990; cf. Cooter's chapter on the body in Cooter and Stein 2013). Embodiment also became a key concern, pioneered by Barbara Duden in her ground-breaking *Woman Beneath the Skin* (translated into English in 1991). Drawing on patient narratives in the casebooks of an eighteenth-century German physician, Duden found that women's bodily experiences reflected a humoral understanding of the body (flows and stoppages) and a close relationship between mind and body. Over the last twenty years this field has burgeoned, with scholars such as Cathy McClive (2002) exploring the uncertainty of pregnancy and Micheline Louis-Courvoisier identifying precise bodily sensations and their overlap with emotions (Louis-Courvoisier 2019). These histories of bodily experience and emotions have implications for how we can understand material, rather than discursive, bodies. Indeed, it has been suggested by Iris Clever and Willemijn Ruberg (2014), building on the work of Annemarie Mol (2002), that a material turn can enable us to look at bodies beyond discourse. Materiality can no longer be ignored. Take, for example, pain and emotions. In the eighteenth century, each could be located in body or mind (or both) and might even have materiality, able to move from place to place within the body (Smith 2008; Bound Alberti 2010).

Not all historians of medicine followed Foucault uncritically; rationalist for the most part, they long remained wedded in various ways to progress-minded notions of social change and medical intervention (as per Spary 2011: 82). Some, like Roy Porter (1990) – one of the most influential historians of the British Enlightenment and medicine – famously opposed Foucault's provocative views on madness on would-be archival grounds. Many other historians, however, dodged confrontation, opting instead for increasingly fashionable anthropological theories and searching for the different cultural 'meanings' of health and disease – a fashion that was rooted in the 1970s and which had deeply influenced early socio-cultural history. It was through anthropological authors that a new focus on non-European and popular European cultures emerged among cultural historians of eighteenth-century medicine. The shift towards cultural meaning has highlighted the different expressions of pain and suffering, disease conceptions, interests in drugs, and food as medicine – including in domestic settings. Such topics have come to be considered as existing either apart from or alongside elite 'white' and Western rational healing theories and practices (for recent examples, see Breen 2019; Chakrabarti 2010; Paugh 2017; Seth 2018). In the 1980s and 1990s, cultural historians' enthusiasm for other disciplines also brought about new interest in the material and visual worlds of medicine, particularly how objects and images affected the way medicine was practised and knowledges were altered. All such interests, if not Foucault-inspired, came to be Foucault-related. In the long run, his theories of power and knowledge influenced all those who were not necessarily keen on his 'histories'.

There are many reasons for the initial resistance of historians of medicine to Foucault. These need not be gone into here (they are reviewed in Stein's introduction to the Renaissance volume, 2021). What is more important historiographically is the gradual acceptance of postmodernism within the Enlightenment cultural history of medicine. As history-writing always reflects the times in which it is written, this gradual acceptance had reasons 'external' to the discipline. Foucault's fluid model of power/knowledge fitted with the socio-cultural, political and economic changes in the Anglo-American world in the 1980s and 1990s (Cusset 2008). This was the time of the emergence of a global neoliberal culture in which older models of power (often modelled on socialist models of power) were increasingly undermined by the daily realities of a rising consumer culture focused on individual choice. In history-writing, too, the individual replaced concern with the social. By the mid-1980s, Roy Porter, also a leader in the *social* history of medicine, was already concluding that within the English context, the medical Enlightenment was profoundly individual: it was neither imposed by a central authority nor reflected in better medicines (Porter 1985: 59). E.C. Spary took this further. Calling the search for medical Enlightenment a 'red herring', she situated the contested site of the Enlightenment in the human body; medical knowledge was inherently political, with considerations of how different bodies should be understood or treated creating a 'moral geography' for the era (Spary 2011: 93).

The winds of change are inexorable and historians, in their time and at their own pace, always accommodate to them. One can be fairly certain that pandemics, economic collapse, climatic disaster and whatever else the future holds for us will eventually find their way into the writing of history, and into the cultural history of medicine no less. Nothing is fixed, despite the aspiration of British Museum's *permanent* exhibition in its Enlightenment Gallery. Indeed, in August 2020 the British Museum announced that it had rehomed its bust of Sloane. It had literally taken Sloane off his pedestal to place the bust in a new display, which drew attention to the links between slavery and collecting. Some complained that the museum was erasing Sloane or rewriting history – an irony, given that Sloane's role in the development of the museum (and his bust) were suddenly more visible than ever. But so, too, more visible was the role of slavery in collecting, which at long last moved into public view. Even permanent exhibitions can be changed as stories need retelling.

The essays in this volume take up subjects that are now at the cutting edge of research. They build upon the tropes and disciplinary borrowings of the cultural history of medicine in its recent past, not least upon the methodological and epistemological accomplishments of the postmodern demystification of the Enlightenment. But they also refine and extend, questioning former lines of inquiry and interpretive angles which they briefly synthesize. All of them register Enlightenment medicine as a moment of transition when older practices and understandings were remade and/or resisted within a wider culture of shifting ideas, practices and experiences. For certain, they reach beyond Alexander Pope's *man*-centric conception of the Enlightenment. Through their very titles, chapters on animals, food, environment and objects de-centre the figure of the man of imperialist history's past, especially that of the heroic white man. They stress, rather, consumption, commodification, measurement and utility, indicating all the while the slippages between categories made up, applied and given different meaning in different contexts – whether state-building, global trade, reason or utility. The other chapters, on authority, disease, experience, and mind and brain, entirely leave behind the old emphasis on individual triumph and professionalization, state institutions and so on. In them we confront, among other things such as gender and race, the meaning of convulsing bodies, the experiences of internal bodily (e)motions and the imagination in relation to reason, respectively. We see how medical authority was brought into being through the cults of classification and categorization, and how that authority was meted out in new terms, explanations and treatments and new locations (e.g. the twang of nerves that replaced the flow of humours and, more generally, relocations from the body to the brain). But such transformations were never complete; they were always fragile and open to various kinds of resistance. We witness in these chapters the extensive overlap between emotions, body and physical experience, putting the intense embodiment of illness or emotion at odds with the ideals of reason.

Such interests permit a return to Sloane-like figures, not because they were 'important' or 'influential' in their times, or even because their study enables us to clear away some shadows around the connections among the practice of medicine, collecting and identity (Smith 2019). Nor is it simply that Sloane-like activities can elucidate a range of cultural historical approaches to eighteenth-century medicine. Importantly, we can now better appreciate the point made by Andrew Cunningham and Roger French in 1990 about how medical professionals like Sloane utilized enlightened practices and knowledge to extend their social and political power (Cunningham and French 1990). The Enlightenment in medicine was not all about intellectual shifts towards secularism and rational thought, as in the emergence of medical philanthropic endeavours like hospitals, Cunningham and French emphasized. This point can be crucial when considering how bodily experiences were shaped at the time, as in Anne Vila's consideration of how French ideas about sensibility were created in medical literature and narrated in fiction (Vila 1998), or Hisao Ishizuka's study of the way in which a new model of the body in Britain (fibre-woven) intersected with medical practices and shaped the cultural phenomenon of nervous sensibility (Ishizuka 2016). If we look beyond its monolithic conception, the Enlightenment becomes a tool for comparison, enabling us to consider how ideas, practices and beliefs played out in different places for individuals, professional and lay. But above all, the chapters that follow allow us to better see how Enlightenment figures like Sloane were bearers of particular orderings of the human and natural worlds, which they dreamed of universalizing. They facilitate a view of how Enlightenment science and medicine effected changes in understanding not only of the human and natural world but also of the self. As the Enlightenment emerged as a moment of transition in medicine when the old might be remade and the new resisted within a milieu of shifting ideas, practices and experiences, so it is that through these chapters we can experience much the same, historiographically speaking. In the final analysis they contribute to a self-awareness of our own historicity.

NOTES

1. Indeed, in his analysis of science and slavery, Andrew Curran (2011: 216–24) identifies how racial inferiority was built into the system of Enlightenment thought. The optimistic scientific knowledge, such as classification, with its social utility in France, resulted in blackness becoming a categorizable 'thing'. Africanness became embedded within the bodies, rather than a mark of culture, a process that reflected Europeans' brutal treatment of enslaved people. See also Londa Schiebinger (2017, 2007) and Suman Seth (2018).
2. Not all scholars bought unquestioningly into the idea of the medical marketplace. Some, such as Brockliss and Jones (1997) looking at France, questioned the applicability of the model beyond England. Others, such as Gentilcore (1998) looking at Italy, emphasised the greater importance of religion.

CHAPTER ONE

Environment

ERIN SPINNEY

INTRODUCTION

In Enlightenment thought, health and environment were inseparable entities. For patients and practitioners alike, eighteenth-century medicine continued to draw on ancient Hippocratic medical theory, which situated health firmly within the environment; as *Airs, Waters, Places* put it, people's 'constitutions and habits follow the nature of the land where they live' (Lloyd et al. 1978: 168). The connections between environment, health and medicine shaped perceptions of new colonies, as well as everyday life and death (Wear 2008: 451; Harrison 2010: 4). Hospitals and grand homes were constructed according to principles that assumed interaction between health and the environment, while new technologies, such as mechanical ventilators, were developed to regulate indoor environments and their permeable access to the outside world (Arnold 2013: 1; Jankovic 2010: 1–2; Stevenson 2000: 165–70). Efforts to control the built environment of the hospital and the ward represent, in many ways, a continuity of ideas between the Enlightenment and the nineteenth century. Moreover, the Anglo-centric story chronicled here is just one part of a wider story of European medicine, with similar experiences in the Iberian- and Franco-Atlantic worlds as medical practitioners and natural philosophers engaged with questions of race, environment and physiological difference (Cook and Walker 2013; Gómez 2013; Curran 2011; Schiebinger 2013).

This chapter examines the built hospital environment to consider the interplay between health, disease and environment in the Enlightenment world. By looking at British military and naval institutions in the Greater Caribbean climatic (or torrid) zone – a region understood by military commanders and

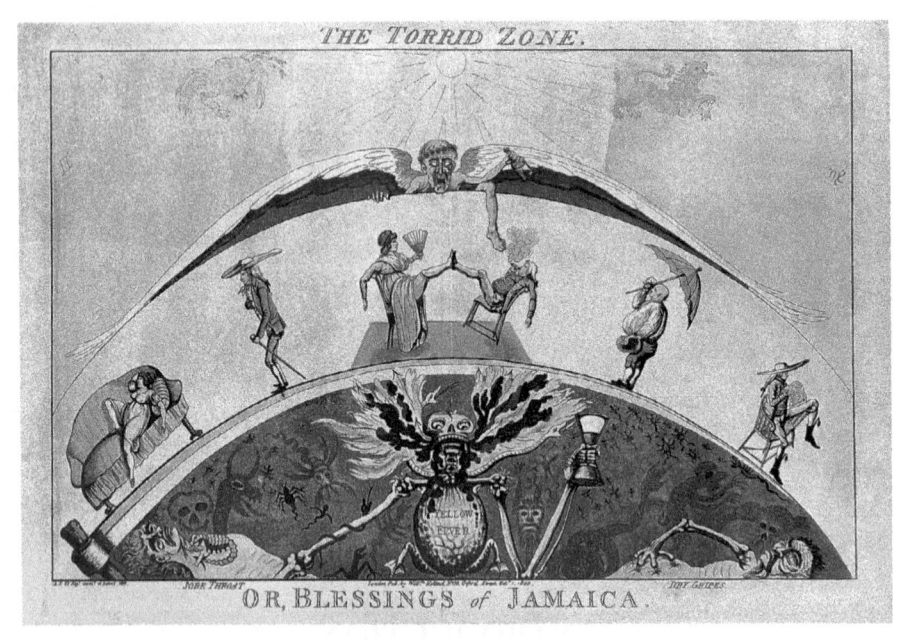

FIGURE 1.1: *The Torrid Zone, or, Blessings of Jamaica*, by Abraham James, 1800. The Wellcome catalogue describes this as a parody astrological diagram, which juxtaposes the languorous noons with the hells of yellow fever, dual aspects of Jamaican settler experience. Credit: Wellcome Collection, London/Public Domain.

medical practitioners to be deadly – it becomes possible to identify the process of constructing environmental medicine (Hogarth 2017: 11; Seth 2018: 16). The way in which military and naval medical officers understood bodies – whether their own, patients' or nurses' – was framed by environmental and cultural imaginings. Their assumptions about bodies were, in turn, reinforced by naval and military policies; such state and imperial policies ensured the continued prioritization of the connection of health and environment in medical and lay thought (Hogarth 2017: 1–4; Seth 2018: 17). The Enlightenment quest for environmental improvement to ensure good health was entwined with concepts of race and class and permeated the lives of everyone living in the torrid zone (see Figure 1.1).

DEFINING ENVIRONMENT

Our present-day understanding of environment as a category pertaining to the natural world is a construct of the mid-twentieth century, a word designed to showcase the interaction between humanity and nature, often in a negative way (Cronon 1996). An early modern definition of environment was not primarily concerned with either nature or the natural world. Rather it denoted the surroundings of an object, which could include – but did not necessarily constitute – the body of a human being, as well as the act of being encompassed or surrounded (OED). An Enlightenment conception of environment is more easily transferable to the built environments of hospitals and hospital wards, where indoor surroundings were environments in their own right, although these environments could and did communicate with the outdoor world. In this chapter, I consider environment as the interaction of the human body with its surroundings; the air we breathe, the clothing we wear, the temperatures we endure and nature in all its facets (Jørgensen and Sörlin 2013).

The indoor/outdoor environmental division was a product of the eighteenth century. As historian Vladimir Jankovic has shown, it was only when indoor comfort became possible for most Britons that the 'dichotomy . . . between the medical qualities of indoors and outdoors' could exist (Jankovic 2010: 1–2). This dichotomy made it possible to control the air, to make spaces healthier, prevent disease from occurring and spreading, and create an environment designed to promote healing. As Jankovic argues, ventilation became an important medical issue; if foul air was a cause of disease, then one could prevent disease by ensuring clean air (Jankovic 2010: 13). Unhealthy air was even thought to emanate from unclean objects, especially bedding and clothing that had absorbed the sweat of the body or some form of disease contagion (see Figure 1.2).

Historian Margaret Pelling teases out the idea that the difference between the concepts of contagion and infection depended on the medium of entry into the body, noting that contagion directly came from contact, while infection indirectly came through water, air or contamination. But the concepts of

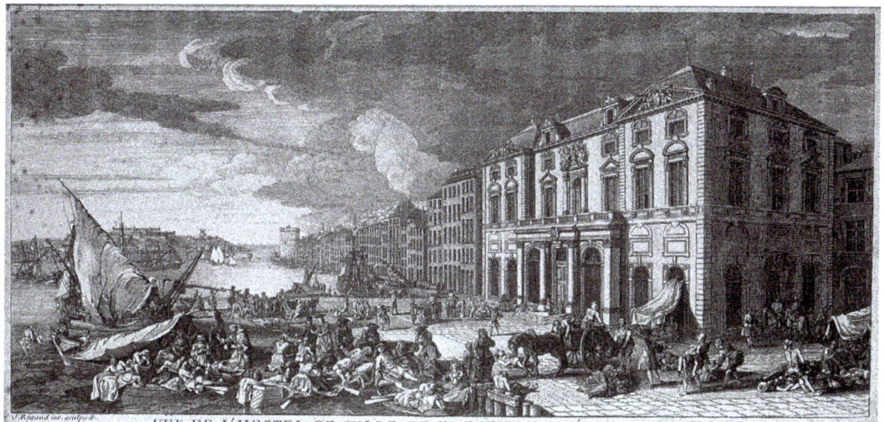

FIGURE 1.2: The port of Marseille during the plague of 1720, etching by J. Rigaud after M. Serre. Note not only the proximity of individuals to contagious objects and people but the dark air over the city. Credit: Wellcome Collection, London/Public Domain.

contagion, infection and miasma overlapped and their meanings changed over time (Pelling 1993: 309–10). By the second half of the eighteenth century, the term 'contagion' could be applied both to an inanimate object (like dirty linen) and to a characteristic of the air or environment (Pelling 1993: 311; DeLacy 1999). Historians Alison Bashford and Claire Hooker (2001: 4) summarize the dual nature of contagion as connoting 'a *process* of contact and transmission, and a substantive, self-replication *agent*' (original emphasis). Within an eighteenth- and early nineteenth-century framework, the concepts of contagion and miasma (bad air) can be viewed as complementary rather than contradictory (Bashford and Hooker 2001: 19, 21; Stevenson 2000: 159; Hamlin 2014b: 26). The foul environment could both create contagion and act as its method of transmission to the sick (see Figure 1.3).

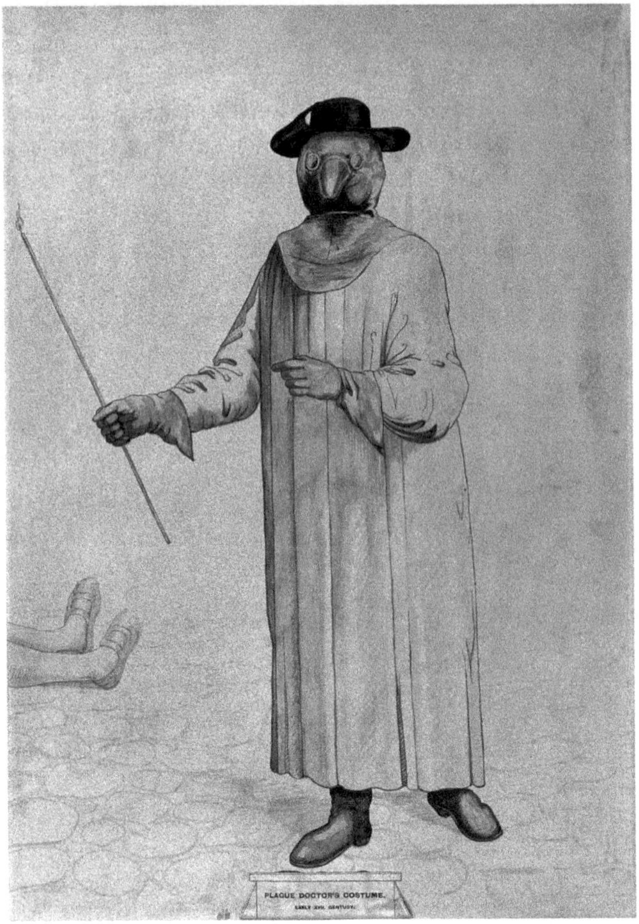

FIGURE 1.3: A physician wearing a seventeenth-century plague preventive costume. The characteristic beak could hold fumigation materials to prevent the breathing in of the plague contagion. Credit: Wellcome Collection, London/Public Domain.

Cultural construction underpins the complex relationship of climate, disease and immunity in medical thought during the Enlightenment period. Europeans shaped and reshaped their conceptions of tropical disease environments to fit their culturally conceived worldviews of climate and race (McNeill 2010; Seth 2018). In certain instances, as shown by Mart A. Stewart (2002) and Simon Newman (2013), the physical landscapes of tropical regions were altered to conform to European cultural perceptions of agricultural productivity. Historians, in their writings, have highlighted the cultural perceptions that form the relationship between race and disease in the Greater Caribbean. Beginning with Philip Curtin's work on the disease environment in nineteenth-century West Africa, historians have focused on either debunking or proving the commonly held belief that tropical regions were the 'White Man's Grave' (Curtin 1961: 94). While some quantitative studies of European settler and slave populations have shown the deadliness of the West Indian tropical environment (Sheridan 1985; Dobson 1989; Burnard 1999), Kenneth Kiple (1984) has discussed what he perceived as the biological foundations of slavery. The use of a cultural lens also elucidates what Gary Puckrein has characterized as the 'climate-race-health nexus' (Puckrein 1979: 180). The concept of race was itself culturally constructed in the long eighteenth century (Wheeler 2000; Wilson 2003), and informed major British military decisions. This included the formation of the West India Regiments (Buckley 1979, 1998), the reliance on black troops and pioneers in various local capacities (Voelz 1993; Braisted 1999; Bolster 1997), and the medical treatment of non-European bodies in a military context (Churchill 2012a; Saakwa-Mante 1999). As this chapter discusses, military medical practitioners like William Fergusson and Robert Jackson – both discussed below – constructed racialized medicalized understandings of black and white bodies with reified contemporary cultural interpretations (Hogarth 2017).

CREATING HEALING ENVIRONMENTS

Healthy hospital design began with the selection of suitable surroundings, through the choice of location for the hospital. Marshes were thought to be especially dangerous because of the odours produced in such regions (Bashford and Hooker 2001: 20). Swampy wetland regions had long been connected to illness in the minds of ordinary people and medical practitioners (Dobson 1989, 1997; Rutman and Rutman 1976). The unhealthiness of marshes was due to the putrefaction of decaying matter, the smell of which would then enter the air (Harrison 2010: 76–7; Brown 2008). Smell could also be connected to eighteenth-century social conventions, wherein a healthy body and environment was either deodorized through bathing and ventilation or improved through the application of sweet-smelling fragrances (Brant 2004). In this sense, the same dangers of marshes could also emanate from any location where large numbers of the unwashed masses congregated. Urban regions, therefore, were to be avoided whenever possible as locations for hospitals. Even urban hospitals tended to be placed on the outskirts of the city to retain some of the healthy benefits of the countryside (Arnold 2013: 106–7). This placement benefited the town in another way, too, as the most dangerous feature of contagion was that it could be formed simply from the congregation of sick people. As medical writer William Buchan put it (1772), hospitals by their very definition could 'become nests for hatching diseases' that might spread to the surrounding town. The decision to locate hospitals on the outskirts of urban areas or in the countryside was advantageous for the sick in the hospitals and for the urban residents.

In 1805, army regimental surgeon Robert Jackson (1750–1827) detailed the difficult balancing act performed by military medical practitioners in selecting a hospital site: 'The site of the hospital under consideration, while such as is judged to be healthy in itself, ought to be so chosen in position as to prove convenient for the execution of business, commanding, by its local advantages, the easy conveyance of such means as are useful or necessary for hospital purposes' (Jackson 1805: 111). Yet while the ability of the site to act as a hospital easily accessible to the sick may have been the overriding concern when selecting a location, other factors needed to be considered. Hospitals, according to Jackson, should be on dry ground and constructed to allow for ventilation, as well as being sheltered with a 'cheering prospect of the surrounding country' (112). They needed protection from excess wind and access to clean water. If any of these were unavailable, it was ventilation that Jackson deemed to be what 'hospitals indispensably require' (115). He elaborated on the primacy of ventilation in an expanded edition of his book in 1824:

> It was often proved, in the history of the late war, that more human life was destroyed by accumulating sick men in low and ill ventilated apartments, than in leaving them exposed in severe and inclement weather at the side of a hedge or common dyke. It is fit that the military officer mark this fact and bear it in mind; and it is also fit that he bear in mind, that churches and palaces are less proper receptacles of military sick than barns, hovels and open sheds.
>
> —Jackson 1824: 542

Just as John Pringle (1707–1787), the founder of environmental military medicine, had complained in 1753 (22–3), Jackson blamed the lack of ventilation for the death of sick and wounded soldiers.

Pringle's experiences as a regimental surgeon during the War of Austrian Succession in the 1740s led him to treat the causes of army diseases as an important consideration when it came to thinking about the military environments of camps and hospitals. Putrefaction of animal matter and unhygienic camp environments fostered the growth of diseases from scurvy to typhus (Charters 2014: 24; Stevenson 2007: 241). A well-ventilated environment was the first necessity for a patient's cure in a military hospital. 'Pure air being of the utmost consequence in the cure', Pringle wrote, 'the physician can never be successful in full hospitals unless every ward is kept sweet by a ventilator' (1752: 289). If expensive ventilators could not be procured, Pringle believed, 'the next expedient is to lay the sick, if numerous, in churches, barns, or ruinous houses' – locations that would provide a permanent state of ventilation (289). The use of ventilators quickly fell out of fashion for regimental military hospitals, due to their expense and the difficulty of transporting them, but Pringle's ideas about the ideal characteristics of military hospitals continued to be espoused by subsequent generations of military medical officers (Stevenson 2007: 242). Indeed, as *Instructions to Regimental Surgeons* (1808) shows, mechanical ventilators returned to use at military instillations – if not hospitals – by the nineteenth century. The surgeon, for example, was to routinely inspect the barracks for contagions and to ensure that 'Ventilators or Air-barrels be not shut or obstructed' (40).

Building on the foundation of sound hospital design was the proper and adequate use of ventilation within the built environment. The first step in ventilating was to prevent overcrowding the hospital wards and to separate patients by symptom or disease. William Fergusson (1773–1846) believed that separation was important to prevent contagion from 'human effluvia, more particularly from bodies under a State of disease'. This would aid recovery by ensuring 'the advantages of ventilation, discipline repose and attendance' (RAMC 210/3). Wherever possible, Fergusson believed, sources of contagion should be removed from sick wards; in Article 4, he noted that this included the too-common piles of 'foul linen of the Sick' that awaited laundering (RAMC 201/3). Negligence in providing adequate medical care or necessary medical establishments had the potential to turn the course of war, as surgeon William Pallison described in a letter to Rear Admiral Pringle dated 21 February 1798 ('Sick and Hurt Board, In-Letters and Orders', ADM/E/46). Cape Town Hospital had been so overcrowded, 'without the smallest ventilation', that the sick sailor sent on shore 'had not only to contend with the disorder he came on shore with, but a floating contagion which must naturally arise from the complication of diseases cooped in so small a space'. In Pallison's estimation:

> many very valuable lives [were] lost last winter all for the want of an Hospital to receive them, and in fact they were allowed to die on board of the different Ships at the very great risque of spreading Contagion throughout the Fleet, and had I not been fortunate enough to get the Government Stables,

unprepared as they were, for the reception of the Sick, I am certain many more would have been added to the list of Mortality.

Whether eighteenth-century medical care could have saved the lives of these men is in many ways unimportant. Both medical practitioners and naval administrators believed that such deaths were preventable with the prevention of contagion; failure to provide a healthy environment came at great expense to Britain, humanity and the naval service.

The inclusion of sections that discussed the importance of ventilation in popular eighteenth-century medical guides, like William Buchan's *Domestic Medicine* (1772), suggests that these views were part of the wider lay understanding. Buchan highlighted to his readers the potential dangers to health of 'unwholesome air' as 'few are aware of the danger arising from it'. People might pay attention to diet, but they ignored 'what goes into the lungs' (92). Overcrowding in places like churches and assemblies – part of everyday life – was dangerous, especially 'if the air has not a free current' (93). Characteristically blunt, Buchan summarized that 'if fresh air be necessary for those in health, it is still more so for the sick, who often lose their lives for want of it' (98). Medical practitioners, whether military, naval or civilian, agreed on the importance of ventilation and fresh air to patients recovering from surgery.

The responsibility of nurses for ensuring that ventilation could be achieved within their wards was a part of their nursing role from the inception of the naval hospitals. The XIII Article of 'Regulations respecting Nurse and Other Servants of the Royal Hospital' (1760) stipulated that in fever, flux and small pox wards 'a small Chick of the upper part of some one or more of the Windows is constantly to be kept open so as at Night gently to move the Flame of a Candle when standing on the table' (439–40). Physicians were to ensure that nurses followed ventilation requirements on their wards. The *Instructions for the Royal Naval Hospital at Haslar & Plymouth* (1808) codified that physicians 'are to take great care that the wards be at all times properly ventilated' (ADM 106/3091: 55). Similarly, Ward matrons at the naval hospitals were 'frequently to visit' unoccupied wards within the hospital 'to see that they be clean, well ventilated, and in all respects fit to be furnished for the reception of Patients' (ADM 106/3091: 203–4). The continual monitoring of nurses' conduct to ensure adequate ventilation in occupied and unoccupied wards emphasizes the crucial medical role of nurses.

During the first half of the eighteenth century, nurses were seen by many medical practitioners as failing in their ventilation duties because of ignorance. Physician William Fordyce (1724–1792), for example, blamed 'silly nurses' for prolonging inflammatory diseases by their 'officious and mistaken care' – closing windows and bed curtains around their patients, which 'depriv[ed] the patient of cool air' (Fordyce 1773: 151). Pringle recommended in 1752 that military hospitals should be placed in churches and run-down buildings, as in such structures 'neither they [the patients] *nor their nurses* can confine the air' (289, my emphasis). A built hospital that might encourage human error in ventilation, for Pringle, was worse than having sick soldiers in the open air and exposed to the elements. But military and naval medical practitioners had another way of ensuring that nurses opened the windows of their wards. In the first volume of *Observations on the Means of Preserving the Health of Soldiers* (1780), physician Donald Monro (1728–1802) drew on the advice of naval physician James Lind (1716–1794), who had recommended the benefits of purifying smoke fumigation. 'These steams and smoke, which are inoffensive to the lungs', Monro wrote, corrected the bad quality of the air and (better yet) would 'make both the patients and nurses desirous of opening the doors and windows for the admission of fresh air' (103). Ward fumigation could also be achieved by less obtrusive means. In 1813, the Irish Medical Board, for example, recommended sprinkling vinegar in regimental hospitals daily (*Instructions from the Army Medical Board of Ireland*, 1813), while decades earlier Buchan had suggested using lemon juice or 'strong vegetable acid' to purify sick rooms (*Instructions from the Army Medical Board of Ireland* 1813: 10–11; Buchan 1772: 98–9).

It was not necessarily ignorance, however, that caused nurses to close windows; the comfort of their patients (or their own) could also have played a role in the decision. Some medical practitioners, like Gilbert Blane (1749–1834), believed that neither nurses nor patients wanted fresh air because it cooled the room and created cold draughts (Brown 2011: 67). Blane, who was the former physician to the Channel Fleet, had a solution to maintain comfort while providing ventilation. He believed that the intake of fresh air needed to be near the ceiling. As such, opening windows at the top to allow a cross breeze 'will be perfect; for the sick are thereby sheltered from direct streams of cold air, and the recent and vitiated exhalations from the living body having, by their warmth, a tendency to ascend, are effectually dissipated' (Blane 1822: 137–8). Cross-ventilation was easier to procure at Haslar, a royal hospital, with its long open wards, but with this increased ventilation came the risk that contagious or foul airs would spill from one ward to another. Even so, cross-ventilation was seen as a feature of hospitals designed in the pavilion model, like Plymouth (Jankovic 2010: 77; Stevenson 2000: 184). Although many medical theorists believed that hospitals demanded a greater flow of air then other spaces, it was not to compromise patients' comfort (Jankovic 2010: 79). Lind, for example, observed in 1778 that ill patients, especially in fever wards, did not complain about fresh air and wide-open windows 'as long as they had sufficient bedding' (334–5). Convalescents, however, perhaps as they were more aware of their surroundings (or as they were not confined to their beds), quickly complained of cold (334–5). Regardless of patient preferences, fresh air and ventilation were seen as key to preventive medicine and speedy recoveries. Nurses working within the wards created a built environment designed to foster healing through cleaning, purifying and ventilating hospital spaces.

RACE, IMMUNITY AND WEST INDIAN NURSES

Hospital design, location and capacity for ventilation were even more important in tropical conditions than in Britain, although the work of nurses was much the same. This was a challenge to naval, military and Company officials throughout the empire. Medical practitioners like Gilbert Pasley, employed by the East India Company, claimed that hospital design in hot climates needed particularly careful consideration, as tropical climates were more likely to cause putrefaction (Harrison 2010: 79). Increased scrutiny over the location of hospitals seemed to be rewarded, as in the case of the relocation of the Jamaica Naval Hospital from Port Royal to New Greenwich in 1744, which briefly saw an increased number of men returned cured to their ships (Crewe 1993: 42–5). However, the original hospital was rebuilt at Port Royal in 1753 owing to the difficulty in transferring patients from their ships and the continued presence of tropical fevers. Yet another new hospital in Port Royal opened in 1756, this time away from the lagoon: a feature intended to prevent desertion, which ended up plaguing the original location with miasma (Stevenson 2000: 234). In September 1815, Fergusson used the same standard to judge the healthiness of the barracks at Fort Bourbon, Barbados:

> The barracks at Fort Bourbon, on the hill, appear to be healthily situated – the ground being high enough to be beyond the influence of the bad air from the ravines below and at too great a distance from the Lamentine marshes to feel their effects – still they are not perfectly healthy – The force of the trade winds, suddenly chilling the body, often induces bowel complaints, and they are not exempt from fevers of the ordinary remittent type, such as arise from marshy exhalations.
>
> —RAMC 210/3

Although the situation for the barracks was deemed to be suitably healthy, the hospital was 'inferior and unworthy . . . without separation from the different classes of sick'. Even the most carefully selected location could be thwarted by inferior hospital design.

Temperature regulation was a key concern for hospitals established in tropical climates, and changes in temperature present in West Indian hospitals were one explanation for high sickness rates (Crewe 1993: 42). Military medical practitioners reacted with surprise, however, at the correlation of increased ventilation during the summer months with continued levels of sickness. Recounting his experiences in the West Indies in the 1790s, William Lempriere (d. 1834) remarked on the difficulty of the summer months in a tropical climate.

June to September was a dry and well-ventilated time of year because of 'the sea breezes prevailing with great regularity, purity, and force' and the heat causing people to open their windows and doors. Although summer should have been 'unfavourable to the production of contagion', somehow it was also when tropical fever was most prevalent (Lempriere 1799: 26).

Lempriere's surprise highlights the universally favourable medical opinion of the benefit of ventilation within all hospital spaces. However, as he had discovered, open windows in the West Indies let in more than just fresh air. Promoters of tropical ventilation also needed to consider the problem of how to deal with mosquitos. Physician William White believed that the combination of perfuming the air and the use of window fans, rather than open sashes, would curb mosquitos (Jankovic 2010: 84).

Early modern conceptions of tropical diseases and the ways to prevent them were tied to the concept of seasoning (Hogarth 2017: 52–4; Seth 2018: 4–6). Seasoning, or acclimatization, was the period of tropical sickness that all new arrivals to the islands underwent before adapting to the climate of the American south-east or the West Indies (see Figure 1.4). This concept was tied to the neo-Galenic and neo-Hippocratic humoral and constitutional understandings of disease, which prevailed into the early nineteenth century (Hamlin 2014a: 61,

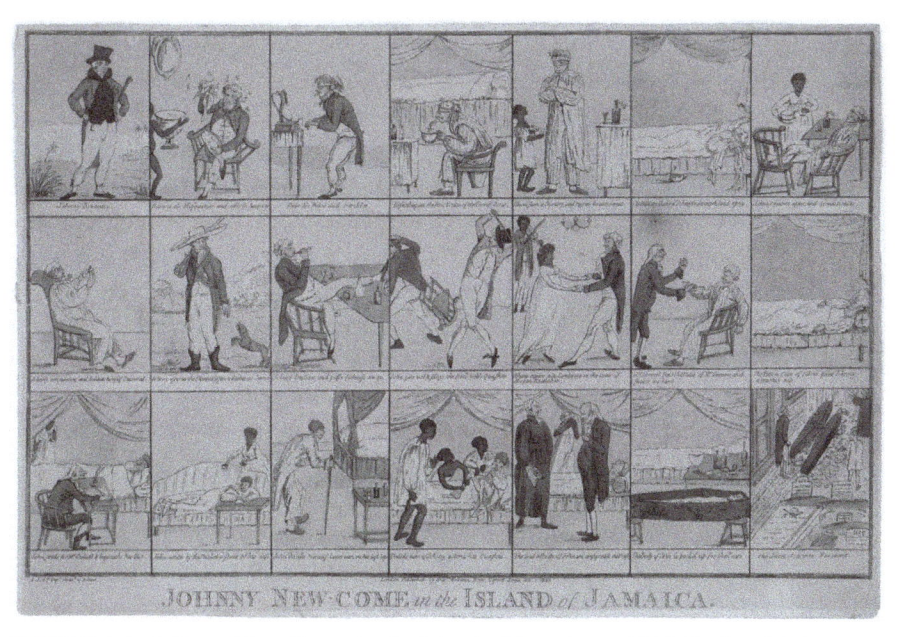

FIGURE 1.4: Johnny New-Come in the Island of Jamaica *c.* 1800. In the eighth pane, 'Johnny convalesces and believes himself Seasoned', before yellow fever takes hold in pane 14. Credit: John Carter Brown Library, Brown University.

109, 181; Wear 2000: 187). Spanish and Portuguese travellers in the fifteenth and sixteenth centuries first described the importance of seasoning and the effects of tropical diseases on strangers to the climate (Klein 1988: 41–3). British medical authorities such as physician Hans Sloane (1660–1753) drew on these earlier understandings. Sloane, for example, detailed the potentially deadly effects of tropical fevers in the first volume of his *A Voyage to Jamaica* (1707) and outlined his view of acclimatization:

> A great many were of opinion that this Fever was what is call'd the Seasoning, that is to say, that every New-comer before they be accustomed to the Climate and Constitution of the Air in *Jamaica*, are to have an acute Disease, which is thought to be very dangerous, and that after this is over, their Bodies are made more fit to live there, with less hazard than before; and this is not only thought so in the Island, but in *Guinea*, and in remote Eastern parts of the World.
>
> —xcviii

Once they were seasoned, Fergusson suggested in 1815, soldiers 'ought to be made capable of labouring under the midday breeze', although they would also need to increase gradually their ability to labour in the hot climate (RAMC 210). The climate was a problem for European bodies, as well as disease.

When it came to African and Indigenous peoples, however, the concept of seasoning changed over the course of the eighteenth century. Initially, it was widely thought that they were exempt from the tropical acclimatization process and its accompanying illness (Warren 1997: 33; Klepp 1994: 500). However, as the century progressed, there were increased references to African slaves both enduring the seasoning process and suffering from tropical fevers (Newman 2013: 80, 220; Hogarth 2017: 34, 53). The seasoning process, nonetheless, was thought to be less severe for African slaves than for Europeans. The necessity for the process itself befuddled planters, who assumed that the climates in Africa and West India were the same. In *Practical Rules for the Management and Medical Treatment of Negro Slaves, in the Sugar Colonies, by a Professional Planter* (1803), Dr Collins noted that when enslaved people were moved between islands, regions or estates, they underwent a process of seasoning; he could not understand the causes for why 'bad effects do ensue, even where the temperature is perfectly equal' (57).

The belief that African and Creole slaves were the only people capable of working in the West Indian climate led to their fatigue duties, or hard labour, such as hospital construction and the transport of regimental stores ('Jamaica (Pay Lists)', ADM 102/461; Buckley 1979: 2, 1988: 99; Voelz 1993: vi). The idea that Africans were best suited to performing labour in the hot climate persisted into the late eighteenth century and was responsible for the creation of the West Indian Regiments in the 1790s. Historian Suman Seth (2018) ties the late eighteenth-century resurgence of 'discourses that asserted the innate capacity for Africans to labour under environmental conditions that putatively made it impossible for Europeans to take their place' (21) to anti-Abolition sentiment in the West Indian medical community. Even while military medical practitioners increasingly recognized that black soldiers were also affected by tropical fevers (Clark 1797: 2–3), Fergusson reported in 1815 that the black Regiments were healthy 'with the exception of the White Officers' (RAMC 210).

At the same time, black nurses were particularly valued in tropical climates, as black women were assumed to be least affected by the fevers. The melting-pot effect of the West Indian disease environment, as discussed by historians Mary Dobson (1989: 270–1) and J. R. McNeill (2010: 44–5), suggests that African and Creole enslaved people only developed resistance and immunity to malaria and yellow fever if they survived a mild bout of either disease. In 1788, army physician John Hunter (1754–1809) observed that 'The negroes afford a striking example of the power acquired by habit of resisting the causes of fevers; for, though they are not entirely exempted from them, they suffer inevitably less than Europeans' (24). Occurrences where black nurses caught yellow fever were discussed with great surprise. Naval surgeon Blane reported in 1785 the (apparently) only eighteenth-century case in military or naval medicine of a black nurse dying of yellow fever: 'It has been said, that it never attacks either the female sex or Blacks. This is in general, though not absolutely true; for I knew a Black woman, who acted as nurse to some men ill of this fever at Barbadoes [sic], who died with every symptom of it' (398–9). This case continued to be referenced more than twenty years later in medical treatises (Dancer 1809: 82). The belief that black people were, with rare exceptions, immune contributed to the selection of black nurses to work in military and naval hospitals and justified their necessity in a civilian context. Due to their perceived immunity, black women were sold as sick nurses for 'great prices', with the citizens of Philadelphia 'over-bidding one another' during the yellow fever epidemic of 1793 (Jones 1794: 8).

People believed that exposure to yellow fever could make anyone – including Europeans – immune to the disease in future. Writing in 1822 about a yellow fever epidemic in Cadiz (1797), Blane explained that 'both Spanish and English selected their [sick] nurses from among those who had had [the disease]' (310). The concept of differential immunity was so pervasive that, according to Blane, those who had fallen victim during the 1797 outbreak did not fear another outbreak in 1819. Rather, they 'shewed no fear or alarm and were not anxious either to quit the city nor to have recourse to seclusion with a view to avoid it'. The extent to which Blane's ideas about European immunity were shared by other military and naval medical practitioners is unclear, given that he did not publish until many had been dismissed from service after the Napoleonic Wars.

However, the only radical aspect about Blane's theory of immunity was that it did not depend on a climatic constitutional adaption; instead, it was related to individual experience with the disease (Hamlin 2014a: 51, 225).

The same understanding of racialized medicine meant that the ideal hospital nurses in the West Indies were African women, not European. In the early eighteenth century, difficulties with transporting and seasoning nurses and matrons from Britain may have also contributed to the racialized belief in the suitability of black women for these roles. Early hospital instructions for Jamaica issued by the Sick and Hurt Board stipulated that local nurses employed in the naval hospital should speak English and that a European woman should be brought from England to act as matron. Yet Campbell, the hospital contractor, found it challenging to contract for an English nurse. The minutes of the Sick and Hurt Board further show that even when the contractor managed to procure an English woman willing to undertake the voyage to the West Indies, she died soon after arriving in Jamaica. Campbell was unable to contract for another (Crewe 1993: 28–9).

Naval medical practitioners also recommended that black nurses should care for those suffering from yellow fever. In 1798, Elliot Arthy, a naval surgeon in Jamaica, explained how 'indigent negro women' provided care to seamen 'labouring under the most violent attack of Yellow Fever' (41). One unnamed nurse, as Arthy described, had attended the sick 'with the most affectionate and unremitted care and attention, night and day, as well as provided them with sustenance, and such other little necessaries and comforts as sick persons require, until they were quite restored to health' (42). For her trouble, though, she was left 'incumbered with a debt' for her purchases of food and medicines; according to Arthy, this took her a long time to discharge (42). Although Africans were thought to be vulnerable to yaws, smallpox and leprosy – diseases that did not affect the European settlers so much – the black nurses were seen to be immune to the diseases that were the deadliest to Europeans. In addition to yellow fever, this included malaria, typhus and scurvy (Lempriere 1799: 25; Dobson 1989: 289). By the second half of the eighteenth century, enslaved people were also inoculated against smallpox, meaning that they would be able to work in smallpox wards without contracting the sickness (Long 1774: 275–6).

In spite of heavily entrenched culturally constructed assumptions, the reality of immunity was far more complex. Many West Africans would have been exposed to the yellow fever virus, thus gaining lifelong immunity, before being enslaved and transported to the West Indies. Such immunity was not universal and depended on having lived in a region where yellow fever was endemic (McNeill 2010: 44–5; Desowitz 1997: 99). The same immunity would occur in the West Indies among European settler, slave and Creole populations if they survived a first exposure; indeed, many would have experienced the disease as children without showing symptoms (McNeill 2010: 45). With the exception of those West Africans and their decedents who had the genetic sickle-cell trait, neither Europeans nor Africans could acquire immunity to malaria (McNeill 2010: 53). Instead differential resistance would be gained from regular exposure to the disease, which lessened or hid the illness entirely (McNeill 2010: 2, 53, 252). The only real certainty when it came to immunity, then, was the Europeans' culturally constructed assumption that enslaved Africans and Creoles had an innate immunity to certain diseases.

When inspecting hospitals in October 1815, William Fergusson also thought highly of the work undertaken by black nurses during an outbreak of dysentery. He recommended that they be used permanently at the Barbados general hospital:

> While superintending the treatment of those people, I was led to an improvement in the Servants department of the hospital, which I shall do my utmost to establish on a permanent footing, I mean the introduction of Black creole nurses, instead of white Soldier orderlies or even Soldier's [sic] Wives to attend on the Sick. I was satisfied there were of great use latterly, in attending upon those of their own colour amongst the recruits that fell ill after they arrived at Barbados, and I am sure that in the white wards they will prove far better nurses than either of the two Classes just mentioned.
>
> —RAMC 210/2

It was likely that Fergusson's views on the benefits of using black nurses were framed by his own experience as a victim to yellow fever during the St Domingo expedition of 1815 (Fergusson n. d.; Hogarth 2017: 73). Fergusson went on to write in his autobiography, published posthumously by his son, that black nurses 'make the best sick nurses in the world' and that 'nothing can exceed' a black nurse's 'vigilance and tenderness'. Moreover, he believed that Creole nurses enjoyed nursing more than any European woman 'and it is to be regretted they should not always succeed in obtaining the place they are so well calculated to fill' (1846: 63–4). Fergusson's depiction of black nurses aligns with the culturally constructed 'mammy' image of the eighteenth and early nineteenth centuries, which depicts the black woman as happily subordinate to whites. This subordination included a willingness to nurse children and the sick (Simms 2001: 882). Culturally, some enslaved women were conceived of as the ideal nurses, not just for their immunity but also due to how they were viewed by British and Anglo-Caribbean populations. Whether the motivation behind Fergusson's views on black nurses was cultural, medical, based upon his personal experience or a combination of these things, he continued to advocate for the importance of their universal labour in the West Indies.

CONCLUSION

The relationship between the European body and the tropical environment was portrayed in medical treatises and military reports as unfavourable and potentially deadly. One possible way to change the balance of power was to ensure that sick and injured sailors and soldiers received adequate fever nursing. The choice to hire black nurses for West Indian military and naval hospitals was based on the climatic understanding of health and disease, which were integrated into cultural norms. These women were perceived to represent the most valuable commodity of all: freedom from tropical fever. Yet while the selection of these women emphasizes how contemporaries viewed the suitability of the African and Creole body for work in the West Indian climate, the work they were asked to do in military and naval hospitals was similar to that asked of other nurses throughout the Atlantic world. The impetus to create hospitals that would be healthy locations relied on the connection between the body of the sick soldier or sailor and their environment. Such built environments were primarily created through the work of nurses: the cleaning of bodies, bedding, clothing and wards, and adequate ventilation through mechanical or natural means. The military and naval dependence on black nurses adds another dimension to the familiar tale of black labour benefiting European colonial rule in the West Indies, while situating that narrative within cultural and environmental understandings of medicine.

CHAPTER TWO

Food

E.C. SPARY

What is a food? This question preoccupied both medical practitioners and their clients in the age of Enlightenment. Renaissance traditions of dietetics, deriving categories and frames of reference from the classics, persisted after 1700. But they were supplemented by new kinds of literature and practice that conferred new meanings upon healthy eating, hunger and appetite. Perhaps the two most salient transformations lay in the emergence of food chemistry and in the politicization of medical involvement with diet. These innovations responded to rapid transformations in the diets of elites and poor people alike, provoked by an increasing availability of, and dependency upon, foreign and prefabricated foods (Gentilcore 2015; Thirsk 2007; Briesen 2010). One result was the emergence of entirely new kinds of medical expertise over food and diet, increasingly reliant upon laboratory knowledge and also increasingly integrated into practices of governance. These changes occurred first and most completely in what Michel Foucault (1977) dubbed the 'disciplinary spaces' of early modernity, such as prisons, hospitals and workhouses. The new field of alimentary chemistry depended upon trials in such spaces for its legitimacy.

The remarkable thing about these transformations, however, was that they were a product far more of the spread of general concerns with self-regulation among eighteenth-century elites than of any top-down imposition of dietary reform by the state. It was in their self-appointed capacity as instructed members of society, increasingly wedded to programmes of public order and social hygiene, that physicians and chemists embarked upon the reform of diet and the revision of classical dietary precepts. That is, what we think of as the defining characteristics of Enlightenment – order, regulation, rationalization, measurement, improvement and education – produced new dietary relationships with governance, mediated by medical and scientific practitioners. Such effects as these changes had within households were mediated by print and industrialization. In this sense, the history of food and diet serves as a topos for bringing some well-known approaches developed within cultural history since the 1980s, and centring upon print culture, communication and symbolism, into conjunction with histories of science and medicine.

At the heart of this conjuncture should be a history of power, as Michel Foucault recognized in addressing other aspects of the history of medicine. How, we may ask, did knowledge experts insert themselves into wider debates concerning the distribution of food resources throughout societies? This chapter will argue that they did so by redefining what counted as 'food' in fundamental ways which fitted middling literate agendas of social management and bodily order. In the process, medical and scientific knowledge offered efficacious ways of discounting a wealth of symbolic meanings and practices already surrounding diet in Western culture, and bringing official dietary prescriptions and policy into line with elite preoccupations with order and self-governance. Viewing this transformation across the eighteenth century is useful for several reasons. Firstly, this period marked an intensified shift in physicians' authority, from the management of the individual regimen of wealthy clients to political acknowledgement of doctors' role as experts over public diet (Jewson 1976; Coleman 1974). Secondly, the social transformations accompanying industrialization increased concerns about the production and distribution of food resources, as well as the relationship between diet and labour. Trials of dietary experiments within hospitals, prisons, workhouses and navies in the eighteenth century would be rolled out as general policies for the public management of food resources in the early nineteenth (Orland 2014; Treitel, 2020; Milles 1995). This chapter will scrutinize some of the processes driving this resignification of 'food', in which medical authority over the body was transformed simultaneously with the emergence of a new programme of scientific investigations into the nutritive value of foodstuffs. In many ways, this programme laid the foundations for the nineteenth-century nutrition science to which our own dietary understandings today continue to be indebted. And if the eighteenth century seems to produce a kind of alimentary expert who still looks familiar today, it is worth recalling how many other familiar practices of consumption also developed in this period, including industrial and ready-made foods, mass dependency on imported foodstuffs and the proliferation of disciplinary spaces where dietary requirements were to be met as cheaply as possible. Both concerns about the implications of these sweeping changes for societies, and attempts to define basic needs, responded to these phenomena.

PECCADILLOES OF THE MODERN DIET

Dr John Arbuthnot's *Essay concerning the Nature of Aliments*, first published in 1731, serves as a useful starting point for exploring the changing landscape of medical knowledge about food. Arbuthnot coined a whole new vocabulary for the medical properties of foods, contributing some 150 terms to Samuel Johnson's *Dictionary of the English Language* (1755). These ranged from 'acescent', meaning 'a tendency to sourness or acidity', 'arid' and 'coction', to 'constipation', 'nutriment', 'perspiration' and 'plethora'. However, he also generated many other neologisms along the way: 'abstemious', 'abundant', 'bamboozle', 'characterize' in the sense of 'mark with a stamp', 'constitution' in the sense of 'bodily frame' and 'extravagance', but also 'fair' in the sense of 'just dealing' and 'privacy' in the sense of 'great familiarity with'. In fact, it is quite surprising just how much Johnson's dictionary depended upon Arbuthnot not just for words relating to food and health, but also for terms connoting trust, credit, equity, luxury and necessity, intimacy and embodiment. As will be seen, these moral themes dominated eighteenth-century debates over food and medicine.

An acquaintance of Isaac Newton and Samuel Pepys, the Scots mathematician was well connected in Augustan England. Appointed physician extraordinary to Queen Anne, he numbers among the Scriblerians – an associate of Swift, Pope and Gay, bending literary talents to satirizing the Tory party (Ross 2004; Aitken 1892; Arbuthnot 2006). A more representative figure of the British literary Enlightenment is hard to imagine. His book on diet would be reprinted four times in English (1732, 1733, 1736 and 1756), and twice in French (1741 and 1756). It represented foods in chymical terms, going beyond an ancient tradition of writings derived from humoral theory.[1] In the eighteenth century, Hippocratic-Galenic humoral models of the body still held widespread sway among medical practitioners and their clients, not only around Europe but across large parts of the world, in India, China and the Ottoman Empire. In this classical tradition, medical knowledge about food fell under the rubric of dietetics, which in turn was a branch of hygiene, that part of medicine devoted to the maintenance of health (Albala 2002; Mikkeli 1999; von Engelhardt 1993).

Regimen, or the hygienic management of everyday life, was a practice for which lay elite individuals expected to take personal responsibility. It covered six non-naturals: the surrounding milieu (airs and waters); sleeping and waking; motion and rest; substances applied to the body; substances ingested; and substances excreted (Emch-Dériaz 1992a; Niebyl 1971). Although dietetics only addressed one of these six aspects, such was its importance that diet remained virtually synonymous with hygiene for the first three-quarters of the eighteenth century. Only in its final decades did this situation change, as new chymical research upon the air, as well as preoccupations with personal cleanliness and climatic or effluvial causes of disease, led to more environmental

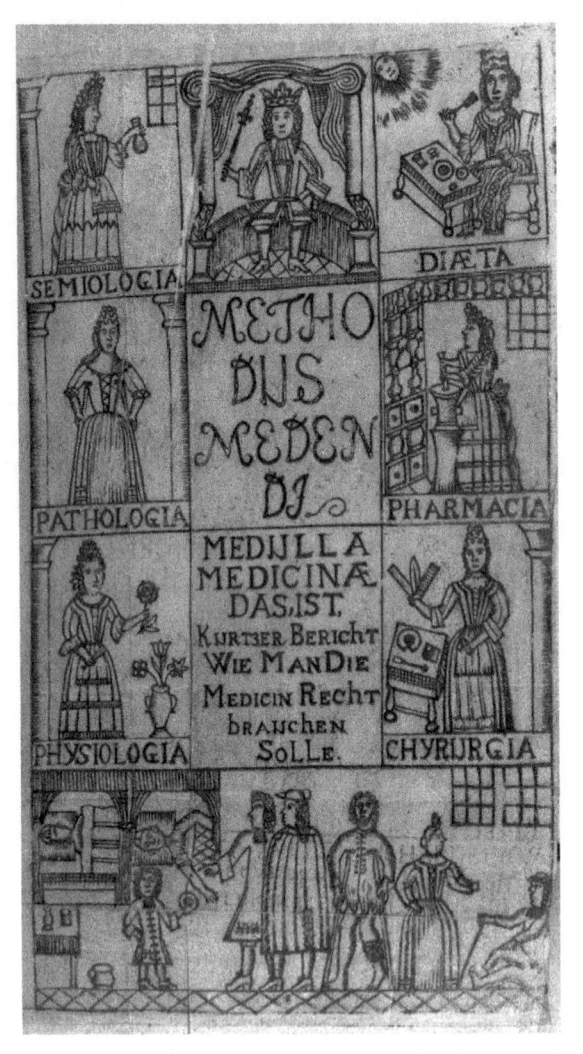

FIGURE 2.1: Diet in the classical repertoire: a German health manual of the early eighteenth century. Helena Aldegundis de Baden, *Methodus medendi. Medulla medicinæ, das ist, Kurtzer Bericht Wie Man Die Medicin Recht brauchen solle*, Warendorff: Ch. Nagel, 1702, frontispiece. Credit: BIU Santé, Paris.

definitions of hygiene, closer to what we understand by the term today (Wear 2008; Miller 1962).

Dietetic manuals were widely owned by literate elites through the sixteenth to eighteenth centuries. Many, though not all, were written by university physicians. Although overall studies of the genre worldwide are lacking, we can extrapolate from different European locations to state with some confidence

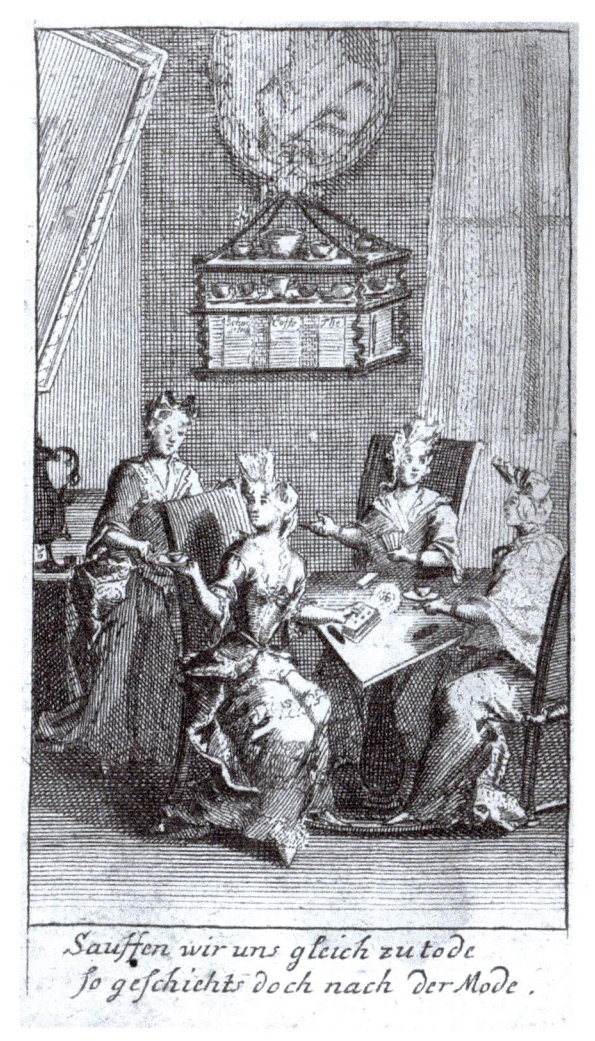

FIGURE 2.2: A German view of the dangers of coffee drinking for health: 'Sauffen wir uns gleich zu tode / so geschichts doch nach der Mode' (Let's just drink ourselves to death, as long as we're being trendy), from D. Duncan, *Von dem Missbrauch heissinger und hitziger Speisen und Getraencke*, Leipzig: J. F. Gleditsch, 1707. Credit: Wellcome Collection, London/Public Domain.

that a high proportion of elite readers relied on classical dietetic precepts mediated by a university-trained medical professional to make choices about their daily diet (Cavallo and Storey 2013; Albala 2002; Williams 2012; Bonnet 1983; Reinhardt et al. 1993; Turner 1982). These precepts centred upon the claim that each individual possessed a unique constitution or temperament, dominated by the balance between the qualities of their humours: wet, dry, hot

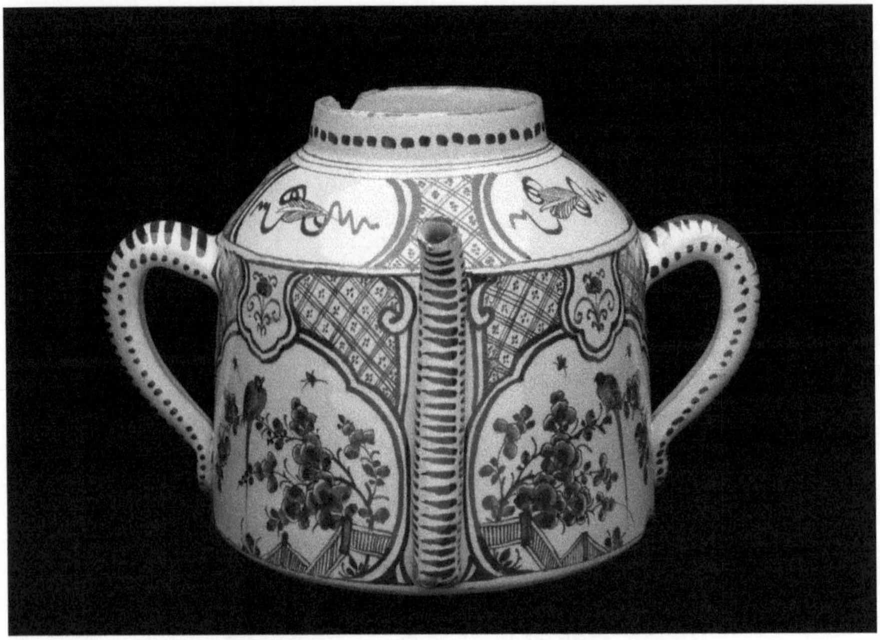

FIGURE 2.3: An early eighteenth-century Dutch posset pot with Chinese decoration, used for serving a mixture of spiced milk or wine and breadcrumbs to invalids. Credit: The Science Museum, London/Public Domain.

and cold (Bartoš 2015; Albury 1998). Lay readers of dietetic manuals were exhorted to know their own constitution and then to avoid eating foods which could shift it further from the ideal. Someone of phlegmatic temperament, dominated by moist cold humours, would be well advised to consume hot and dry foods like spices or fried dishes; by contrast, in the gut of a bilious person these same hot foods might be 'powder kegs', in the words of the Jacobite physician Daniel Duncan (1705: 14), a professor at the famous French medical university of Montpellier.

There was no singular 'healthy diet' in the eighteenth century in the way that we would understand it today. Each foodstuff possessed unique humoral qualities, and bitter disputes erupted among medical practitioners over how to classify new foods and drinks entering European diets within the humoral system, and which were most appropriate for particular social groups, genders, ages or occupations. Their clients were also intensively involved in this process, since the home was the main locus of cure. Kitchens and stillrooms doubled as spaces for preparing remedies, household receipt books routinely juxtaposed medical and culinary receipts, and new foods often first entered the European diet as medicines (Leong 2008, 2013). The boundary between foods and medicines, eating and healing, was thus blurred.

The iatrochymical approach of Arbuthnot and his generation of doctors did not so much jettison this humoral model as tack on a new dimension centred upon the balance of acids and alkalis in the consuming body. 'No person', Arbuthnot (1731: 82) opined, 'is able to support a Diet of Flesh and Water without Acids, as Salt, Vinegar, and Bread, without falling into a putrid Fever'. His Continental contemporaries, chymical physicians like Johann Joachim Becher, Georg Ernst Stahl and Friedrich Hoffmann in Germany, or Louis Lémery in France, likewise published chymical explanations of foodstuffs. Their writings circulated the learned world; Hoffmann's Anodyne or Drops, a compound of three parts spirit of wine and one part ether, made consumers all around Europe happy when it entered official pharmacopoeias. This chymical research underpinned various fashionable diets in the middle years of the century, such as the 'lemonade diet', based on the principle of correcting the acid–alkali balance in the body (Hufbauer 1982). Considerations of hot or cold, wet or dry, did not vanish from this chymically oriented work, but they received far less emphasis in dietary advice.

Chymistry was only one of several medical doctrines to challenge the dietetic status quo during the eighteenth century. *An Essay of Health and Long Life* (1724), read even more widely than Arbuthnot's essay, and written by a fellow Newtonian, Dr George Cheyne, spoke to a new constituency of consumers concerned about modern lifestyles as a cause of ill health (Guerrini 1986, 2000). The backdrop to such concerns was an enduring theme in scholarly works: the decline in vigour and longevity of the human race since the Biblical episodes of the Fall and the Flood (Palmer 1991). In the eighteenth century, these Renaissance worries about corporeal decline were revived in a large literature on new diseases such as vapours that, it was claimed, were emerging in consequence of changing dietary practices. Eighteenth-century eaters lived through what has been dubbed the 'nutrition transition', when traditional habits of consumption shifted in ways that can be documented even in the archaeological record (Cessford 2017: 171). Ale and beer gave way to coffee, tea and chocolate; herring and oatmeal ceded to white bread and tea; sugar and spices brought from great distances to European markets, largely by the Dutch, shifted from princely treasures to occasional luxuries, then necessities (Otter 2012; McCants 2007; Walvin 1997; den Hartog 1995; Cullen 1992; Teuteberg and Wiegelmann 1972). As the taste for spices and exotic beverages like tea, coffee and chocolate burgeoned, the prospect of whole societies become dependent upon foreign foodways alarmed leading doctors like Jean-Baptiste Chomel in Paris, leading him to rehearse an older suggestion that 'in a state of health we can find herbs and fruits at home which suit us just as well as Tea, Coffee, Pepper, Ginger &c. . . . in a word, one could demonstrate that France encloses within her bosom or on her frontiers all that is most necessary and useful to the health of her inhabitants' (Chomel 1712: unpaginated; see also Spary 2004; Cooper 2007). The worry about alienating

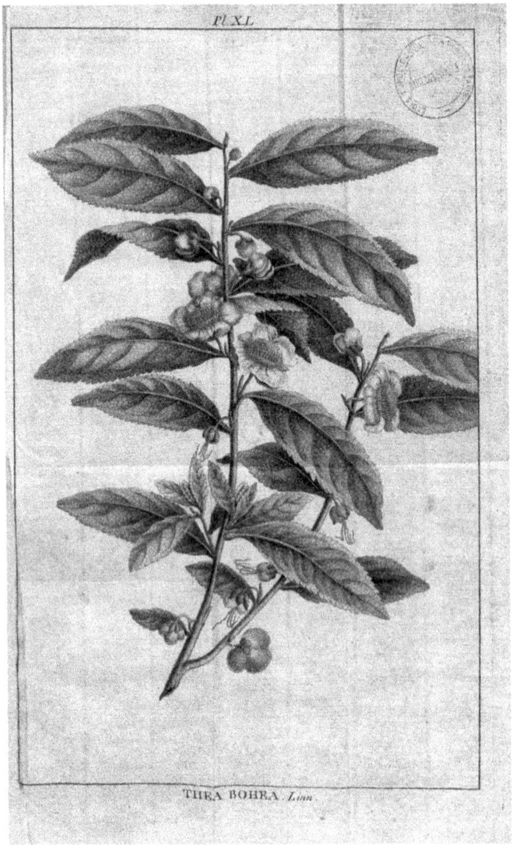

FIGURE 2.4: Thea Bohea, depicted by the Lotharingian physician botanist Pierre Buc'hoz, *Dissertations sur l'utilité et les bons et mauvais effets du tabac, du café, du cacao et du thé*, Paris: de Bure, 1788, plate XL. Buc'hoz was a strong advocate of indigenous substitutes. Credit: BIU Santé, Paris.

one's own body by consuming foreign foods – and foreign climatic influences along with them – led European colonists to depend on supplies of imported food shipped from the metropolis to the colonies at vast expense (Earle 2012).

Such concerns addressed profound questions of identity that accompanied the emergence of the nation-state and the expansion of European colonial empires. When French cuisine was taken up in other European countries like England, Germany and Russia after 1700, anti-French sentiment provoked adverse commentary on the new fashion. Yet eighteenth-century physicians railed largely in vain against the Frenchification of polite diet and table manners (Mennell 1996; Paston-Williams 1993). As an anonymous 'High-German Doctor' mocked in 1720 (285):

> I have often thought of my dear Parents Advice, never to aspire beyond *Butter-milk* and *Potatoes*; but once getting into a Gang of *Stage Highway-Men* who liv'd prodigally upon the *Spoils* of the *Nation*, I soon found the *Sweets* of *Plunder,* and, by degrees, brought my Palate to relish *French Ragoo's* and Forc'd Meats.
>
> —original emphasis

Criticisms were directed against French cuisine for two reasons: firstly, with its emphasis on blending, flavouring and disguising foods, it was viewed as a form of artificiality and deceit, producing fake pleasures. Secondly, as part of a luxury lifestyle, French cuisine was harmful not only to the individual's body but also to the health and morals of the whole nation. The acquisition of new tastes for new goods was seen as having irreversible effects upon the fabric of the body and the health not only of the individual but of society as a whole. Diseases such as the vapours, hypochondria, gout or consumption were explained as a product of the enervation of modern bodies by bad eating habits, particularly the embrace of such foreign and luxurious foods (Guerrini 1999a; Jonsson 2005; Rousseau 1976; Porter 1993, 1994; Wagner 2013).

Changed tastes were particularly troubling in countries without maritime empires, which in the eighteenth century included much of central, northern and eastern Europe. Here exotic consumption tended to be seen as particularly excessive and unhealthy. After Sweden lost its colonies to Russia in the early eighteenth century, political power was seized by the reformist Hats party in 1738. It was to the Uppsala physician Carolus Linnaeus that the Hats turned in an effort to make postcolonial Sweden self-sufficient in plant resources (Koerner 1999). Physicians and apothecaries waded into the debate over whether indigenous substitutes like chicory root could effectively replace exotic foods and drugs like coffee (Ball 1991: 19). Such attempts to argue for the medicinal equivalence of local foods with exotic imports might, however, be sceptically received. A contributor to the newspaper *Gothaische gelehrte Zeitungen* (26 July 1775: 483) denied that any 'among the products of German soil can be ranked equal to foreign coffee in respect of goodness'.

It was also hard to reach agreement as to which scientific techniques were the most reliable predictors of the healthfulness (or otherwise) of unfamiliar foods. From the time of Robert Boyle onwards, in the late seventeenth century, scientific practitioners had used chymical analysis to investigate the medical and nutritive properties of foodstuffs. Although analysis remained an active field of enquiry throughout the eighteenth century, it was not generally viewed as offering any firm evidence for the relationship between chymical and nutritive or health properties of foods until later decades, when solvent analysis enabled the isolation of the nutritive principle of meat, bread and milk (Orland 2010; Spary 2014). Chymical analysts – mostly apothecaries and physicians –

also struggled to find a secure way of predicting toxicity, despite extensive experimentation upon ergotic rye, potatoes and other foods (Stroup 1985: 51–3; Fink 1990). Botany was an important resource: in an article on the aubergine, much used in Islamic cuisine, the editor of a French medical newspaper, the *Gazette de Santé*, concluded that its membership of the genus *Solanum* rendered it unsafe to eat (10 October 1776: 159–60). But neither discipline offered an agreed-upon means of adjudging the health effects of new and exotic foods.

Anxieties about the management of the self in this globalizing world were widespread among European elites. Reacting to the extensive public expenditure upon foreign goods, many reformers, spearheaded by physicians, proposed radically alternative lifestyles centred on the rejection of modern diet. Similar concerns may be found as far back as the Roman Empire, in the attacks of Horace or Cicero upon the lavish lifestyles of their political opponents; repurposed in the eighteenth century, they lost nothing of their political sting, nor their framing of eating's future in historical terms, as a choice between bad modernity or antique purity. In his *Primitive Physick* of 1747, for example, John Wesley, the founder of Methodism, advised his readers to 'Abstain from all mixt, all high-season'd Food'.[2] For Immanuel Kant, professor of philosophy at the University of Königsberg, leading a healthy philosophical life meant avoiding tobacco, coffee, spices and meat. Kant was a close reader of dietetic works, who regularly sent dietary recommendations to his fellow philosophers. His remarks came in the context of a reflection upon mortality provoked by the recent demise of the Jewish philosopher Moses Mendelssohn (Roth 2015: 204ff).

The conjuncture is a resonant one. A couple of years earlier, in 1784, the Prussian king Frederick the Great had proposed a prize essay question on the subject 'What is Enlightenment?' The two answers which remain the definitive contemporary definitions of that term were, of course, those written by Kant and Mendelssohn (Kant 1784; Mendelssohn 1784; Foucault 1991). The emphasis of Enlightenment upon secular improvement meant that, increasingly, even philosophers moved away from a focus upon learning as a route to understanding the Christian life after death, and instead addressed their efforts to the medical resolution of dietary problems in the here and now.

BODIES OF RADICALISM

Claims that modern society was eating itself to death – as vocal as those of our own time – not only underpinned scepticism about modern cuisine and exotic foods, they also led to a resurgence of interest in classical vegetarianism, and encouraged a view of body weight as a measure of virtue and fitness. Cheyne's weight of 450 pounds did not stop him becoming one of the high priests of the cult of 'low regimen', an ostentatiously anti-luxurious diet, and in this guise he fielded hundreds of letters from readers of his books eager to lose weight. In a time before the invention of the calorie, it is interesting to consider what counted as a healthy diet in the view of this doctor. For the fundamental characteristics of 'low regimen' were strongly moralized. It was to be 'plain', 'simple' and 'spare'. Eaters were exhorted to practice 'temperance' and 'abstemiousness' (Guerrini 2000; Berry 2014; Briesen 2010: 27ff). Other physicians recommended the milk diet, which framed milk as a pure and simple food capable of correcting luxurious and artificial diets packed with spices and richness (e.g. Pomme 1767: *passim*; Wilson 1993). That is, the reform of diet went beyond health to moral goals allied with those of the temperance movement that was beginning to demonize spirituous drink. The adoption of low regimen was a good way to signal middling lifestyles and conduct as rational, orderly and measured. These values were then contrasted with the perceived wastefulness and lack of control over the body's needs, desires and actions deemed characteristic of both the upper and the lower social orders (Brennan 1988; Clark 1988; Smith 2002).

Cheyne's work was widely read, but also widely attacked. Many critics preferred to remain anonymous. One, purporting to be a Fellow of the Royal Society (*Remarks on Dr. Cheyne's Essay on Health and Long Life* [1725?]: 15), disputed Cheyne's central claim that dieting and temperance guaranteed good health: 'I have known Persons of the exactest Temperance, who delighted in Pudding and Roots . . . and yet these very Persons were eat up with the *Scurvy*'. Dieting remained a controversial practice, and its political roots were apparent to contemporaries. The navel-gazing of the European literate elite was manifest in its focus upon the relationship between health and obesity. A Renaissance device known as the Sanctorian chair, which sank as the eater consumed more food, putting the table out of reach, knew a revival in the eighteenth century as readers sought to quantify their dietary sins (Albala 2005; Dacome 2001, 2012).

Treatises on 'static medicine', in which health was directly correlated to body weight, were published around Europe by doctors like Martin Lister, Giorgio Baglivi, James Keill and Denis Dodart. These elaborations of an earlier static tradition featured in numerous editions of Sanctorius's original work, often with a national flavour added, such as Keill's and Dodart's measurements upon British and French bodies respectively (Noguez 1725; Lister and Baglivi 1742). Yet self-weighing was not as self-evident as it appears to us in hindsight. Consensus had first to be produced over *how* obesity should be correlated to health: for example, whether scales or measuring tapes were the best way to quantify portly eighteenth-century gentlemen. Moreover, despite the modern appearance of an obsession with body weight, the causes of obesity were understood very differently before the invention of the calorie. For those desirous of reducing, the Paris physician Charles-Gabriel Le Clerc recommended occasional draughts of vinegar, abstaining from drinking altogether, purgatives and 'the frequent use of women' (Le Clerc 1719: 232). Eighteenth-century

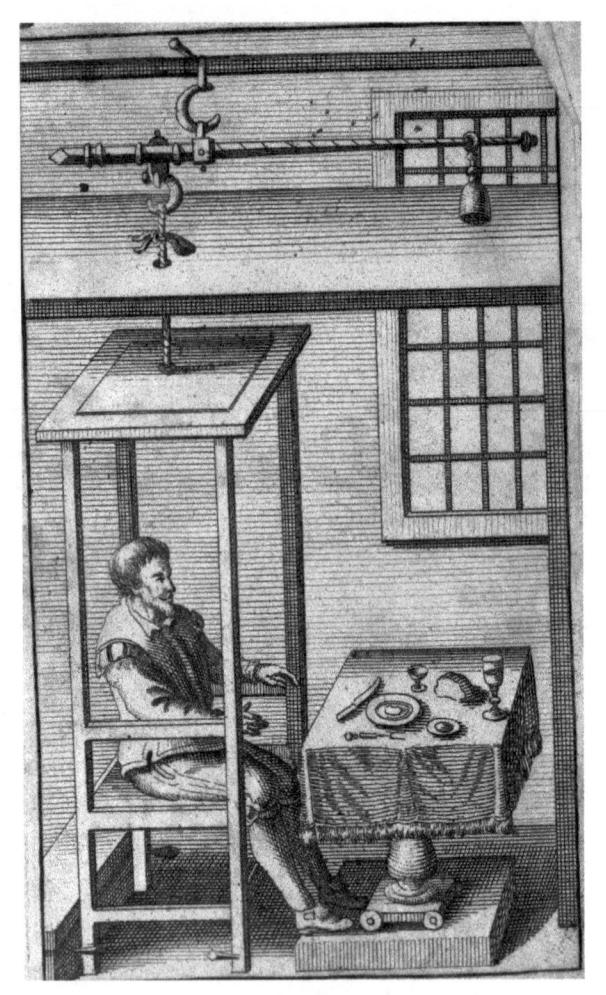

FIGURE 2.5: Sanctorius on his scales, pictured in an eighteenth-century edition of his *De statica medicina: aphorismorum sectionibus septem comprehensa*, Leiden: Widow of Cornelius Boutesteyn, 1713, frontispiece. Credit: BIU Santé, Paris.

authors made little distinction between fat and muscle. Rather, excess weight was seen as a consequence of excess consumption of nutritive substance. Concerns about body weight were, accordingly, more closely tied to worries about the inequitable distribution of nutritive resources through society (Spary 2014; Stolberg 2012; Fischler 1993).

Similar moral themes were apparent in medical debate over vegetarianism, a more radical programme of dietary reform that recruited supporters throughout the eighteenth century. Scholarly yearnings for a lost dietary Golden Age peppered editions of Ovid's *Metamorphoses* and Porphyry's *De abstinentia*. As Antoine Banier, a French royal academician, asseverated in his 1732 translation

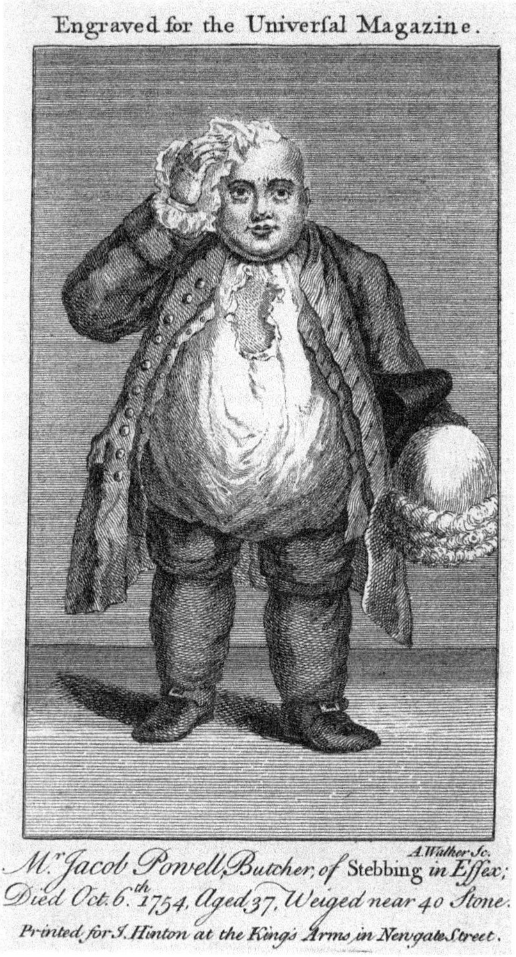

FIGURE 2.6: Jacob Powell, butcher, of Stebbing in Essex, depicted in the *Universal Magazine* after his death in October 1754 at the age of thirty-seven, weighing nearly forty stone. Credit: Wellcome Collection, London/Public Domain.

of *Metamorphoses* (III, book 15, 215; Guerrini 1999b), at 'that happy time . . . man did not sully his mouth with the blood of Animal . . . Whoever it was that . . . introduced the custom of eating Animal flesh, opened the door to all sorts of crimes at the same time'. The famous Florentine physician Antonio Cocchi's (1743) *Del vitto Pitagorico* backed up the moral argument with a detailed account of the health benefits of vegetarianism. An advocate of Newtonian cosmology, Fellow of the Royal Society and classical scholar in his own right, Cocchi commanded scholarly respect. Inscribing himself within the tradition of static medicine, he gave anatomical justifications for the claim that vegetables were the natural human diet. However, his advocacy of the vegetable diet met with an equivocal reception around Europe.[3] Probably the main reason for this was the link between vegetarianism and political radicalism (Guerrini 2012a; Stuart 2007; Spencer 1993). The basis for increasing – though always modest – elite support for vegetarianism over the century was its association with social critique. If in the 1750s the Genevan philosopher Jean-Jacques Rousseau was being caricatured as a lackey to the rich who went on all fours like an animal, keeping a lettuce in his pocket, by the 1780s both Rousseauism and vegetarianism had become fashionable among the reform-minded young nobility in France (Spary 2012). During the turbulence of the 1790s, the connection between vegetarianism and political radicalism became ever more apparent. Percy Bysshe Shelley's post-Revolutionary *Vindication of Natural Diet* (1813), heir to the kind of reformist agenda espoused by Cheyne and Wesley, eloquently critiqued modern capitalism's effects upon the twin bodies of the citizen and the nation (Morton 1994).

Traditional dietetic advice correlated elite status with refinement. To eat 'coarse', 'rough', 'harsh' or 'raw' foods was to alter the body, approximating the elite eater to the common one (Eden 2008: 4–20; Watts 2011). This was the basis of many objections to vegetarianism. To those arguing that cookery played an important medical role by purifying and exalting foodstuffs, low regimen, with its embrace of humble diet, seemed to threaten both the health and the social standing of elite bodies, even more so the vegetable diet with its insistence on coarse roots and earthy foods. The issue came to a head in debates over 'economic bread' in 1770s to 1790s France. Economic milling, which bulked out flour supplies by leaving in some of the bran, was a technique devised by entrepreneurial millers and sold to the French Crown as a way to make the grain supply stretch further. But when medical commentators issued stark warnings about the concomitant loss in nutritive virtue of the staple food, economic milling lost favour with the government (Kaplan 1996; Spary 2014).

The presence of doctors and apothecaries as advisors to legislators in such debates over the food supply during the later eighteenth century points to a sea change in the public and political status of medical accounts of food. Cocchi's book (1743: 57–8) heralded this shift in no uncertain terms in its claim that a lack of vegetables caused scurvy. He invoked the disciplinary space of the college as evidence of his assertion: 'In Italy . . . the symptoms of scurvy have been seen to increase or diminish in strength in accordance with the more or less frequent use of fresh plants. This is what occurs in some communities or colleges, where boarding students are often deprived of this nourishment out of an unwise economy.' Cocchi's remark is interesting for two reasons: firstly, because it highlights the regulated collectivity as an experimental space for testing a hypothesis as to the cause of scurvy; secondly, because it raises the larger question of what foods were in fact required for good health, and how far doctors could claim to be able to pronounce on general as opposed to specific dietary laws.

Cocchi's claims about scurvy also touched a nerve in contemporary statecraft. By mid-century, European colonialism was developing apace. Voyages, whether naval or commercial, became ever longer. Maritime powers – Genoa and Venice, the Hanseatic League and the Baltic seaports, as well as England, Sweden, Russia, France, Spain, Portugal and the Netherlands – competed for distant goods. Scurvy was a significant obstacle to successful global trade and exploration, and also to victory in the many wars fought at sea for control of distant colonies. From the Seven Years' War onwards, many spaces of European conflict were far removed from Europe itself: in Goa or the Antilles, in the Mascarenes or the Moluccas, and in North and South America. The administration of such distant spaces meant that scurvy prevention was a matter affecting maritime supremacy and therefore of national concern. The French government hired a doctor to mine the travel account of Captain James Cook for details of his anti-scorbutic measures.[4] The ship, in the age of long-distance maritime exploration, became an important space for experimenting on the connection between diet and health, where new techniques of food preservation, substitution or preparation proposed by savants – such as an anti-scorbutic carrot preserve proposed by the Portuguese academician João Jacinto de Magalhães in 1772 – were trialled by ships' surgeons and reported upon to ministers around Europe (McBride 1991; Lawrence 1996; Harrison 2013; Spary 2009).[5] Some of these techniques, including canning, stock cubes and 'nutritive powders' that were claimed to concentrate the food principle in a small compass, were also fundamental developments of early industrial food production (Goody 1997; Mennell et al. 1992; Shephard 2000; Stead 1991; Thorne 1986).

FROM PERSONAL REGIMEN TO IMPERSONAL REGIMEN

The interest in solving collective as opposed to individual health problems became a growing priority of medical and scientific practitioners in many parts of Europe over the course of the century. The internationalism evident in attempts to tackle scurvy also extended to other kinds of problems, understood to be essentially hygienic in nature, that were resulting from processes of urbanization, industrialization or imperialism. Here the example of Benjamin Thompson stands out. Thompson was born in Massachusetts, the son of an American merchant of modest means who married a wealthy woman. Having fought for the Loyalist cause during the American Revolution, he was rewarded with a top post in the Georgian army and ennoblement as Count Rumford in 1791, before relocating from England to Bavaria as advisor to Elector Karl

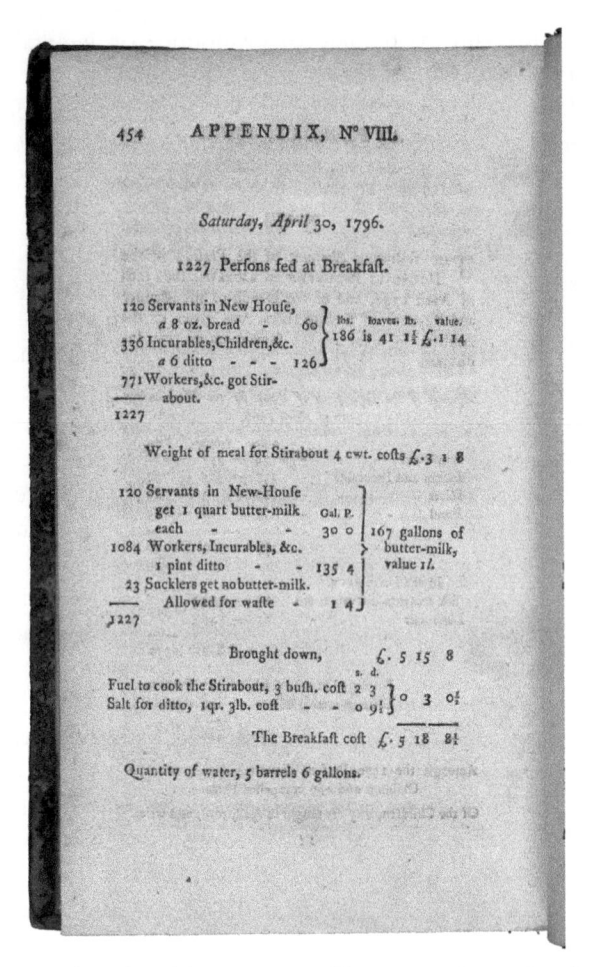

FIGURE 2.7: Quantifying breakfast. Benjamin Thompson, Count Rumford, *Essays, Political, Economical, and Philosophical*, I, London: T. Cadell Jr, 1796, 454. Credit: Wellcome Collection, London. Permission had to be sought for this image through the Wellcome Archives. This one is not an image on their website.

Theodor. His interest in the science of heat led him to design new measures of efficiency for running Bavarian workhouses frugally and productively, which extended to diet.

Rumford (as he now was) used his experimentation in Munich as the foundation for workhouse reform proposals which he touted around Germany, England and France during the 1790s. In his view, these experiments pointed to 'the very small quantity of SOLID FOOD, which, when properly prepared, will suffice to satisfy hunger, and support life and health; and the very trifling expence at which the stoutest, and most laborious man may, in any country, be fed' (Rumford 1796: 195–6; Sherman 2001). Rumford's priorities accorded well with Central European programmes of medical police and cameralism. The former practice extended administrative oversight to the exercise of hygienic policies and the collection of health data – including on diet – across an extended territory. The latter was the new science of governance and increase of state resources (Carroll 2002; Rosen 1953, 1974; Wakefield 2009; Sechel 2003). Certainly Rumford's agenda encompassed more than good health alone; he aimed to convert the poor from a burden on the state into productive members of society, and to terminate begging. Even though Rumford was not medically qualified, the health claims underpinning his projects found wide support in the European medical and scientific community. In particular, his view that diluting food did not dilute its nutritive value was avidly seized upon by administrators and scholars. In a striking passage that seems to suggest that deception and artifice had a role in these rational projects for the quantified management of food consumption, Rumford (1796: 195) concluded that:

> The nutritiousness of a soup, or its power of satisfying hunger, and affording nourishment, appeared always to be in proportion to its apparent richness or palatableness ... I constantly found that the richness or QUALITY of a soup depended more upon a proper choice of the ingredients, and a proper management of the fire in the combination of those ingredients, than upon the quantity of solid nutritious matter employed; – much more upon the art and skill of the cook, than upon the amount of the sums laid out in the market.

Rumford's was not a lone voice. Eighteenth-century medical literature was full of reported cases of human bodies nourished by water alone, or air, or nothing at all (Hollis 2001). Although one might suppose that such reports would number among the first casualties as Enlightened knowledge spread, in fact the governmentalization of temperance ensured that the converse happened: ever more sophisticated scientific and medical explanations were generated to accommodate such reports. In turn, these explanations served to justify cost-cutting when it came to feeding the poor or distributing limited food supplies, whether in hospitals or in whole nations. In Paris, the apothecary Antoine-Augustin Parmentier (1781: 2–3), promoting the potato as a substitute for wheat, commented that:

> We daily observe ... that in the foods which make up a meal, not everything is substantial, not everything converts itself equally into chyle; one need only live in an environment charged with nutritive corpuscles, to acquire a stoutness that is not always obtained from eating foods. Brewers, Butchers, Starch-makers, Cooks & Pork Butchers seem to owe that freshness & good health which distinguish them from the other artisans to the plant or animal vapours circulating in the atmosphere of their workshops.

Since Parmentier went on to become a nutritional advisor to the French king Louis XVI, then later to successive Revolutionary governments (where he was also responsible for setting up a national chain of soup kitchens), we can see how priorities of temperance and austerity characteristic of the low regimen movement were, by the turbulent end of the eighteenth century, percolating from the self-scrutiny of Enlightened elites into government policy and poor management. Canny rulers like Frederick the Great of Prussia could solve multiple problems at once. After 1779, many luxury foods, including coffee, were subject in Prussia, a non-colonial power, to some of the highest taxes in Europe. The king employed several hundred disabled poor, immediately dubbed *Kaffeeschnüffler* or 'coffee sniffers', to detect smuggled coffee being roasted in Berlin households, thus employing the poor, enforcing low regimen and policing tax revenues at one stroke (Müller 1997: 412).

From such examples, it is easy to discern some salient shifts in the relationship between food and medical authority over the course of the eighteenth century. Healthy diet was becoming a general preserve of government in the attempt to turn populations into productive resources (Foucault 2007: 1–4). Knowledge experts who could pronounce on medical matters were allying themselves with governments to promote social hygiene programmes around Europe. Medical attempts to define and quantify healthy diet, or to make definitive pronouncements as to the healthfulness or otherwise of individual foods, were becoming enrolled in structures of statecraft.

Such initiatives developed across a number of fronts over the course of the century. Contemporary programmes for the collection of information about national health, known as medical police, gave ample space to food and diet. The rationalization of the food supply was seen as central to the maintenance of public order by rulers and administrators around Europe, as well as to the measurement, management and improvement of populations (Winston 2005; Quinlan 2007). Concerns about the circulation, distribution, reproduction and shortfall of nutritive resources coloured not only social hygiene but also political economy, chymistry, agronomy and cookery. Food thus spanned the personal and the political domains, while precepts of self-regulation increasingly entered policies for the governance of whole societies. It is no coincidence that the end of the eighteenth century produced the *Essay on the Principle of Population* of Thomas Malthus, the English clergyman who argued that population growth would inevitably outstrip the food supply (Malthus 1798; Bashford and Chaplin 2016).

One consequence of medical police was the progressive medicalization of ordinary life around Europe. The rational management of the food supply was one of the areas in which physicians like Samuel-Auguste-André-David Tissot interested themselves. Between the 1760s and the 1780s, this Swiss doctor moved from writing health manuals which advocated austerity for his rich corresponding clients around Europe, to proposing poor relief programmes in his home canton of Lausanne. Between times, he worried about the waste of nutritive substance from the bodies of feckless masturbators; his campaign against onanism would have long-lasting effects upon European males over many generations (Emch-Dériaz 1992b; Stolberg 2000). Tissot's interests mirrored a wider gearing-up of elite authors towards the secular resolution of societal problems, combining the centrally organized gathering of observations with the implementation of programmes of management of land, bodies and resources. Medical definitions of what counted as the true nutritive principle, and how much of it each category of body required, were central to all debates about how and to whom food resources should be distributed.

In reflecting upon how to provide a healthy diet for all of society, reformers took the models of temperance and self-restraint that elites were constantly exhorted in dietetic manuals to command, and multiplied them across the social spectrum. There was widespread interest in organizing for the poor a dietary programme centred around temperance and self-restraint. These were skills of bodily self-management that, elite authors claimed, poor eaters were unable to master for themselves or wilfully avoided in favour of fashionable luxury foods. Efforts to hamper the lower orders from consuming above their station underpinned the extension of older mechanisms of sumptuary legislation to new foods. In many German towns, for example, coffee consumption was prohibited to the poor (Heise 1987: 39 ff). In traditional elite dietetics, the emphasis had been on the infinite variety of individual constitutions and upon self-knowledge; medical clients were expected to learn about, then cater to, their own temperament as it changed over their lifetime, from youth to old age. The needs of the state were otherwise. Rulers, ministers, administrators, and military or naval commanders sought a one-size-fits-all solution to administrative headaches such as feeding ever larger armies, efficiently outfitting ships for long-distance voyages and managing the budgets of hospitals, prisons, workhouses, barracks and schools, as well as addressing the management and increase of the food supply to prevent food riots. That is, all the many disciplinary spaces that sprang into life as a direct result of eighteenth-century attempts to organize, rationalize and make useful the bodies of the poor, the idle and workers imposed their own logic of nourishment, which was rather different from the individualistic emphasis of dietetic manual authors and their clienteles.

A precondition for accomplishing the Enlightened extension of statecraft to the body was the establishment of a universal model of dietary needs applicable to all. In matters of poor management, individualized regimens were superseded by medical and administrative claims about universal dietary requirements. While rations had been used in hospitals, armies and navies from the start of the century, it is only by the 1770s that we begin to find cost-efficiency entering the equation where the management of whole populations was concerned. The results of physicians' and apothecaries' trials of experimental diets in disciplinary spaces such as hospitals, prisons or workhouses were used as evidence of the quantity of nourishment required to sustain life, as well as of the extent to which good health really required certain staple foods with particularly high symbolic value, such as bread or meat (Thoms 2005).[6] In times of crisis, when such foods were lacking, it was to medical experts that states turned to offer alternatives and pronounce on the health effects of new foods like the potato. Although this advisory role is insufficiently studied, in many countries such practitioners made claims before government and in the public press about the chymical, medicinal and physiological effects of alternatives when normal food supplies ran short (Abad 2006). Chymists in particular profited from growing demand for food expertise in every domain, from naval supplies to health foods to soup kitchens. Such activity would become ever more prominent over the course of the nineteenth century, but already in the closing decades of the eighteenth, medical practitioners were contributing to programmes for the rational management of public diet.

Techniques of medical bureaucracy that worked on shipboard (say) seemed to offer plausible solutions to many of the problems of urbanization and poor diet associated with industrialization. Physicians and apothecaries were active as investigators – both evaluators and inventors – of preservation techniques, including freezing, canning, drying and extraction (Teuteberg 1995, 2007; Forbes 1958). The concerns of Enlightened elites for moral and social order underlay the increasing prominence of medical practitioners as government advisors in creating food policy. It is also important to stress that elite bodies continued to benefit from a more personalized medical experience. Food and medicine remained closely linked within the household, allowing scope for affluent consumers to define their own 'healthy diet' or simply to reject medico-scientific arguments.

CONCLUSION

Eighteenth-century dietetic advice often appears distinctly at odds with our views today. Fresh fruit and dietary fibre, for example, were widely condemned as health risks before 1800. The young woman at Den Haag in the Netherlands who 'was cured of a Dropsie by eating a great Quantity of Cherries', on the advice of the Dutch doctor Herman Boerhaave, only featured in so many editions of his *Aphorisms* (e.g. 1735: 371–2) because her cure challenged humoral standards of good dietetic practice and supported Boerhaave's chymical inclinations. Yet, despite many changes in the knowledge and availability of foods since the eighteenth century, in fashionable tastes, culinary techniques and eating habits, our diets still invisibly enshrine many humoral claims of the past; we add oil and vinegar, traditional correctives of cold and wet foods, to salads and we fry fish, a heating practice in Galenic culinary manuals. As ever, diet and health are highly complex systems of practice, threaded through by a range of different priorities: local cuisines, new fashions, personal tastes and medical recommendations vie with one another to produce the diet that we eventually consume. This was equally the case in the eighteenth century. Most elite people still followed rules obeyed by their parents and grandparents, but even contemporaries acknowledged that diets were changing with the advance of colonial empires and global trade. Many poor people remained at the mercy of an irregular food supply, although where circumstances allowed, they too embraced new food fashions and understood their own bodies in terms of humoral theory. Scientific and medical experts joined forces with governments around Europe to document and then reform diet and the food supply. They began in small managed disciplinary spaces like workhouses and hospitals; but by 1800 they were integrated as advisors to states attempting to administer large-scale problems of the food supply, on the basis of their authority over what counted as a 'healthy diet'.

The question of whether medico-scientific interventions in the food supply had measurable effects upon the health of poor consumers during the eighteenth century remains unanswerable. Besides perennial issues of absent or inadequate data, among the insuperable problems confronting attempts to quantify diet by the light of today's dietary standards are the fact that eighteenth-century reformers had markedly different understandings of the 'healthy diet' from those of modern historians. Their ventures into national food policies marked the first moment when medical practitioners had to articulate universalizing claims about the body's true dietary needs, and therefore the first historical moment when recording what people ate became more than a matter of writing individual case histories. Their universal truths of human dietary requirements were, however, articulated under particular political circumstances: industrialization and the 'nutrition transformation', the demands of war and imperialism, and the increasing globalization of consumption. Nineteenth-century physiological and nutritional experimentation by doctors like François Magendie, Claude Bernard and Justus von Liebig would build upon these politics of self-restraint that dominated later eighteenth-century debates about food and health. If solvent chymistry had centred upon a rather undifferentiated account of 'the' nutritive substance, around 1800, understandings of an adequate diet would fragment in response to a coupling of vivisection experiments with chymical analysis. chymistry-physiological enquiry in laboratories led to the invention of food groups, and eventually of the calorie as a unit of nutritive value, through the research of first French, then German chemists (Kamminga and Cunningham 1995; Stahnisch 2004; Holmes 1975; Cullather 2007; Treitel 2008; Neswald et al. 2017). But the establishment of chymical and medical authority over public nourishment antedated all of this.

Both the convergence of attempts to quantify dietary requirements with new needs to manage working bodies, and the moralization of consumption and body weight, are trends that underpinned the emergence of a new science of nutrition and continue to underpin our public discourse about diet today. When scholars embark upon the history of food, or even of individual foodstuffs, in the eighteenth century, therefore, the mutability of the very category 'food' in social, medico-scientific, political, commercial and culinary discourse means that they must scrutinize the fine-grained allegiances and agendas of their protagonists with care (Harris 2004; Fogel 2004; Newman 1995; Rotberg and Rabb 1985; Vernon 2007). It is not enough for the cultural historian to approach the 'meaning' of foods by simply collating a series of discussions over time. Rather, we need to acknowledge that multiple, sometimes conflicting, accounts of food and nourishment coexist in any given culture, and that each has profound implications for access to, or the meaning of, particular foods. These contestations warrant analysis and explication, for – perhaps more than any other aspect of human agency – food connotes the entanglement of power and knowledge that makes up culture. Its eighteenth-century history highlights some significant transformations in the relations of authority and expertise structuring that entanglement in the Western world.

NOTES

1. 'Chymistry' is the term proposed by Principe (2007) to denote the broader horizons of chymical practice up to the end of the eighteenth century, embracing medical chemistry as well as artisanal pursuits.
2. Bardell (1979) shows that Cheyne was an important source for Wesley's views. See also Wallace (2003). For similar agendas in Switzerland and France, see Bonnet (1979).
3. E.g. reviews in *Avant-Coureur* (1762: 477–81); *Gazette de Santé* (1773: 5).
4. Archives nationales de France, Mar-G 179: letter, Achille-Guillaume Le Bègue de Presle to Antoine de Sartine, naval minister, Paris, 22 February 1777.
5. Archives nationales, France, Mar-G 179 (76); Mar-D^3, dossier 5.
6. On the food crisis produced by industrialization, see Muldrew (2011). On work, waste and nourishment, see Wise and Smith (1990); Simmons (2015). On institutional diet, see Thoms 2005.

CHAPTER THREE

Disease

LINA MINOU

INTRODUCTION

This is a chapter on eighteenth-century disease, as seen through a connection to emotion in the cultural context of the period. The connection between emotion and disease is not new. Indeed, as Theodore Brown observes, in surveying the history of mental disease, the interest in how emotional factors contributed to 'somatic disease onset or exacerbation can be traced from antiquity through the nineteenth century' (Brown 1993: 450). Brown calls the doctrine of the non-naturals (the factors associated with preserving or restoring health which included the passions) the 'longest standing tradition of mind-body connection in Western medicine' (451). 'Deeply felt emotions', he explains, 'could either exacerbate already existing somatic disease or help precipitate previously inapparent physical disorders' (439). A part of this chapter is devoted to emotion as a contributing factor to disease, as described by Brown. However, my analysis also considers emotion itself as disease. Firstly, I focus on specific emotions and their patho-physiology in historical context. I then shift from particular emotions to cultures of emotion, specifically the culture of sensibility and how it influenced attitudes to disease. In so doing, I aim to show the multiple ways that emotion and disease were linked in the period, a complex association that went beyond the mind/body connection.

The discussion is influenced by the rise of the history of emotions as a field of research (Plamper et al. 2010; Eustace et al. 2012; Plamper 2015; Boddice 2018). Historians of emotions contend that, rather than being a stable psycho-biological category, emotions change over time. Thus, the emotional past itself can, and should, be the subject of historical analysis and interpretation.

The way this is to be achieved, though, is a subject less agreed on. Historians of the emotional past have access not to the felt experience of emotions, but only to their expression. They have access to emotional vocabularies of the past, emotion words and discourse about emotions. Barbara Rosenwein is a pioneer of the field who introduced the concept of 'emotional communities' – the various topoi of expressing, sharing and policing emotion. This concept redressed previous reductive conceptualizations of historical emotional life, which had depicted it as following a linear trajectory towards refinement (Rosenwein 2006). Rosenwein herself emphasizes the role of language as a discovery tool. 'Emotional communities', she writes, are delineated by 'common discourse, shared vocabularies and ways of thinking that have a controlling function, a disciplining function' (Rosenwein 2006: 25).

The element of control and power in the expression of emotion is central to William Reddy's conception of 'emotional regime' (2001). Reddy's work is unique in its capacity to bridge essentialist models of emotion, mainly expressed in neuropsychology, and anthropological readings that maintain emotions are culturally and historically contingent. Reddy's 'emotives' is an analytical term that allows both for essentialist, stable, qualities in emotion and for the possibility that their meanings and expression are historically and culturally relative – and thus subject to change. Reddy's account of emotion also highlights the political aspects of emotion. His notion of an 'emotional regime' can be thought of as a dominant 'emotional community' in Rosenwein's terms (Plamper et al. 2010: 256). As such, an 'emotional regime' is connected to authority and the political hegemony of any given period, with the capacity to shape what is acceptable in terms of emotional expression and to create 'emotional suffering' for those who do not align with it.

It is clear from the above that the history of emotions has similar objectives to cultural history – indeed, that the former is part of the latter. If cultural history is concerned, in the words of Mary Fissell (2004: 365), with the 'making of meaning . . . how people in the past made sense of their lives, of the natural world, of the social relations, of their bodies', then the history of emotions comes to ask what life, in the context of these negotiations, felt like. In this sense, the history of emotions is not a wholly new field of enquiry but a different lens for the history of experience. The cultural history of medicine has been attuned to sufferers' experiences, with studies of illness considering the patients' lived experiences. A good example is Alanna Skuse's account of cancer in the early modern period (2015). The account reveals that what had previously been considered as figurative descriptions of symptoms were actually part of the physical and emotional experience of illness for the early modern patient. In addition, disease itself is a highly emotive experience, pointing to the ways that medical and emotional pasts are interlinked.

Despite this, medical historian Fay Bound Alberti finds that contemplating the role of emotion in medical theory and practice is not straightforward. Alberti notes that most studies are concerned with power dynamics rather than emotions in the medical encounter (Bound Alberti 2006: xiv). She further notes that following Roy Porter's appeal to explore 'history from below', to focus on personal experiences of illness or the relationship between patient and practitioner (Porter 1985; Bacopoulos-Viau and Fauvel 2016), medical historians have tended to use social history approaches. Alberti's edited volume on *Medicine, Emotion and Disease* (2006) decisively focuses on patients' and physicians' attempts to make sense of emotion from the eighteenth century to the 1950s. Her own contribution to the volume traces the shift from a physiological model of emotions, with the heart and the vascular system at its core, to one centring on the brain and nervous system. She recognizes this shift as an important step in the scientific redefinition of emotions as quantifiable and measurable experiences (Bound Alberti 2006: xix). Her account examines the 'bodily nature of affect', in pre-laboratory medicine, as well as the 'circumstances in which empathy and compassion became a desirable aspect of the medical encounter' (Bound Alberti 2006: xviii). My analysis also elucidates the emergence of the desirability of compassion in healthcare as part of the cultural reform and the reform of emotions brought by the eighteenth-century culture of sensibility.

My approach does not seek to separate itself from the objectives of cultural history in search of a sole focus on emotions. As shown above, this separation may be not be entirely possible. I am, however, indebted to a series of premises that derive directly from the field and the work of the scholars discussed above. Firstly, by being formalized as a field of study on its own, the history of emotions advocates for taking emotions seriously. This is particularly important with regard to medicine, as even in contemporary medical settings emotions can be viewed with suspicion due to a 'scientistic ideology that only affords meaning to what can be measured and controlled' (de Zulueta 2013: 88). Taking emotions seriously enhances our understanding of pre-modern medicine and provides context for the trajectory that led to current tensions between emotions and professionalism in medicine. A good example of this is Michael Brown's recent study on emotions and surgery in the eighteenth and nineteenth centuries, which rectifies the image of surgery as a field of practice that requires dispassion – a persistent assumption in both scholarship (Payne 2007) and society. Brown's study reveals the complex role of emotion in surgery, made all the more significant in an era before anaesthesia when the practitioner was confronted with immense pain that could not be managed effectively (Brown 2017).

Secondly, the history of emotions revolves around the theme of change (Bound Alberti 2006: xv). Recognizing that emotions are not stable entities and change over time is important because it can help trace the reciprocal relationship between medical theory and conceptions of illness on the one hand and the production of emotional concepts on the other. For instance, humoral theory – the paradigm under which health consists in the systemic balance of the four humours in the body: blood, yellow bile, black bile and phlegm – dominated Western medical thought for centuries and was, as physician and medical historian Michael Stolberg comments, 'a major source of emotional concepts and expressions in the early modern period' (Stolberg 2019: 113). In what follows, I read the relationship between emotion and disease in the context of major transitions in medical thought and cultural shifts of affect in the period both preceding and during the eighteenth century. I refer to major transitions in physiology that can be traced from humoral medicine, in which diseases were conceived primarily as systemic fluid misbalance, to a mechanical medicine that explained the body as a collection of fluids, with vessels that worked harmoniously in health and malfunctioned in disease. From mid-century onwards, the nervous body of sensibility emerged, with nerves – disordered, weakened or affected – becoming predominant explanatory concepts and mediators in illness.

In terms of cultural shifts, I take 'Enlightenment' to be a meaningful category in two ways. One is that the culture of sensibility, the major instigator of emotion reform in the period, is rooted in the works of moral theory philosophers such as Lord Shaftesbury, David Hume and Adam Smith. The philosophical framework underpinning Enlightenment ideals made carefully managed emotion the foundation and guide to justice and morality (Frazer 2010). This was reflected in the prominence of the social emotions in the period and the change in social mentality that they signify. The culture of sensibility that flourished in the period, especially towards the middle of the century, posited that the sensible self was capable of being sensitized to respond with empathy, by being 'educated' into taking positive social action as a result of emotion. Sensitization could be achieved by exposure to sights of distress, whether fictional or real. Distress, in the form of suffering from disease, became part of this aesthetics of suffering and moral edification. The culture of sentiment can be seen as a dominant emotional discourse and as such linked to structures of power and social aspirations in the period.

The second way in which 'Enlightenment' is meaningful as a term here relates to medicine and its progressive professionalization. The period is characterized by the systematization of medicine and the emergence of physicians and surgeons as expert professionals. Their methods were increasingly more homogeneous than the heterogeneity of voices that had characterized medical writing and diagnosis previously (Geyer-Kordesch 1995: 114). In addition, the philosophical framework of the Enlightenment made improvement of health a socio-political ideal: 'Medical images – diagnosis, therapy, regimen – were central to the sociopolitical visions of the *philosophes*; and integral to more secular and materialist images of the future, the improvement of health under the guidance of a wise medical profession became highly influential' (Porter 1995: 3). This contrasted with the early modern period; when healing was a pluralistic enterprise, there was a more formalized approach to treating disease that made physicians' voices more prominent. The discussion is also sensitive to continuities that persist despite these major transitions. Discussing the medical revolution that led to mechanism, Andrew Wear remarks that 'the new philosophy did not, and could not, alter traditional rational ways of thinking about the illness and the effects of medicines – although the terms in which the explanations were couched, of course, did change radically' (Wear 1989: 319). Moreover, the making of the 'sensible' body, in the middle of the period, instead of signifying a radical break with the past, led to a holistic view of disease that brought medical concepts of the past (the non-naturals) to the fore again.

Thirdly, the 'history of emotions' approach has direct methodological implications. As discussed above, language is prominent for the historian of emotions. Work in the field has significantly expanded our notion of what constitutes an 'emotion word'. We have come to recognize not only that fixed emotion words, such as anger or fear, can differ in meaning in the past but also that the affective vocabulary of the past can include more varied terms than these. In turn, this insight has enhanced our understandings of the vocabularies of disease in the past. For instance, Lisa Smith points to the overlap between mind and body in eighteenth-century medicine and the 'inseparability between physical and emotional suffering' (Smith 2008: 459) and reveals how emotional states could be symptoms of disease. Significantly, she also identifies terms such as 'heaviness', or 'uneasiness' – terms bearing emotional valence in the period – as being part of the vocabulary of physical disease (Smith 2008). In addition, we have become more attuned to the persistence of affective elements in the discourse of disease in the past. Meegan Kennedy's study on case histories of cardiac disease in the nineteenth century shows that the experience of the disease was described in romantic terms, despite the increasingly clinical character of its management (Kennedy 2014). Finally, my own previous study on early modern envy demonstrates the overlap between physical and affective language in the discourse surrounding the emotion. The language was not simply metaphorical, but was reflective of the connection between envy and black bile, a toxic humour, and to disordered digestion, which affected both the physical and mental nourishment of the body (Minou 2017).

In this chapter I also focus on the discourse about emotions in the past in order to show the interrelationship between emotion and disease. More specifically, I draw on the discourse of anger in popular medical writing of the period to show how emotion is linked to pathogeny – that is, how it can contribute to or exacerbate physical disease. I discuss the discourse surrounding envy to show how emotion can be linked to pathology, even being considered wholly as disease. The sources I refer to are pre-1800 works on domestic or popular medicine, which offered advice on either the preservation of health or the management of common diseases. They usually contained references to the passions, and their effect on the body, in the tradition of the non-naturals. As

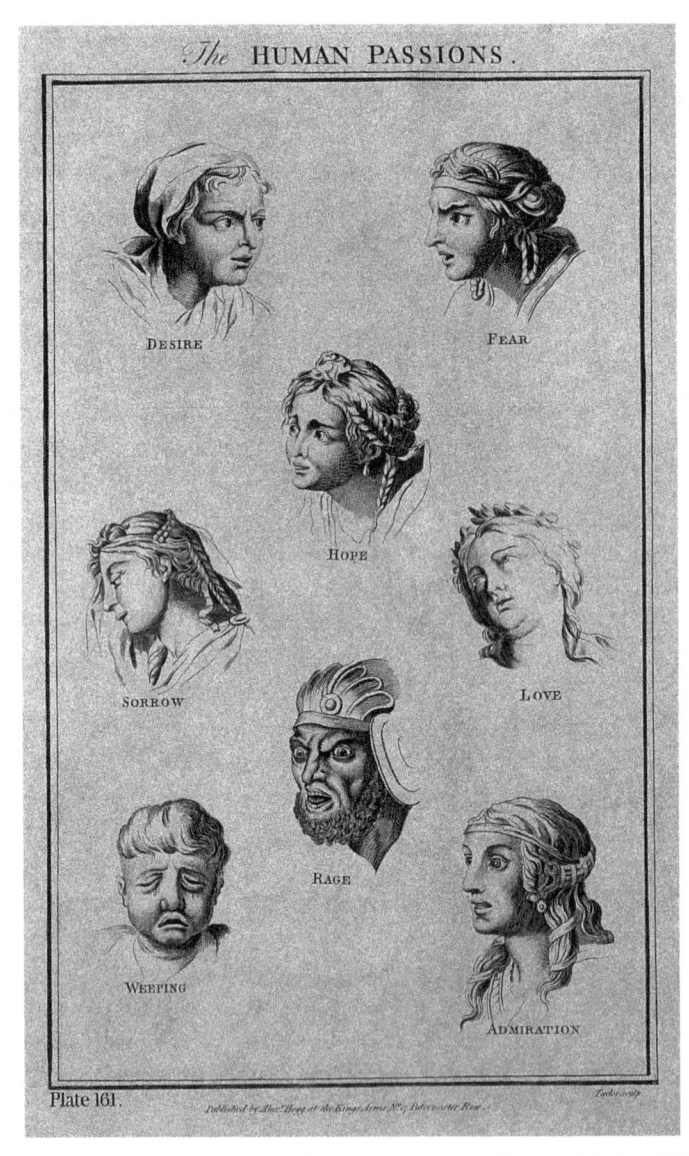

FIGURE 3.1: Eight heads depicting the human passions, etching by Taylor, 1788, after C. Le Brun. Le Brun's depiction of the passions is supported by his theory of the passions, which is set out in his *Conférence de M. Le Brun sur l'expression générale et particulière* (Paris: E. Picard, 1698). Credit: Wellcome Collection, London/Public Domain.

the century progresses, specialized works on the effect of the passions on the body begin to appear, such as William Falconer's *A Dissertation on the Influence of the Passions upon Disorders of the Body* (1788), and these are also included in the discussion. Moreover, as my period of interest also spans the early modern period – in order to showcase the patho-physiology of emotion under the humoral model – I also refer to works of a spiritual nature, such as sermons.

Finally, I concentrate on the significance of compassion in the emotional discourse of the period to show how attitudes to disease can change according to the dominant emotional paradigms operative in the period. In this later part, I am concerned with the prefaces of popular medical publications. Following Gerard Genette's work, I am conscious of these sections as 'paratexts' serving a function (Genette 1987). More specifically, I view the preface as best hypostatizing Genette's conception of a paratext as 'a zone of transaction: a privileged place of a pragmatics and a strategy, of an influence on the public' (Genette 1987: 2). Inspired by Genette's work, other scholars have paid attention to the potential for interpretation afforded by paratexts and their dynamic position as spaces for the construction of authorial identity, their function in establishing the work as a whole and its reception, and their contexts of patronage and authorial status (Smith and Wilson 2011; Rennhak 2011). However, most such work centres on early modern texts or is mostly concerned with the prefaces of literary texts.

By contrast, I find the prefaces of medical works of interest not only as spaces for the negotiation of an authorial identity in a competitive medical marketplace (Jenner and Wallis 2007), but also as spaces affording opportunity for the expression of emotion. Prefaces usually include a statement on the part of the author or translator regarding the necessity of the work, driven by an increasingly competitive medical marketplace and the need to establish one's authorial reputation within it. Often, the works provide accessible definitions of disease and advertise their public benefit. Many medical writers profess their expertise and differentiate their publication from similar books by distinguishing themselves from the other 'impostors' or 'empirics'. It is in this rhetorical space – which negotiated disease as a concept and its experience in the form of symptoms and complaints, and also addressed the person experiencing it – that references to emotion can be found.

EMOTIONS AND DISEASE UNDER THE HUMORAL PARADIGM

This section focuses on how envy was pathologized in the early modern period and beyond. With its origins in the seven deadly sins and its potential for social disruption, envy was seen as a paradigmatically pathological passion, defined only in the negative. The discourse around this passion was, in essence, a discourse of 'disease' involving metaphors of consumption and corrosion. Most negative passions were associated with bodily effects that could threaten disease. However, envy was associated with the most grievous diseases, especially those that worked insidiously to destroy the body.

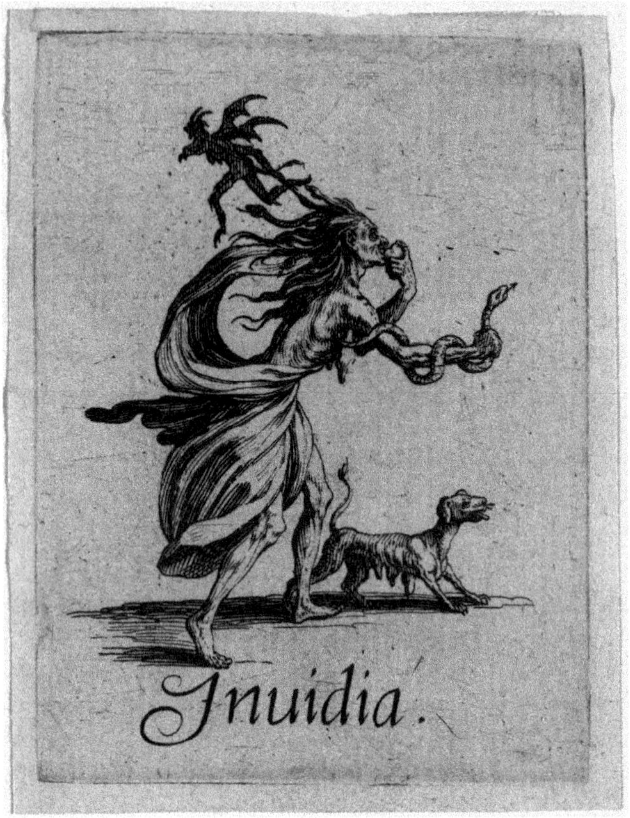

FIGURE 3.2: Jacques Callot, *Envy*, c. 1620. Credit: The Metropolitan Museum of Art, New York, Bequest of Edwin De T. Bechtel, 1957.

In 1616, Thomas Adams defined envy as a 'consumption' and a 'languishing disease in the body'. He went on to describe the effects of it for the person experiencing envy in language that was blended, encompassing both spiritual and physical terms:

> Envy fitly succeeds anger, for it is nothing else but inveterate wrath. The other was a franticke fit, and this is a consumption; a languishing disease in the body, the beginning of dissolution, a br[ea]ching of the vessell, not to be stopped till all the liquor of life is run out . . . this spiritual sicknesse is a consumption of the flesh also, and a pining away of the spirits.
>
> —Adams 1616: 18

This description was followed by enumeration of symptoms, or signs associated with it, that were purely physical such as 'a pale face without blood', 'leane body without any juice in it', 'black teeth' and a 'heart full of gall' (Adams 1616: 20). The basis of envy's pathology in the humoral model lay in its connection to the humour of black bile – the most toxic and malign humour of all (Siegel 1968: 258). The symptoms associated with it reflect this connection, but the description of envy given above extends beyond this association. References to 'consumption', 'languishing' and 'pining away' suggest a slow and horrifyingly certain decay of the body to the point of fatality.

Early modern cultural discourse about envy borrowed from the medical vocabulary to convey the dangerousness of this passion. The threat of fatality, terrifying physical signs and the misery of such a pathological affective experience were discernible tropes. One of the most enduring images of envy in the early modern period derived from literary tradition; the portrayal of envy in Ovid's *Metamorphoses*. The poet presented envy as a gruesome creature, with 'sallow cheeks', 'shrunk body' and bosom 'green with bile' (Ovid 1986: 47). Early modern literary representations of envy added to Ovid's image. To exemplify envy, Joshua Poole listed such terms as: 'pale', 'lean', 'swelling', 'lean-fac't', 'cancr'd', 'viperous', 'poisonous', 'black-mouthed' and 'snake-haired' (Poole 1972 [1657]: 89). This kind of imagery was immediately recognizable to the early modern mind as signifying physical disorder (see Figure 3.2). For instance, references to 'leanness' and abnormal colour served metonymically to denote disease, while 'swellings' and the adjective 'cancr'd' directly suggested grievous illnesses such as cancer. The most usual terms used to describe the effects of envy on the body centred on the notion of 'wasting away'. Envy, Jonathan Blagrave (1652–1698) wrote, 'pines [the envier] away, eats his heart, consumes his bones, wastes his flesh' (Blagrave 1693: 14). Similar language was used to describe the action of cancer on the body. This association was not random, as the illness and the passion shared a common humoral element: cancer was thought to be caused by the stagnation or corruption of black bile in the body (Skuse 2015: 31–3). Envy was perceived as a propensity of those with melancholic complexions – that is, those affected by excess of black bile. Regimens of health often cited this passion under melancholy (Langum 2016: 112; Minou 2017).

The blending of the literal and psychical with the figural and the moral was a large part of the early modern discourse on envy – and, indeed, on the passions and disease. When Levinus Lemnius (1505–1568), a Dutch physician whose work circulated in English, sought to exemplify the dry complexion to his readers he encouraged them to bring to mind the physiognomy and shape of envy, described by Ovid (Lemnius 1576: 69r). Thomas Brooks (1608–1680), a religious author, wrote in 1657 that 'Envious Soules are like the Ravens, that flye over the sweet Garden, and light upon the stinking Carrion' (Brooks 1657: 268). To be envious, Brooks suggests, is to exhibit unnatural behaviour. The reference to offensive smells is more than a striking image. Early modern regimens of health frequently noted that sweet smells, and especially the pleasant air of the garden, were considered beneficial to health because they strengthened and nourished the spirits (Cavallo and Storey 2013: 196).

The specific way in which early modern envy was pathologized summarizes some of the defining characteristics of early modern disease. Unnaturalness and misery are prominent themes. Unnaturalness meant unnatural biological function, manifested, for instance, in the excessive leanness and paleness associated with internal disfunction. It could also be seen in the elements of ugliness and deformity that underlined the diseased person's appearance. Due to the extreme pathological nature of envy, this extended to also include elements of monstrosity, as is seen, for instance, in the combination of literal and figural characteristics – such as 'pale' along with 'snake-haired'. Contingent on its unnaturalness was the notion that to experience this 'diseased' passion was an especially heightened and unremitting form of suffering. Envy, writers admonished, is a 'perpetual torment' and a 'constant misery' and makes the one experiencing it 'the most uneasie creature in the world' (Lambe 1695: 17).

The early modern discourse of disease was markedly heterogeneous and could admit both the body and mind, expressing the agony and terror of disease in terms that differed little from the emotive language of literature. This language was shared by an equally heterogeneous group of people. Falling ill, the suffering associated with it and the search for meaning in the experience was in the realm of both spiritual writers such as Thomas Adams and also physicians such as Levinus Lemnius. Both drew on the same physical signifiers and the same figural imagery to describe the diseased state of envy. This link between the physical and the figural was, as Skuse remarks, a specific 'iteration of the cultural construction of bodily experience' (Skuse 2015: 8) deriving from humoralism and the fact that in the early modern body physical and psychological states were inextricably linked, or what scholars have called medicine at a 'figural/literal cusp' (Hunter 2004). By the end of the eighteenth century, changes in the medical model meant that the pathology of the passions, and also the cultural framework of disease, were expressed in different terms.

EMOTIONS, MOTION AND DISEASE

In 1799, Dr Willich described the effects of envy, which

> deprives those addicted to it of an appetite for food, of sleep, of every enjoyment, and disposes them to febrile complaints; but in general it is hurtful to those only who brood over and indulge in this corrosive passion. For the world contains vast numbers, who show their envy at almost every event productive of good fortune to others, and who yet often attain a very great age.
> —Willich 1799: 592

The novel element in this description in that envy is deleterious under certain conditions only. By the time of Willich's writing, major shifts in physiological understanding had already occurred. The physiology that prevailed in medical discourse towards the late seventeenth century was spurred by the impact of scientific discoveries, primarily William Harvey's discovery of the circulation of the blood (1628), and the influence and impact of Newton's physics. The former broke decisively with Galenic tradition and the notion of the production of the blood in the liver. The latter introduced a concept of dynamics with extensive applications to fields other than physics, including medical theory. Various schools of thought emerged, offering explanatory models of the workings of the body based on scientific principles. Bound Alberti traces this transition and demonstrates how the combined impact of the "iatrochemical approach of Thomas Willis, the mechanical physiology of Pitcairne and Hoffman, the hydrodynamic physiology of Boerhaave, the models of sensibility and irritability of Von Haller, and the neurophysiology of Cullen" created new interpretations of the workings of the body. In combination, they 'facilitated a concept of the body that operated according to distinct laws of motion' (Bound Alberti 2010: 24).

In humoralism, the passions influenced the body through a heart-based and heat-inducing dynamic. Each humour was vested with certain qualities such as heat, coldness, dryness or moisture. The predominance or deficit of a quality affected the systemic balance. In the words of Pedro Gil Sotres: 'the emotional dynamic was triggered by the introduction of heat and spirits into the heart or by their outflow from the heart' (Gil Sotres 1998: 313). A centrifugal or centripetal movement was central to the understanding of the specificities of influence of each passion. Anger, for instance, produced a quick displacement of the spirits and heat away from the heart and towards the extremities of the body in preparation for action (revenge). Studying anger and the mind/body connection under humoralism, Elena Carrera describes unhealthful forms of anger as dangerous because 'this excessive movement of bodily heat outwards could lead to the dissolution of the body's natural heat' (Carrera 2013: 140). In the ensuing modified physiology, the heart – hitherto equated with the seat of the soul and the passions – loses its prominence (Bound Alberti 2010). The body ceases to be a 'vehicle' for the soul and becomes a 'machine', with operations that follow natural laws and can be measured and analysed. This had profound implications for the way in which the effects of the passions on the body were comprehended and articulated, as well as how pathology came to be defined.

Mechanical theories conceived of the body as a closed system of solid parts containing fluids the pressure and flow of which were governed by hydrodynamic principles. Herman Boerhaave (1669–1738), a leading figure in eighteenth-century medicine, defined health and disease in keeping with this model:

> For as the very being of health consists in a moderate, free and equal motion of the blood, or in the equality of pulse and tone of the just temperament and quantity of fluids; so the seat of every disease, and the immediate cause thereof, is placed in the motion, as it is immoderate, obstructed or unequal, by reason of the lost distinction of the pulse and tone of the solids, as also the intemperament and disproportion of the fluids.
>
> —Boerhaave 1715: xxiii

As the passage above illustrates, and as Luyendijk-Elshout (1970: 82–3) notes, in Boerhaave's system of physiology, 'action' instead of function became key. Its action-oriented nature made the circulation of the fluids paramount. Accordingly, health, for Boerhaave, depended on free and unobstructed movement, whereas disease was described in terms of stagnation or constriction in the body, which resulted in unusual or defective motion.

By the end of the century, the effects of internal motion on the nerves in the body were becoming central to explanations of disease. Describing the action of envy on the body in the latter part of the century, William Falconer (1744–1824) wrote: 'Envy is a passion of a rather equivocal nature, being stimulant or sedative, according to circumstances, which is natural enough to suppose, it being composed of passions of an opposite kind, namely, sorrow and anger' (Falconer 1788: 19). The 'equivocal' nature of envy was recognized in early modern discourse as well. Thomas Adams, for example, noted that envy was a passion encompassing anger, calling it 'an inveterate wrath'. However, where Falconer uses the terms 'stimulant' or 'sedative' to describe the physical effects of these passions, Adams uses 'franticke fit' and 'consumption'. This latter pair of terms is notable in that it uses conditions to exemplify physical effect, by way of analogy. The former pair of terms makes use of physiological properties. The words 'stimulant' and 'sedative' encapsulate the concern with acceleration or retardation of the fluids and the proper tension of the solids. The language suggests a concern with interior physical action: action affecting parts of the body that could be stimulated – particularly the nerves. Such terms reflected the new vocabulary being used to articulate the pathology of the passions. The new concept of health was based on regularity of motion, shifting away from humoral properties and stemming from scientific principles.

While this change seems radical enough to create significant breaks with the past, there were also continuities with the early modern period. Anthony F. M. Willich, for instance, a medical writer of the late eighteenth century, still found that the 'happiest' physical state' was to be in 'a moderate degree of gaiety' (Willich 1799: 579). (See Figure 3.3.) His description echoed the long-established tenet of preventative care that existed in earlier health regimens. In a recent study of the genre of health regimens, Sandra Cavallo and Tessa Storey conclude that the emotional state most beneficial to the organism was neither

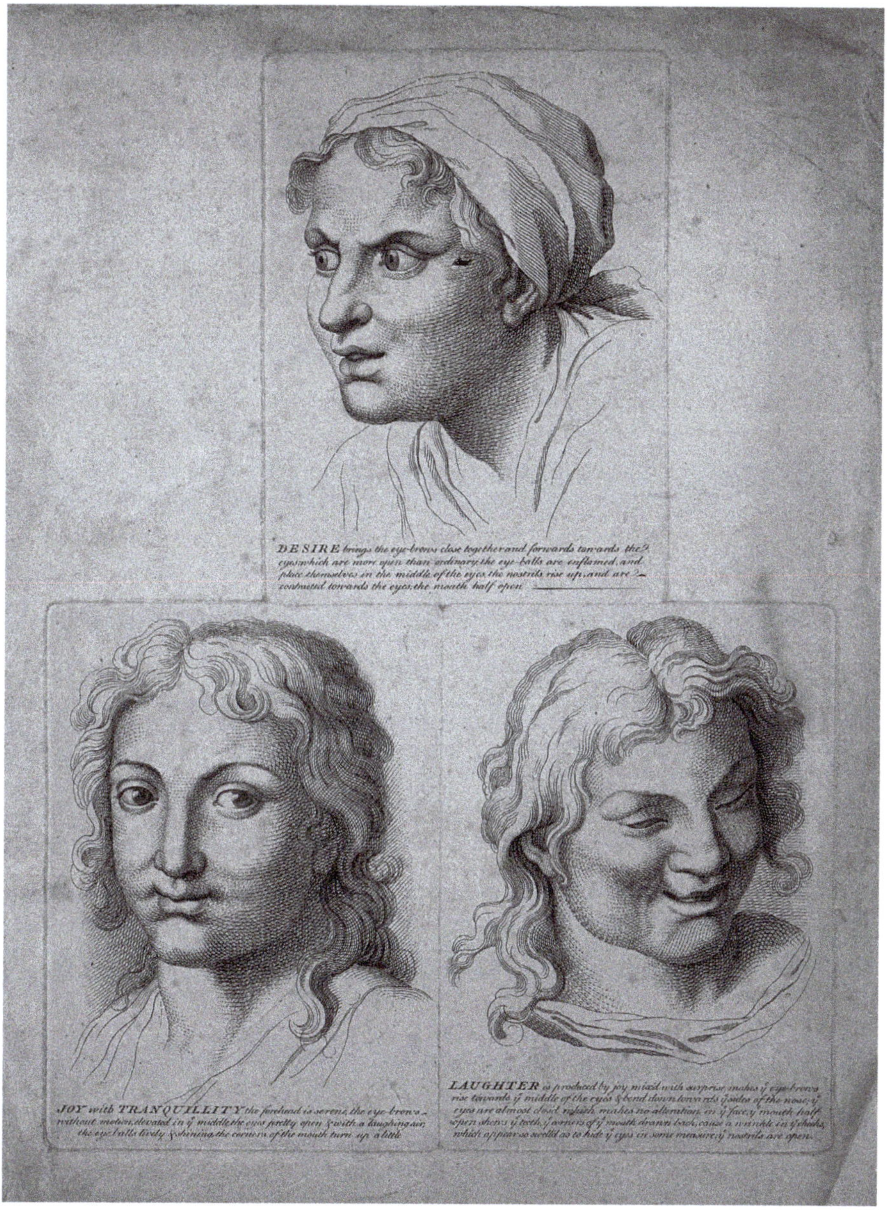

FIGURE 3.3: Face showing peaceful joy – a mix of serenity and liveliness. From engraving after C. Le Brun of three faces: expressing desire and peaceful joy, and laughing. Credit: Wellcome Collection, London/Public Domain.

negative (such as anger) nor emphatically positive (such as joy), but was a state of balanced contentment found in 'cheerfulness'. In cheerfulness 'the spirits travelled around the body in a calm, peaceful, but purposeful way – distributing natural heat evenly throughout the body' (Cavallo and Storey 2013: 183). For Willich, 'gaiety' allowed for 'the circulation of the fluids and perspiration [to be] carried on with proper vigour; [and] thereby obstructions [to be] prevented or removed' (Willich 1799: 580).

Thus, long-established tenets of physiology remained operative in this period, even though they were expressed in different terms. For instance, although the bodily effects of passions were explained differently, the passions were still utilized in healing according to the old principle of curing by contraries. As Stanley Jackson, a psychiatrist and medical historian of psychological caring practices, puts it: 'whether the language is that of too warm and too cool passions, or excess of circulatory motion and deficit of circulatory motion, the theme of excited passions versus subdued passions persists' (Jackson 1990: 167). The idea of a contrast came into play during treatment, with the healer attempting to arouse a contrary passion in order to restore balance in the organism (Jackson 1990: 167). The psychosomatic aspect, then, persisted in eighteenth-century medicine, as well as the notion that systemic balance was integral to health.

SENSIBILITY, NERVES AND DISEASE

Scientific change does not necessarily imply a linear break with past conceptions of disease. However, there are aspects of disease that can be seen as distinctive of this period, particularly the prominence of nervous diseases. The focus on nervous disorders can be tied to the rise of sensibility, along with its emphasis on nerves and the properties of irritability and sensibility as the vital principles in explaining biological function. 'Sensibility' was a quality of physiological origins before the term and concept acquired cultural currency. Extensive experiments by Albrecht von Haller (1708–1777) showed sensibility to be the unique property of the nerve fibres of being able to perceive stimuli and was separate from the quality of the muscles of being able to contract (irritability). Any part of the body that was rich in nerves was, consequently, endowed with great sensibility. Haller's model was very influential for medical theory, leading to the prominence of the nervous system in conceptions of the body, health and disease. Health could be expressed now as the 'balance between the nerves' sensibility and the muscles' irritability' and disease as an 'excess or deficiency of these qualities' (De Renzi 2004: 188).

Other scholars contest this neurocentric account, arguing that in the shift away from the fluids in the body and towards the behaviour of the solids as explanatory tools in physiology and pathology, historiography usually omits the significance of the 'fibre body'. Hisao Ishizuka argues for the prominence of 'fibre medicine' in the early part of the century. With fibre as the minutest meaningful solid of the body, Ishizuka shows that the living body was conceived not as physically dense but as an organized whole of delicate fibres interwoven together (Ishizuka 2016). The fibre body was flexible and fragile; disease or therapy centred on such notions as the vibration, proper tone and elasticity of the solids. Such an enhanced understanding of the medical landscape of the period is welcome, but what matters to the present discussion is the fact that both fibre medicine, as Ishizuka names it, and the usual neurocentric account essentially posit a complex and delicate body with heightened susceptibility to external stimuli. Accordingly, the passions now threatened a different kind of disorder. Bernard Lynch (d. 1745) dedicated a section of his *Guide to Health* to the passions and affections of the mind from the viewpoint of the physician. He explained that the harmful influence of the violent passions of the mind brings about 'great disorders' by 'universally stimulating, irritating, and twitching the nerves and fibres, in such a manner as disturbs their natural contractions' (Lynch 1744: 316)

Conversely, the benefits of the passions to the body also reflect this changed understanding. The notion of beneficial instances of anger was present in humoralism, but this was to counteract coldness (Carrera 2013). Lynch, quoted above, also allowed for a positive effect of anger, but its usefulness now consisted in 'stir[ring] up a brisk circulation of the languid fluids in a cold and phlegmatick constitution' (Lynch 1744: 316). In his treatise on diseases, William Forster also acknowledged anger as a curative force, as by 'agitating the animal spirits and making their motion stronger and freer obstructions capable of hindering the actions of the nerves could be removed' (Forster 1745: 113). John Burton (1710–1771), writing on the non-naturals, noted that 'Anger and joy keep the fibres in their natural tensions, assist the secretion and derivation of spirits to all parts of the body, and consequently promote circulation and digestion' (Burton 1738: 338).

The two sections above demonstrate that the period understood disease in different terms to the previous era. Willich's sober description of the effects of envy, cited above, shows a language of pathology that was characteristically devoid of hyperbole, a long way from being at the 'figural/literal cusp' of the early modern period. Moreover, the section on anger's physical harm and benefit illustrates a different vocabulary of physiology and pathology. This operated not by complex metaphors and analogies between the body and the macrocosm, as we see in early modern descriptions of envy-as-disease, but by reference to the physical properties, such as tension and vibration, of the solid parts of the body among which fibres and nerves were particularly meaningful. As such, the eighteenth century is confirmed as a pivotal moment in the making of medicine as a scientific practice which tends towards the clinical – that is, towards dispassion.

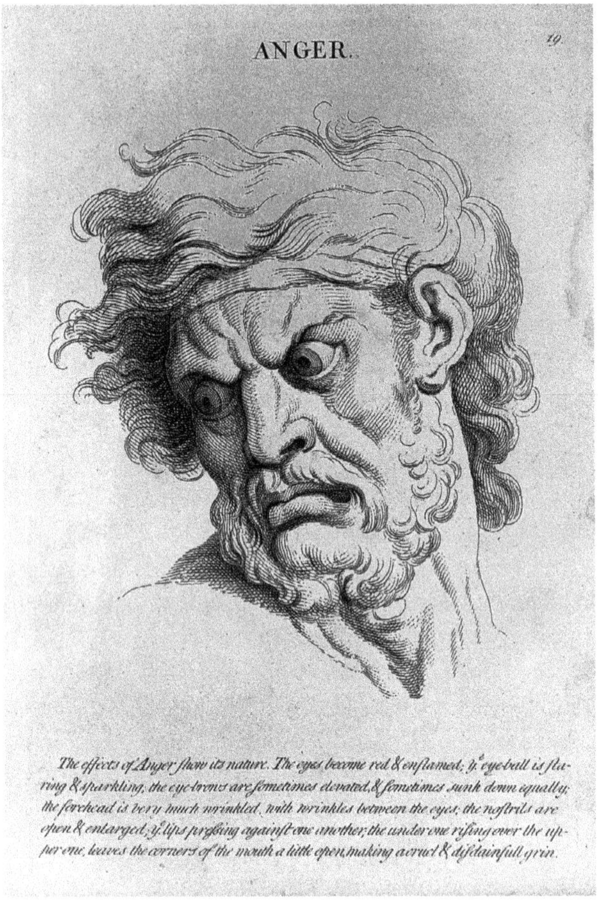

FIGURE 3.4: Face showing anger, Charles Le Brun, 1760. Representing the various passions of the soul. Credit: Wellcome Collection, London/Public Domain.

However, these sections also attest to continuity. In their attempts to identify the specific ways that passions affected the body and how they linked to disease, medical writers followed a psychosomatic view of disease. Even the most consequential change in the physiology of the time – the focus on sensibility and the nerves – was not radical enough to result in wholly different constructions of disease. As Heather Beatty points out, 'the emphasis on sensibility and the rise of the nerves as agents of the vital principle invited a strongly holistic view of disease, whereby external impressions, emotions, and environment could physically affect the body through nervous sensation' (Beatty 2015: 14). Indeed, what was distinctive about the period is to be found less in pathology and more in attitudes towards disease, which reflected a cultural emphasis on social emotion.

EMOTIONAL LANGUAGE AND DISEASE

Popular eighteenth-century medical texts referred to emotion in a way reminiscent of the cultural discourse of sensibility. The connection is discernible, for instance, in the various emotive words that were associated with symptoms of disease and even in definitions of the term 'disease' itself. Prefaces of popular medicine treatises are a rich source of information regarding this change in the vocabulary of disease and will be discussed here as 'privileged' and strategically important rhetorical spaces. Crucially, prefaces, beyond their function as paratexts as identified by Genette (1987), are the only space within medical works where personal expression is afforded to such an extent. The rest of the work is devoted to information, knowledge, deductions from principle and allusion to medical authorities. Only the preface affords extensive opportunity for the author's own voice to be used, and as such it is suited to affective language. However, these instances of affective language should not be seen as spontaneous. Rather, I see them as instances of strategic alignment on the part of medical authors with the dominant emotional discourse of their time.

To begin with, the concept of disease within these prefaces is distinguishably different from early modern conceptions centred on unnaturalness. Disease was, of course, still a preternatural condition, but authors tend to explain it in terms devoid of the hyperbole and terror of the early modern era. Often, there is a marked confidence on the part of the author in the ability to provide an explanation of bodily function and to define disease as the way in which this is disrupted. In turn, such definitions emphasizing ease of function influenced the understanding of disease and its symptoms. William Forster explains health as the state in which a person has 'a power to perform human actions with ease, pleasure and perseverance' (Forster 1745: preface [7]). 'But', he continues, 'if a person is unable to perform these actions, if he feels uneasiness, pain, or soon grow weary in performing them, we say he is sick, and we call this condition a disease' (Forster 1745: preface [7]). As the terms 'ease' and 'uneasiness' enter definitions of disease, there is, in parallel, a growing use of such vocabulary on the part of the sufferers of disease. Drawing on medical consultation letters to study eighteenth-century pain, Lisa Smith unveils an array of emotive terms that described various forms of physical suffering; significant among them is the use of the term 'uneasiness', a word used to describe primarily mental agony, but equally applied to physical symptoms of disease (Smith 2008: 463–4).

Understanding disease in such terms also had consequences for the way both the physician and the patient were represented. When the objective is to define disease as a medical concept, descriptions are pragmatic and dispassionate. Boerhaave's definition of health and disease above is a good example of this. Within popular medicine texts, there were also pragmatic descriptions. For instance, disease might be described as an 'affection' of the parts of the body that results in disrupted function. However, popular medical treatises quickly dispensed with definitions to move into practical advice and in so doing, they introduce emotive terms that refer to the disease itself, the patient experiencing it and the medical practitioner whose role it was to offer relief. Terms such as 'uneasiness' were flexible enough to denote a precise symptom, or an abstract, general feeling of indisposition. Commonly, medical authors referred to any kind of disease as 'distress' or 'misery'. Certain diseases might be singled out as the 'most deplorable' due to their physical impact – or due to their status as 'fashionable' (such as nervous diseases). The symptoms of a disease might also be 'deplorable'; there was even reference to 'deplorable ulcers' (Allen 1749: 215). Amid talk of 'uneasiness', 'misery' and 'distress', the figure of the sick person emerges as a 'sufferer': an individual in a 'deplorable state', 'miserable' and in need of relief. The shifting language highlights suffering and epitomizes the growing cultural concern with social emotion.

By mid-century, sensibility gained popularity that exceeded its origins in physiology. Physicians debated Haller's doctrine, with its separation between sensibility and irritability and their strict localization. Some theorists suggested that sensibility was not a localized quality, but was in fact widespread throughout the body. Underlying the debate was a concern with the relationship between individual organs and the organism. More precisely, medical authors were concerned with how autonomous organs could become organized bodies (Gaukroger 2010). Questions about sensibility were central to medical and philosophical questions about living organisms, physical sensations and emotions. As Beatty (2015: 24) points out:

> In the eighteenth century the relationship between philosophy and medicine was unquestioned by both physicians and philosophers: both subjects offered rules for proper living; and the interdependence of the soul and body meant that medical and philosophical prescriptions were equally important. In this vein, emotional and medical sensibility belonged as much to the philosophers as it did to the pathologists.

Emotional sensibility came to define the eighteenth century and could be understood, in the words of Graham Barker-Benfield, as a 'particular kind of consciousness, one that could be further sensitized in order to be more acutely responsive to signals from the outside environment and from inside the body' (Barker-Benfield 1992: xvii). Within this framework, the capacity for social emotion was a manifestation of individuals' sensitization to their environments and was elevated in cultural consciousness. As Ute Frevert suggests, 'sympathy, or the ability to empathize with suffering and pleasure, the capacity for fellow-feeling, became a cardinal human virtue in the eighteenth century, a means for the good and maintenance of society' (Frevert 2014: 13).

An extended capacity for sympathy also appears in the language of relief from disease. Treatises that appeared at the beginning of the century echo earlier tenets of disease as human fate. There was a recognition of the limitations of medicine in relieving the torture of disease, and a resignation towards mortality. References to compassion usually indicated divine compassion. 'Man being born to die', wrote Peter Paxton in 1701, 'there must be changes or diseases where we in vain implore the help of medicines' (Paxton 1701: preface). Writing in 1739, on the diseases that afflict human bodies, Theophilus Lobb noted that it is 'an instance of God's compassion and goodness that we have relief from torture and misery' (Lobb 1739: preface [x]) in the form of medicine.

By mid-century, though, there was a marked difference in the vocabulary surrounding relief from disease. It had become the mark of human compassion to strive to relieve disease. In 1763, the physician Samuel Clossy noted optimistically: 'there's scarce any disease of the parts, or the whole system that will not admit of some relief, which every humane man will endeavour to administer' (Clossy 1763: ix). In 1765, the translation of Tissot's *Advice to the People* circulated with a note in the preface that emphasized that it was the 'natural feelings of humanity that dispose us to advise remedies for the poor sick' (11). In 1779, the physician William Rowley prefaced his book of remedies for various diseases by stating that 'humanity dictated me to the necessity of the present publication, as numbers are daily suffering under ravaging complaints' (Rowley 1779: preface [2]). Medical authors repeatedly made the point that it was compassion towards the sufferer that incited them to action.

Afforded the opportunity for personal expression in the prefaces to their texts, medical writers assumed both an authorial and a professional identity and negotiated a different place within the hierarchy of agents of cure. As Hannah Newton has shown in her study of processes of recovery in early modern England, the physician was placed in a hierarchy of recovery below 'God' and 'Nature'. The physician was either a 'servant' of nature or a 'co-governor', but his role was constantly defined within this framework (Newton 2015). In eighteenth-century popular medical texts, the opportunity for authorial expression and the use of sentimental language allowed the author to identify as a specialist in professional terms and as a person of social capacity. By defining disease as suffering, medical writers claimed both the knowledge to relieve it and the sensitivity that motivated them to do so. They could thus assume the role of the sensible practitioner.

This complex identity extended beyond the remit of medical knowledge and assigned to, or demanded from, the physician additional skills that had resonance within the Enlightenment context. Anne Vila, in her study of Enlightenment pathology, shows how the making of the sensible body delineated a highly specified image of the Enlightened attending physician who possessed not only knowledge but also the interpretative powers to properly decipher the subtle signs of the body (Vila 1998: 61–2). As physiological sensibility became more than the property of the nerves, it increasingly defined complex bodily systems. Moreover, its correlation of nuanced psycho-physiological reactions with instances of distress created a new image of the skilled physician: someone who was acutely perceptive and attuned to the sensible body. Simultaneously, the cultural currency of sympathy and of the social emotion – in combination with the Enlightenment ideal of improved health – completed the image of a healer who was not only knowledgeable but also caring and compassionate. The physician now more than ever ceased to be an 'enabler' of nature when administering care and became a social figure who could claim both a professional status (as the holder of scientific, sober knowledge) and a social role (as the compassionate administerer of care).

Characteristically, the phrase 'compassionate care' entered the language surrounding disease. Sentimental language became part of formal, organized charitable action to relieve disease. 'Of all circumstances that affect the mind of the man with compassion', noted a 1743 sermon on encouraging public infirmaries, 'no one seems to touch it so nearly, as the seeing our fellow-creatures labouring with diseases, and even perishing under them for want of proper and timely assistance' (Maddox 1743: 26). The same publication termed sufferers of disease as those 'miserable objects' that 'excite our pity'. In many prefaces, patients were styled as 'miserable objects', 'wretched victims' and 'unhappy sufferers', thus creating an aesthetics of suffering that reflected sentimental norms. Underpinning this kind of affective language was a change in social mentality which marked the eighteenth century. The change was manifested in the philosophical discourse that made social emotion, in the words of Norman Fiering (1976: 196), 'insistently natural' and instigated humanitarian action that made the relief of disease an issue of public care. As Spierenburg's study of the progressive abandonment of public executions has established, the period was a defining moment in the social capacity for sympathetic identification. Spierenburg argues that in this period suffering, even when occurring within the sanctioned social system of judicial punishment, becomes rejected because the sufferer is increasingly recognized as a fellow-creature (Spierenburg 1984: 185).

Evidence of this increased capacity for sympathetic identification can be found in instances where compassion was called for to replace previous attitudes in the context of medicine. Those who suffered from the 'hypochondriac' disorder, commented William Buchan, 'though they often be made the subject of ridicule, justly claim our highest sympathy and compassion' (Buchan 1774: 66). Evidence of change in affective attitudes is also found with regard to diseases carrying social stigma. This was especially true of venereal diseases, the sufferers of which were seen as causing their own demise through 'guilty' and 'criminal commerce'. Treatises on venereal disease, representing a substantial part of all medical publications in the period, offered medical advice out of compassion not for the sufferers themselves but, as a mid-century publication noted, for the blameless victims, the spouses and companions of those affected (*The Family Magazine* 1741: 425). By the end of the century, though, the absence of compassion for these 'unhappy objects' began to be a cause for concern (Hodson 1791: 66).

This does not mean that compassion in eighteenth-century medical context can be understood as thoroughly uniform or singularly optimistic, any more than it can in the cultural discourse of compassion overall. Even though compassion was valorized in the period, there were heated debates about who, and what kind of suffering, should elicit or deserved compassion (Frevert 2016: 83). In addition, by the latter part of the century the culture of sensibility drew criticism and was seen as too close to affectation rather than being sincere emotion (Ellis 1996). Showcasing this ambiguity, a medical commentary of 1776 deemed compassion 'unseasonable' in the context of surgery, advising that the patient's friends should never be admitted to the operation 'lest they disturb' the procedure with 'their cries' (Swieten 1776: 147). The moment of distrust of compassion revealed here is suggestive of the suspicion of the capacity of emotion to overwhelm and cause disorder, inherent in the discourse of sensibility. It is also interesting, however, that this tendency to lose control of emotions is ascribed to the 'friends' of the patient and not to the surgeon, suggesting perhaps that expert practitioners can attain the subtle balance between emotion and ordered performance. However ambiguous, the significance of compassion to the medical culture of the period is distinctive. At the very least, the fact that medical writers needed to acknowledge it and draw a line between compassion and the demands of their profession evidences its relevance to medical practice and its particular resonance within eighteenth-century culture.

CONCLUSION

Spurred by insights from the field of the history of emotions, this analysis has viewed emotion as culturally dependent and subject to change, and disease as a broad category extending beyond biological ailments. It has considered the dynamic of their connection by focusing on envy, anger and compassion: each one an affective term that reveals something different about notions of pathology. The language of envy intimates pathology in the extreme, connected not only to disease but to fatality. As I have argued elsewhere (Minou 2017), having a solid basis in the biological, the essential function of this language is apotropaic. Envy was denounced as a particularly threatening passion within early modern social hierarchy because it stemmed from displeasure with one's own position relative to the position and possessions of others. Anger could also be a subversive passion threatening violence and discord, and in need of control (Rosenwein 1998). Thus, it traditionally exists in 'healthful' and 'unhealthful' forms (Carrera 2013) which were, in their turn, exemplified differently according to the dominant medical model. Finally, identification with compassion in a strategically functional and meaningful authorial space, such as the preface of a medical publication, spells also identification with the dominant emotional discourse of the time.

Through these emotions, I have reflected on change and continuity in the medical model and problematized a linear view of medical progression towards clinical objectivity and dispassion, in line with other scholars such as Fay Bound Alberti and Michael Brown. Moreover, I have expanded upon the usual correlations between culture and disease as perceptible in the culturally contingent nature of certain pathologies – for example, in historical diagnoses of hysteria or monomania. Taken together, the sections above show pathology and disease as entangled with the politics of emotion; they were flexible categories tied to culture in multiple ways. Pathologized emotion is not only manifested as deeply felt, bearing the capacity to overwhelm a person and to bring to the fore questions regarding the connection of body and mind. Emotion-as-disease, pathologized through medico-cultural discourse, elicits questions about the (dis-)connection of the body and the individual's experience (shaped by the socio-political environment), suggesting a 'diseased' relationship. Conversely, naturalized emotion, as compassion was considered to be in the eighteenth century, intimates a proper and sanctioned form of connection between the individual and their wider socio-political environment, placing their body in a 'healthy' association with it.

CHAPTER FOUR

Animals

MONICA MATTFELD

'In my life', Sunaura Taylor writes,

> I have been compared to many animals. I have been told I walk like a monkey, eat like a dog, have hands like a lobster, and generally resemble a chicken or penguin... I understood that saying I was like an animal separated me from other people. Whether I considered if the statement meant that I was less than human, I don't remember.
>
> —Taylor 2011: 192

Her life-long experiences with animal descriptors and people who attempt to use animal labels in jest and to hurt are common to many people deemed disabled.

History is full of ape girls, wolf men, Darwinian missing links, and individuals like the Elephant Man and the Wild Girl who willingly (or not) became the focus of the public's fascinated and objectifying gaze. There were those who were famed for their animal mimicry abilities or for performing the seemingly impossible, and those who were thought absolutely non-human. Often associated with 'freak' shows, fairgrounds and circuses, those who were labelled disabled were never far away from the animal kingdom. Disability and animality, however, extend far beyond the circus tent's walls. The eighteenth century is full of accounts of 'monsters', the 'unnatural' and the 'defective', while tales of the pigeon-toed, the deaf and the blind, and the amazing abound. A perpetual source of fascinated curiosity, disability was a constant in many people's lives and a relentless worry for many others. The century is one where discourses surrounding disability move from 'superstition' to rational science; however, it is also a century in which the very underpinnings of medical thought and understandings of the human were grounded upon the bodies of, and similarities to, animals.

For example, Stefanie Buchenau and Roberto Lo Presti illustrate the interwoven nature of animal and human in their collection *Human and Animal Cognition in Early Modern Philosophy and Medicine* (2017). As they point out, throughout Western history and throughout the Enlightened eighteenth century, animals have underpinned most avenues of human medical knowledge. Many comparative anatomists, for instance, began their investigation into the human with a 'bottom-up approach' that starts with animals and emphasizes 'homologies between them' and humans (2017: 8). In an approach that was problematic – even 'humiliating' – to many, 'animal bodies had certain practical and epistemic advantages over human bodies'. Indeed, 'Not only were they more accessible to anatomists, but they also presented analogous features in greater variety and in simpler form' (2017: 8). As such, the century's greatest scientists, natural philosophers and medical men looked to animals for answers to questions about humanity, the cosmos and the natural world. For example, Robert Boyle in his search for the movement of blood and an understanding of vacuums and Alexander Monro in his anatomy lectures both relied heavily on animal experimentation and vivisection (Meli 2013; Guerrini 2006). Even the period's (arguably) most influential politico-cultural movement, sympathy, found its physiological roots in animal research (Eichberg 2009).

Encompassing some of the major developments associated with the Enlightenment, the long eighteenth century was a period of scientific innovation, increasing discourses of humane treatment towards criminals, declines in capital punishment and the prevalence of duelling, and the growth of sentiment as a driving force in ideal behaviour. However, as the above examples indicate, it was also a time of thinking beyond the human. As Stephanie Eichberg illustrates in her look at the role of animal experimentation in understanding of human bodily feeling and emotion, when animals are included in history the evident semblance with the animal world quickly destabilizes the anthropocentric absolutism of the Age of Reason (2009: 274–95). Indeed, animals, as this chapter indicates, are not only fundamental to a cultural history of medicine but to understandings of how humans negotiated shifting definitions of humanity and animality. This chapter, then, begins the process of inviting the animal back into history, and it does so through two case studies. The first looks to the period's fascination with invisible 'defects', especially deafness and lack of verbal language, through the early scientific writings of George Sibscota. The second moves to the late century's fixation upon spectacular physical disability and the appearance of Three Monstrous Craws in London's most popular illegitimate theatres. Together, these two examples of the anomalous in the eighteenth century indicate a period of contradiction and eternal liminality. It is a period that endlessly tries to reject the animal in exchange for an anxious claiming of some form of humanity even in the face of its apparent instability. Discourses of the 'monstrous' and the 'defective', then, were paradoxical and problematic for period definitions of human and animal species. The unusual body disrupted the seemingly solid difference between species, while often resulting in simultaneous and opposing views of the self for viewing audiences.

Therefore, the eighteenth century is a period of desire and disgust, love and loathing, and fear and fascination with alternative bodies. This two-edged sword, I argue, stems from the complicated nature of humanity itself and of the constant awareness of the animal in ourselves. Giorgio Agamben's work in *The Open* can help to explain some of this phenomenon. As Agamben, looking to Carolus Linnaeus and his classification system, points out, '*man is the animal that must recognize itself as human to be human*', or in other words, '*Homo* is a constitutively "anthropomorphous" animal . . . who must recognize himself in a non-man in order to be human' (2002: 26–7; original emphasis). Within Agamben's anthropological machine, being human, defining the human against the animal, is a continual process of 'caesura', of making cuts that separate humanity's dual nature (both human and animal together), that reject the animal and construct the human (2002: 38). This is done through a Lacanian mirror stage, in which the human is defined through the recognition of the reflected self image and a simultaneous rejection of the always animal looking back. When gazing at an animal mirror, then, 'man, looking at himself, sees his own image always already deformed in the features of an ape' (2002: 26–7). When one sees the self, one sees the animal in all humans there, looking back, creating an unwanted and uncomfortable awareness of the animal in the human. Compounding matters is the malleable nature of humanity, a species that 'can receive all natures and all faces', according to Linnaeus, as humankind possesses the 'seeds of every sort and sprouts of every kind of life' (2002: 30). Individuals, then, can rise above humanity's animal nature and become perilously human or sink down to the brutes – it is all possible thanks to the face of the animal looking back. Thus, for Agamben, the seeing of the animal self is the process by which 'human' is witnessed, recognized and desperately clutched while the animal is firmly rejected. Agamben argues, for example, that the wild children so fascinating during the seventeenth and eighteenth centuries 'are the messengers of man's inhumanity, the witnesses to his fragile identity and his lack of a face of his own' (2002: 30). The attempts at 'humanizing' and civilizing these children, and the many people of the period thought of as disabled, 'shows how aware they [the witnesses] are of the precariousness of the human' (2002: 30).

However, I argue, the process of negation as the means to define the human was also one of happy acknowledgement, even of welcoming the animal in the self – as Sibscota's work indicates. Defining the human based on rejection, on caesura, was part of his epistemology, but for him defining the disabled meant accepting the animal as part of all humans. For others, defining and understanding the disabled was more violent. For many, I argue, the animal itself fights back against its continual exclusion and works to ensure its continual presence even in the face of its rejection. Seeing the animal within the human, especially within the disabled body, can be alluring, desirable, fascinating and wonderful. The animal in the self draws us in, whether we like it or not, and allows the emergence of the animal face, the 'ape' in the human, to spring forth, imperilling the already precarious nature of the human. Therefore, seeing the wild children, and those with sensory or physical disabilities, was a process of rejecting the animal recognized within their 'monstrous' bodies. It was also, though, about a desire to see, to acknowledge and to feel the quiver of fear such recognition entailed (Todd 1995). Meeting the animal in the human self was exciting, thrilling, desirable and one of the motivations behind the eighteenth century's continual fascination with the different, the odd and the monstrous. At a time of Enlightenment rationalization and the celebration of human exceptionalism (despite medical breakthroughs built upon suffering animal bodies), an uncomfortable realization emerged: that within the eighteenth century's disabled, the animal was always there, lurking, a welcome and worrying message made visible.

DISABILITY AND ANIMALITY

This chapter weaves together two primary fields of study: animal studies and disability studies. These two fields, generally, do not look to each other, as Taylor (2011) clearly indicates, and they certainly do not do so as standard historical method. This situation is much like the history of medicine in general, where, as Woods points out, 'scholars influenced by the "animal turn" have not been drawn to study the history of medicine, while historians of medicine have remained largely unaware of the "animal turn"' (Woods et al. 2018: 13). This chapter, then, is intended to bring these seemingly disparate fields into conversation with one another, while attempting to raise questions about the nature of historical disability and otherness during the long eighteenth century.

The cultural history of animals is part of a growing field of animal studies, a field that takes the presence of animals as central. As Erica Fudge (2006) argues in her much-quoted paper: 'this new history is a history in which we are being asked to look at the ways in which animals and humans no longer exist in separate realms'. It is a history that resists modernity's and the Enlightenment's effects 'in which nature and culture coincide; and in which we recognize the ways in which animals, not just humans, have shaped the past' (2006). Interested in questions of human–non-human relationships, categorization, anthropomorphism and agency, for example, animal studies often explore the concept of 'human' as always also animal. Donna Haraway's theories are foundational for the field and clearly articulate the shared nature of human and animal within history. As Haraway eloquently puts it in her *Companion Species Manifesto*, animals, and for her specifically dogs, 'are not surrogates for theory; they are not here just to think with. They are here to live with. Partners in crime of human evolution, they are in the garden from the get-go' (2003: 5). Animals should not and cannot be divested from human history or understandings of being in the world. However, outside of animal studies, scholars continue to disengage from animals. As a result, animals, until recently, have usually been considered alien or other and relatively separate from major cultural developments.

Likewise, disability studies have also only recently included the non-human animal. First emerging with the 2012 ground-breaking collection *Earth, Animal, and Disability Liberation: The Rise of the Eco-ability Movement* (Nocella II et al. 2012), some scholars are starting to shift their focus towards an ethically and politically motivated stance that deliberately brings together the systematically downtrodden, marginalized and damaged. The book, and the follow-up 2017 collection, *The Intersectionality of Critical Animal, Disability, and Environmental Studies: Toward Eco-ability, Justice, and Liberation* (Nocella II et al. 2017), shifts away from 'traditional' disability studies and moves towards a more inclusive theoretical position that focuses on differing abilities for all. Within this framework, and when it is added to an active interrogation of 'normalcy, ableism, and civilization, in the manner of eco-feminism ... eco-racism ... and eco-colonialism', the previously hierarchical and disparate labels of ecology, disability, and human and non-human become 'truly diverse'. What emerges, then, is a concept of 'interdependent' systems and beings that are 'different – in the most liberating sense of the word' (Nocella II 2012: xiii). Thus, together all beings must be respected as valuable within 'the larger bio-community' (2012: xiv).

However, the activist work of bringing together ecology, animal, human and disability under one theoretical umbrella is not without its discomfort – especially for the study of history (Duncan 2012: 39; Withers 2012: 112–15; Basas 2012). With a lengthy record of derogatorily conflating the Other, the disabled body, with that of the animal as part of the disenfranchising process, acknowledging the animal within disability history has problematic and ethical implications for individuals today. Inviting animals back into disability history, it is feared, may undermine or destroy the long struggle to establish the irrefutable humanity of those deemed disabled while reinforcing historical and ongoing harmful animalizing discourses. Acknowledging the animal in history might just allow its acknowledgement in people today. Indeed, the animal might still be there. Thus, looking to the animal, facing the animal within history, 'might ... betray an unease that querying the "human" might inadvertently allow for a slide to the "animal"' (Walsh 2015: 20). For Walsh, the non-human animal is always there, waiting, in the history of disability, and because of its ubiquitous presence many scholars and disability activists work to reject the animal outright (2015: 20). However, as those who interrogate equally problematic discourses and histories (such as race and 'breed') realize, when discussing animal history you cannot escape the animal in all of its forms (Haraway 2019). Taylor, like Haraway, ventures into the fraught realm of the human and the animal; they enter into 'slippery territory' that is an exploration of dis-abled human and animal oppression, and once present, 'there is no way to discuss animal metaphors without recognizing the atrocities that they have been used for: the rhetoric of Nazi Germany, of racism, of slavery'. Indeed, for Taylor, 'the rhetoric of the sideshow was hardly better, clearly using animal comparisons to support racist ideologies and demeaning and patronizing stereotypes. So why, when so many people, myself included, have felt the negative and hurtful consequences of being compared and associated with nonhuman animals, would I enter this territory' (2011: 196). Why indeed? For Taylor it is an ethical imperative for scholars to call attention to the suffering of both humans and non-humans over time in an effort to improve the welfare and treatment of both oppressed subjects (2011: 196).

For me, entering the 'slippery territory' of the animal within is a means of coming to understand (even at the most basic level) my own disability and position as an individual with personhood alongside other animals. I was recently diagnosed with two allergies: one to rabbits and the other to all artificial fragrances. The animal allergy results in life-threatening asthma attacks, and the fragrance allergy has caused an over-sensitization to all fragrance (natural and artificial) and many synthetic chymicals. I have a dog's nose, one that can scent fragrance at quantities and distances most other humans cannot; I also have an immune system that interprets those scent signals as it does rabbit dander – as foreign invaders. Thus, like that of canines, my view of the world as an individual with a sensory disability in a culture filled with pets and artificial scent is largely dependent on smell, with my sight and world mapping increasingly manifesting as a scent-scape full of dangerous places, people and animals to avoid. Studying the co-mingled history of animals and disability, then, is a journey of the self and my invisible disability, but like Taylor it is also an essential exercise that can begin to scratch the surface of a long, co-mingled history of human and animal. Indeed, as Lennard Davis bluntly states: 'To have a disability is to be an animal, to be part of the Other' (1995: 40). It is a history of the oppressed, the excluded, the weak, the disenfranchised, and it is a co-history of animal and human together, along with the subjugated of all species, that needs to be told as a means of reclamation and empowerment. It is a history that I hope will help, at least in a small measure, to call attention to the shared histories of the repressed alongside the always unstable definition of 'human' that anthropocentrically denies intelligence, life and personhood to so many. Thus, my chapter follows Erica Fudge's and Taylor's arguments that, no matter how uncomfortable, 'we can say that history without animals is unthinkable' (Fudge 2002, 2006).

THE 'DEFECTIVE'

The word 'disability' and the category of 'disabled' are not standard across history. As David Turner argues, 'the "disabled" as a distinctive group, defined in terms of having needs separate from the broader mass of the sick and being entitled to specific welfare benefits – together with "disability" as an umbrella term – are the products of the twentieth-century economic and social developments' (2012: 11). During the eighteenth century they were not terms of identity or group belonging. Instead, the term 'disabled' was infrequently applied during the period. When it was used, it was usually within its legal definition: that of a person who was incapable, or so disabled, of inheriting land or property (2012: 17). It was also used to indicate someone who had lost their able-bodied status (capable, strong, and healthy), or someone who was completely incapacitated through poverty, drink, violence, etc. (2012: 20). In the eighteenth century, then, for both human and animal, 'disabled' and 'disability' were impermanent descriptors of someone who was temporarily unable to perform the duties expected of them.

Other terms for physical impairment were more common during the period and described situations that were frequently permanent. These included 'lame', 'crippled', 'deformed', 'defective', and 'monstrous' (Deutsch and Nussbaum 2000; Davis 1995). However, what and who fell within these categories was remarkably diverse. The work of Sibscota focused on the 'defective' and is the subject of this section. Those deemed defective were usually simple to label, as they often had a sensory impairment, such as deafness or blindness (Deutsch and Nussbaum 2000: 2), as a result of anatomical difference. As Lennard Davis argues, such people afforded unprecedented fascination for philosophers, medical practitioners and the general public to the extent 'that Europe became deaf during the eighteenth century'. The end of the seventeenth century and the beginning of the eighteenth saw the deaf and mute become visible to ableist society, effectively defining them as a unique community of their own (Davis 1995: 51). Before this period the deaf were understood not as a separate group, only as a scattering of individuals who suffered under the widespread assumptions that refused them language, intelligence and often humanity.

At the start of the long eighteenth century, however, the beginning of Enlightenment inquiry asked new questions about the nature of language, the relationships between communication and the soul, and the problematic definitions of human and animal (Serjeantson 2001). Such questions brought the deaf and mute to the forefront of scientific and philosophical debate. Some of the most influential texts of the period include, among others: John Bulwer's *Philocophus* [*The Deaf Man's Friend*] (1648) and *Chirologia, or the Natural Language of the Hand* (1654); George Delgarno's *Art of Communication* (1680); John Wallis's *De Loquela* (1653); William Holder's *Elements of Speech*

(1699) (all members of the Royal Society, as Lennard Davis points out); John Ammon's *Sudus Loquens* [*The Talking Deaf Man*] (1694) and *Dissertatio de Loquela* (1700); Daniel Defoe's *Duncan Campbell* (1720); Abbé de l'Epée's *Instruction of Deaf and Dumb by Means of Methodical Signs* (1776); J. L. F. Arnoldi's *Practical Instructions for Teaching Deaf-Mute Persons to Speak and Write* (1777); and R. A. Sicard's *Theory of Signs* (1782). The eighteenth century became a period of intensive investigation into some of the defining features of humanity, with speech and rationality at the forefront of discussion (Smith 2017; Wolfe 2017). Scholars consistently asked: how did sign language work? How did it relate to Biblical tradition and the long-standing assumption that verbal speech defined the human? What were people to do about the animals from around the growing empire that could talk and were rational (Wolloch 2019; Smith 2017)?

However, while uncertainty was evident in these texts surrounding where the deaf and mute, as ambiguous species, fit within this seemingly uncertain human/animal linguistic field, many authors on the subject sidestep direct engagement with the subject, content to leave that tangled web of contradiction to someone else. Some engage in questions of the soul (Bond 1720: 346), while others simply refer to the rationality of the deaf and mute as 'sagacity' – a term reserved for animal thought processes (William Holder, quoted in Branson and Miller 2002: 83). These authors generally do not ask questions about what was human even in light of the period's new information about (and fascination with) apes, 'savages', wild children and ostensibly rational animals of all types (Wahrman 2004: 132–3).

In contrast, such questions are taken up by George Sibscota in his *The Deaf and Dumb Man's Discourse* (1670). Scholars know very little about Sibscota. Jan Branson and Don Miller (2002: 89) suggest the name was a pseudonym for an unknown author and that *The Deaf and Dumb Man's Discourse* was a translation of an earlier (1660) Latin text included in a collection of medical essays by Anthony Deusing (professor of medicine in Groningen, Holland). Regardless of authorship, though, the text was a learned scientific treatise expressly written as a clear rejection of the implicit animality within previous works on the subject. Sibscota argues for the intelligence, human rationality and immortal souls of the deaf and mute while also, contradictorily, welcoming the animal in as an aspect of all humanity. *The Deaf and Dumb Man's Discourse* is a piece of activism that directly targets the problematic, oppressive and slippery boundary between the human world and the animal. Engaging with period debates on animal and human language (see for example Serjeantson 2001), and working within a long history stretching back to classical works on the subject by Aristotle, Plutarch and Pliny, among others, Sibscota's late seventeenth-century treatise is split into two interconnected halves. The first half unpicks the accepted Western views of the relationship between deafness, the ability to speak, the acquisition of language and the ubiquitous presence of the divine. The second half, *An Additional Tract of the Reason and Speech of Inanimate Creatures*, continues the various themes introduced in the first half, but it does so through an in-depth exploration of animal rationality and the apparent ability of non-human animals to express their internal selves through human-like speech or writing. Throughout the two halves, Sibscota asked what is true rationality, how the image of God differentiates between human and animal, and what are the limits of communication for all beings (human, animal and 'defective').

Sibscota begins his contribution to ongoing discourses on defective bodies by tackling one of the most prevalent beliefs of the eighteenth century: the idea that the clearest demarcation between humans and animals is humanity's capacity for verbal speech (Branson and Miller 2002: 71). Indeed, 'the faculty of Speech (which presupposeth reason) is only bestowed upon Man', Aristotle claimed, and as such 'no other Creature can Speak' (quoted in Sibscota 1670: 49). Such philosophy underpinned other authors' use of 'sagacity' and 'creature' when describing the deaf, and it was used throughout the early modern and modern world to define those with sensory or physical disabilities as lesser than, as not quite human. Those who could hear were thought to be naturally able to speak intelligible language because, within this classical Aristotelian philosophy, speech was a direct result of hearing and rationality. Thus, to be a hearing-enabled person was to be a reasoned creature able to talk (Sibscota 1670: 49). If someone could not hear, however, it was immediately thought, throughout the seventeenth century and into the eighteenth (Green 1783), that such an individual was incapable of verbalizing language. This inability to speak, in turn, evidenced the connection between hearing, speech and rationality. To be deaf was to be 'dumb', and to be 'dumb' was to be an irrational brute.

This Aristotelian tradition was not universal, however. Many eighteenth-century philosophers and medical practitioners took an alternative stance. Taking inspiration from the Plutarchan theriophilic tradition, with its love of animals and firm belief in animal rationality being on a par with that of humans (Preece 2005: chapter 1), influential philosophers like Locke and Rousseau (Davis 1995: 59) argued that animals did have reason (of a sort akin to that of humans) and that they could speak as a result (Serjeantson 2001). Sibscota took inspiration from this tradition and spent much of his *Discourse* refuting Aristotle's teachings on hearing, speech and anatomy (Sibscota 1670: 50, 52). However, when it came to animal rationality he agreed with Aristotle's hierarchical views. While initially unclear about his views on non-human rationality, Sibscota later established not only that 'dumb brutes' possessed 'some *Idea* of Reason, or some kind of ratiocination in them' (Sibscota 1670: 59), but also that they, in many instances, illustrated a unique ability to communicate through speech, body language or writing.

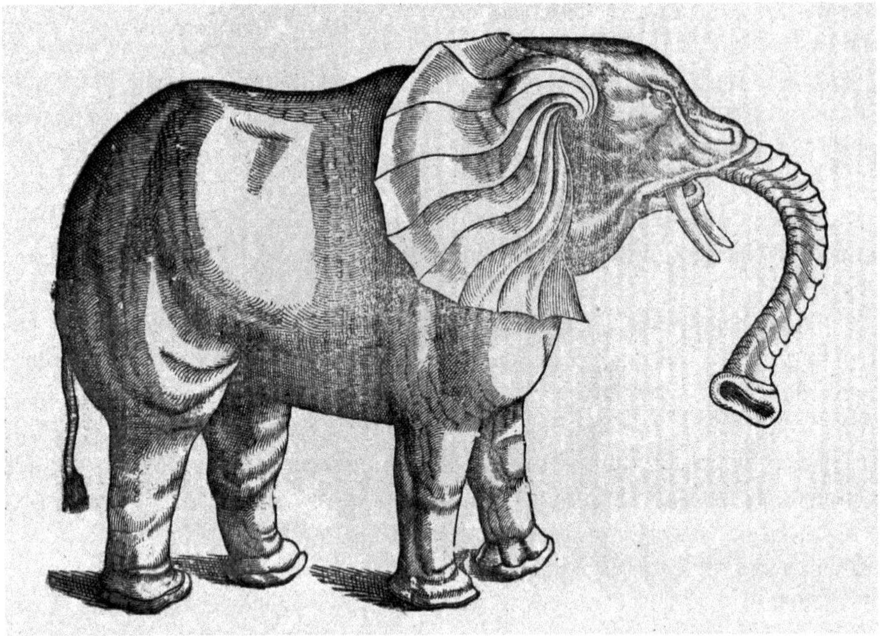

FIGURE 4.1: Woodcut of an elephant, from Edward Topsell, *The History of Four-Footed Beasts and Serpents*, London: E. Cotes for G. Sawbridge, T. Williams and T. Johnson, 1658. Credit: The University of Houston Library, Houston, USA/Public Domain.

Sibscota looked to a variety of animal species and historical sources to illustrate his points, and followed period classification systems that placed elephants, apes, dogs and horses next to humans on the hierarchy of rationality (Mattfeld 2017: 53). Indeed, species as diverse as elephants, sparrows and spiders all expressed reasoned responses and the clear ability to communicate their desires and internal thoughts. For Sibscota, the clearest examples of animal rationality came from elephants and his own dogs. Historically, elephants were believed capable of complex thinking and problem solving, indicating their ideas physically. For example, as naturalist and pioneer medical botanist Garcia de Orta related, elephants were known to understand the verbal wishes of their handlers and to make rational connections between action, inanimate object and falsehood. As Sibscota (referencing de Orta) relates, an elephant handler recalled when one of his elephants asked to be fed at his usual time, the food being late. He showed the elephant that his meal was late because his food bowl was damaged, stating that if the elephant wished to eat, he first needed to take the bowl to the blacksmith for repair. As the story goes, the smith did not mend the bowl well, and upon showing the still-broken vessel to his keeper, the elephant was commanded again to return it to the smith for fixing. The frustrated elephant returned the bowl to the smith, throwing it down 'with a querulous tone', and this time closely monitored the smith as he worked. The anthropocentric smith, disbelieving in animal rationality, desired to 'put a Cheat upon him' and only pretended to fix the holes. But the elephant was not fooled when he took the bowl to the river and attempted to fill it. When the water ran out instead, the elephant, 'being hereupon highly incensed, . . . ran back to the *Brazier*, and bellowed out with a thundering voice'. Chastised, the smith finally fixed the bowl properly. The elephant, however, was 'mistrustful' and tested the bowl in the river again. Only 'when he saw that it would hold, he turns himself to the standers by and shews it, calling them as witnesses to the matter of fact; and so went home' (Sibscota 1670: 53–5). This heavily anthropomorphized account of elephant rationality and verbal communication was further embellished with tales of elephants copying written text from a book and expressing themselves using sounds remarkably akin to human speech.

According to many classical authors and established medical theory, then, Sibscota argued, animals like elephants did not differ from humans in their vocal anatomy, language understanding, communication or rational abilities. Elephants could speak through their trunks using either language systems and 'proper terms' 'with their own kind' or human speech (Sibscota 1670: 64, 65). Indicating an awareness of linguistic communities defined along species lines, while radically undermining the anthropocentric nature of language, Sibscota suggested that such speech acts were remarkably similar to the abilities enjoyed by people with deafness as a 'defect' in the late seventeenth century. As Sibscota states, 'Although the major part of Brutes have no articulate Voice, and so do not make use of Speech properly so called, . . . they express their inward conceptions one with another, and with Men also, by the Gestures, Sounds, and Noises which they make with their Bodies, and such other kind of means; even as Dumb Men use gesticulations and various motions in lieu of Speech, whereby they discourse very significantly among themselves, as well as with other persons' (1670: 66–7). Like elephants, those who were 'deaf and dumb' could, in some instances, verbalize speech, use gestures to communicate and write, making themselves understood to others 'of their kind' and to the wider hearing-abled society.

The communication abilities of deaf people are well documented in Britain from at least the Roman period, with indications that many early modern individuals used effective sign language with others who were deaf or mute and to the wider community (Branson and Miller 2002: 61–2). For example, on Friday 9 November 1666, Samuel Pepys recorded an intense fire breaking out at Whitehall and Horse Guards. News about the fire was conveyed to Pepys and his friend Downing from a 'dumb' but 'cunning rogue'. The boy, well known to Pepys and Downing, 'made strange signs of the fire, and how the King was abroad'. Downing, unlike Pepys, understood the boy and explained to Pepys that 'it is only a little use, and you will understand him, and make him understand you with as much ease as may be' (Pepys n. d. [1666]). According to Pepys, who often mentioned deaf people in his diary (1660–1667), there was nothing wrong with the boy's intelligence and clarity of communication for those who knew his language. It was a matter of 'ease' for the abled and disabled to communicate, including complicated information on the state of a fire and the king's residence.

For Sibscota, such abilities were the same among his elephants, dogs, sparrows, spiders, ants and parrots – at least on the surface. Sibscota's insistence on the rationality and linguistic ability shared between animal and human was not intended to perpetuate the assumption of negative animalization of 'defective' bodies within period discourse. Instead, by placing those who were deaf and mute beside animals, and by approaching the subject through an investigation of animal rationality, Sibscota undermined some of the most insidious reasons for animal and human repression and persecution within ableist society. Through his multi-species investigations into hearing and language, Sibscota claimed similarities between the species – something vehemently denied during the Enlightenment. Close comparisons between animal and human equalized the hierarchy of human exceptionalism to some extent, while allowing for species' differences to become undeniably evident. It also rendered previous authors' erroneous beliefs on the subject ludicrous. Placing the defective beside animals reclaimed animality as a positive attribute for all humans and as an integral component of 'humanity' that should be embraced. In doing so, Sibscota demonstrated how fundamentally different God's beings actually were, placing the deaf and mute firmly on the side of the human. The defining feature of humanity for Sibscota was not speech as most claimed but was located in the interwoven ideas and epistemologies of rationality and theology.

Humans, whether unencumbered by 'defects' or struggling under a sensory deficit, were the only beings capable of knowledge of the divine. Animals, Sibscota argued, *seemed* capable of understanding their world and their place within it, and of expressing their innermost thoughts; however, they were not capable of wider abstract ideas. They could not truly understand God, his teachings or the concept of salvation. The 'Reason of Brutes', Sibscota argued, 'is absolutely different from Humane Reason in its very essence' because it was composed of 'a kind of sensitive or material faculty of the Soul' (1670: 69). Humans also had this element as part of their souls, 'vulgarly called Cogitative in man', but it differed in quality to that of animals as it had the benefit of interacting with a 'rational Soul', or an immortal one. The result was that while animals did have a form of reason, as evidenced by Sibscota's rational menagerie, human reason was 'far more noble and excellent, than the Reason in any species of Brutes can be' (1670: 70). This differentiation between human and animal rationality was not unique to Sibscota (Smith 2017: 135; Wolfe 2017: 152), but it meant that even elephants, who appeared to possess full rational abilities (understanding even the hidden motivations of humans and the concepts of falsehood, time and the self), did not possess 'true' human rationality. Unable to 'conceive any thing of God', elephants and other animals were unable to 'dispute concerning God by the deduction of Causes, or by the successive end, nor by conclusions drawn from the principles imprinted in their minds' (Sibscota 1670: 80). Animals could not learn or comprehend the concept of a higher power or learn of biblical events. Even if they had an immortal soul, animals' lack of true reason and knowledge meant they were unable to gain salvation.

This absence of human-like rationality called into question animals' communication abilities, and those of humans who shared an animal-like 'defect'. Humans, in general, were capable of knowing the divine and achieving salvation through true rationality. The problem, then, was whether those with a sensory deficit, such as the deaf and mute, could learn of God and achieve salvation when they were unable to hear religious teaching in church. Sibscota argued that hearing was not the issue. Countering Aristotelian philosophy, Sibscota suggested that speech, and hence rationality, was not predicated upon the ability to hear. Regardless of whether a person could hear the scripture, they were physically, rationally and spiritually capable of learning because they were human and capable of achieving salvation through literacy.

Other authors who had explored the deaf and mute also came to this conclusion as part of the period's reframing of literacy as the pre-eminent form of communication – replacing verbal speech as the most essential communicative ability (Davis 1995: 61). As Davis states, for many authors at the turn of the eighteenth century (including Sibscota), 'there is little difference between a hearing person and a deaf one in the reading or writing process' (1995: 59). What resulted from this elevation of literacy, and the growing belief in the unconnected and learned abilities of speaking and reading, was the beginning of regular and institutionalized instruction for the deaf and mute. Early educators and language specialists were interested in the nature of language – such as standardized signing alphabets, gaining the ability to read and write, and even, in some cases, to speak – and its connection to knowledge. For them, all humans were given unique language by God, and in its primitive form, sign language was thought to predate the Tower of Babel, making it the 'perfect', originator language (Branson and Miller 2002: 71–2). Sibscota dismissed such notions, stating there was no original language and that it was God's design to have multiple languages, including sign. But like his philosophical compatriots, he questioned Aristotle's views on sound as the basis of language and the truism that verbal speech alone reflected the mind while being 'the source of the soul' (Branson and Miller 2002: 72). For Sibscota, all creatures, human and animal, could communicate by 'signs', produce a voice or make sound of some sort if their anatomy allowed, and some animals (like parrots) could approximate or ape human language (see also Smith 2017). Intelligent, rational speech, however, was the result of the immortal soul and dedicated instruction. For him, and later authors on the subject, the deaf and mute were akin to innocent infants who required time and patience to learn how to communicate, negating the concept that God was only made manifest to those who could hear and speak. All language was Godly, hence all humans, regardless of their ability to verbalize speech, were a product of his divine plan (1670: 37).

It did not matter to Sibscota that humans and animals seemingly shared the ability to read, write and communicate. Such similitude should not lead to any 'humiliation of human sovereignty and uniqueness' in the slide down the human/animal hierarchy (Wolfe 2017: 151), as it was simply a product of shared qualities among all of God's creatures. An inability to articulate speech was no longer an indicator of something unnatural, sinful or animal (Turner 2012: 36); God's plan demanded a human population that was diverse and healthy, like the brute beings around them (Branson and Miller 2002: 82). Within this philosophy, the deaf and mute were categorized as animal in the same way as their able-bodied neighbours: akin in most respects, but fundamentally different when it came to their rational souls. The deaf and mute were simply another form of human equally as capable of reason as the able-bodied. Indeed, and as John Dunton concluded in his 1701 *Post Angel*, those who were born 'deaf and dumb', such as the four children of wool merchant Charles Leane, ought to 'thank God who hath made the Difference' (quoted in Turner 2012: 37).

The argument that the presence of people with sensory or physical 'defects' was part of God's divine plan faded during the eighteenth century, a period 'best understood as transitional' according to (Gabbard 2011: 83–4). The older beliefs in God's plan were replaced by increased medicalization and institutionalization of the defective or deformed body, and a heightened belief that such individuals were distinctly Other to the rest of the human species (Turner 2012; Branson and Miller 2002: 92). Sibscota's work followed this general shift in how defective bodies were constructed, as he worked within a more ancient, religious mindset regarding the deaf as people who could achieve salvation through writing and signing, as St Augustine and the venerable Bede both argued (Branson and Miller 2002: 67–8). However, he was also a fundamental part of the Enlightenment drive towards the medicalization of disability, placing individuals' inability to hear or speak firmly in the realm of anatomical 'defect' or the result of disease. Now, defective people were no longer part of any divine plan; instead, they were ideal candidates for medical intervention, for being saved from themselves and from their aberrant bodies, and for the demonstration of the superiority of rational science and medicine over the human body. For those deemed deaf and mute, such rationalization came in the form of dedicated and increasingly institutionalized language schooling and, for some, a status that constructed them as the epitome of the new literate society (Turner 2012: 37). However, for individuals with visible physical differences that placed them within the categories of 'deformed', 'curious' or 'monstrous', their experiences during the eighteenth century could differ markedly from the experiences of those who were deaf and mute.

THE MONSTROUSLY 'DEFORMED'

Monstrosity and deformity were not neatly definable categories during the eighteenth century. The terms were often interchangeable and connoted someone or something that had deviated from the laws of nature through their own actions, by accident or through other processes (Deutsch and Nussbaum 2000: 2). Often associated with some form of moral corruption, monstrosity disclosed the flaws in the deformed and defective, while monsters 'revealed wither the hidden condition or the future of mankind, biologically and/or morally' (Benedict 2000: 127). They were 'warnings', according to Barbara Benedict; traumatic disruptors of the viewing audience's sense of stable self, for Lennard J. Davis; and 'simultaneously and compulsively fascinating and repulsive, enticing and sickening', for Elizabeth Grosz (Benedict 2000: 127; Davis 1995: 132; Grosz 1993: 56). Monsters, like the animals they were thought perhaps to be, acted as mirrors for the able-bodied to view and construct themselves. As Todd explained: 'Indeterminate amalgams of forms, monsters [like the animal] make us experience a dispersion of identity. They are liminal creatures, straddling boundaries between categories we wish to keep distinct and separate, blurring distinctions, haunting us with the possibility that the categories themselves are ambiguous, permeable' (Todd 1995: 156). They were unsettling creatures, but people of all classes and genders were unendingly attracted to them because of their very liminality – and the attractiveness of witnessing the Other that was so akin to the self. It was all about 'the frisson that comes with seeing how closely the monstrous verges on the normal, the human, the everyday' (Todd 1995: 157).

While the history of disability is much more than the history of 'freak shows', as Taylor makes clear (2011: 196), 'the history of the aberrations of the physical body cannot be separated from this structure of the spectacle' (Stewart 1993: 108). Even with its racist and oppressive capitalist regimes, the exhibition of Othered bodies was an expected aspect of interaction with eighteenth-century 'monstrosity' and a regular feature of a society fascinated by the atypical form (Guerrini 2010: 110–11). As Anita Guerrini (2010) and Paul Semonin (1996) argue, the general public, royalty, nobility, natural philosophers, members of the Royal Society (such as John Evelyn and Robert Hooke), physicians (such as Sir Hans Sloane, president of the Royal College of Physicians) and private collectors were all captivated by the wondrous monsters exhibited throughout London. Indeed, the eighteenth century enjoyed multiple public locations at which the monstrous were routinely made public. From local and national fairs, most famously Bartholomew Fair (Morley 1859), private houses and well-known establishments around Covent Garden and the Haymarket, to the many coffeehouses, illegitimate theatres and the first circuses, the century's popular entertainment economy thrived on physical irregularity (for example, see Moody 2000; Mattfeld 2017). Thus, the many displays of the Othered body are fruitful events through which the construction of monstrosity can be explored.

The many displays of 'monsters' and the 'curious' had the potential to shape the lives of people deemed physically unusual throughout the period (Deutsch and Nussbaum 2000: 1–2). As Rosemarie Garland Thomson argues, displayed, or 'freakish', individuals were placed on a continuum of difference with other disabled people, rather than representing a complete rupture with the Othered position (1996: 11). Exhibited monsters functioned as visible echoes of other 'deformed' people, such as Alexander Pope, Samuel Johnson, Horace Walpole and William Hay (see for example Turner 2012). Monstrosity on display made visible the cultural and medical constructs of the aberrant body, effecting the lives of those who deviated from established bodily and cultural norms. Women were considered malformed men, while eunuchs and hermaphrodites strayed from increasingly strict gender binaries of clearly sexed and reproductive bodies (see for example McCormick 1997; Thompson 2016). Fops diverged from acceptable methods and levels of conspicuous consumption, and hence from ideal masculinity, while those with physical 'abnormalities', such as unusual height, weight, skin colouring or general shape, deviated from the ideal and healthy human body. Even people who were labelled 'ugly', those with scars and those with disproportionate features like large noses were often ostracized for their deformity. The eighteenth century was a period when anomaly of any sort (physical, mental, cultural, social) positioned a person as an Other, as odd, dangerous and monster. It was a period when humanity's ability to adopt many faces, especially Agamben's animal image, was remarkably strong; anyone deviating from the ideal might become animal and deformed during a period that was increasingly concerned with establishing and policing clear hierarchies and binary difference (Wahrman 2004). The eighteenth century was a period of the ubiquitous animal in everyone, but for those deemed monstrous its presence was always problematic – especially when they were placed on display for commercial gain.

One of the most famous examples of the monstrous body on show, and of the popular engagement with discourses of animality that appeared alongside them, comes from the well-publicized lives of 'The Monstrous Craws' (Figure 4.2). In keeping with the tradition of placing 'odd' or 'interesting' people and animals on display within the metropolis (Pender 2000), the Craws originally consisted of three unnamed people, one man and two women. The Craws were shown to the gaze and whims of the London elite starting on Friday 22 December 1786, at 'Mr. Pecket's, Trunk Maker, No. 30, in the Haymarket'. 'JUST arrived from Abroad', declared the newspaper, 'Three Wonderful Phaenomena, wild born, of the Human Species . . . were of a very small stature, being little more or less than five Feet high; each with a monstrous Craw under the Throat, containing

PRICE REDUCED.

To the Nobility, Gentry, and the Curious for inſpecting moſt Extraordinary Human Beings, of the wild Species born.

Juſt Arrived from Abroad,

And to be Seen at Mr. Becket's, *Trunk Maker*, No. 31,

HAY-MARKET,

From Ten o'Clock in the Morning, till Nine in the Evening,

Three Wonderful Phœnomena,

Wild Born, of the Human Species :

THESE are Two Females and a Male, of a very SMALL STATURE, being little leſs or more than *Four Feet High*;

Each with a Monſtrous CRAW

under the Throat, containing within, ſome Three, ſome Four, ſome Five BALLS or GLANDS, more or leſs big than an Egg each of them, and which play upwards and downwards, and all ways in their *Craws*, according as incited and forced, either by their Speaking, or Laughing. Theſe Three

Moſt wonderful wild born Human Beings,

whoſe Country, Language, and Native Cuſtoms are yet unknown to all Mankind, it is ſuppoſed ſtarted in ſome Canoes from their Native Place (believed to be ſome ſtill unknown remote Land of South America) and being after Wrecked, were picked up by a Spaniſh Veſſel, which in a violent Storm, was alſo loſt off Trieſte, in Italy, when theſe Three People, and another of the ſame kind, ſince Dead, were providentially ſaved from periſhing; though, it is imagined, there were more on board of their Species.—At that period they were of a dark Olive Complexion, but which has aſtoniſhingly, by degrees, changed to the colour of that of Europeans.

Theſe Three *truly-ſurpriſing* Beings, have attracted to themſelves the moſt minute Attention, and great Admiration of all the Princes, celebrated Anatomiſts, and Naturaliſts, to whom they have been preſented in Europe, for their Rare, and yet Unknown Species; and not leſs indeed, for their moſt apparent and ſurpriſing Happineſs, and Content among themſelves; moſt endearing Tractableneſs and reſpectful demeanour towards all Strangers, as well for their unparallel'd and natural, chearful, lively, and merry Diſpoſition, Singing and Dancing (in their moſt extraordinary Way,) at the will and pleaſure of the Company

Admittance, One Shilling Each:—

FIGURE 4.2: Handbill advertising the exhibition at 'Mr Becket's, Trunk Maker, No. 31, Hay Market'. Credit: The Trustees of the British Museum, London.

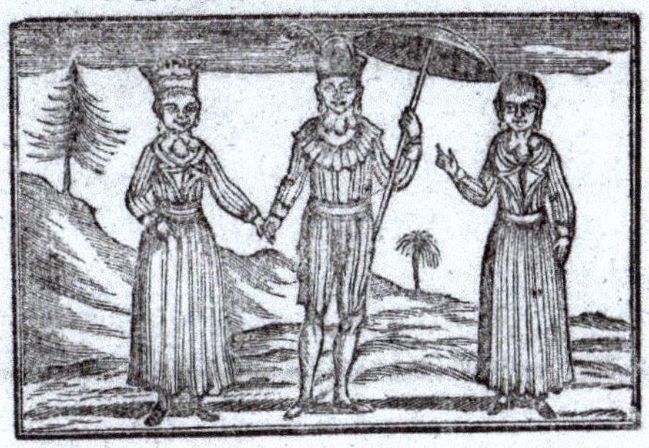

within some three, some four, some five Balls or Glands, more or less big than an egg each of them; and which play upwards, downwards, and all Ways, in their Craws, according as incited and stimulated wither by their speaking or laughing'. The three were of unknown origin and language, but it was suspected they were from somewhere in South America and had made their way to England via Trieste, Italy ('Advertisements and Notices', *Public Advertiser*, 26 December 1786). Going on to eventually show at the Royal Grove (6 August 1787 to approximately 2 September 1787) under the management of Philip Astley, and the Royal Circus (3 September 1787 to approximately 22 December 1787) under Charles Hughes, the Monstrous Craws proved a smash hit. Quickly becoming a household name, the Craws were a particularly popular form of the exoticized, racialized and animalized human attraction.

The Craws' animal-like monstrosity positioned them as 'surprising curiosities' who were 'wonderful', 'astonishing', 'extraordinary' and 'amazing' ('News', *Gazetteer and New Daily Advertiser*, 24 January 1787; 'News', *Morning Chronicle [1770]*, 16 April 1787). They were of particular interest to the general public, the learned medical investigator and the inquisitive natural philosopher. With the eighteenth century's rationalization and medicalization of the anomalous body came a shift in thinking about wonder and curiosity, from the belief in miracles and God's majesty to scientific inquiry. In the seventeenth century, monsters took on a new 'intellectual fascination' that placed them within the realm of acceptable philosophical curiosity and began to demarcate those who were interested in the monstrous for learned inquiry from those of the unthinking mob fascinated by monstrosity's wondrous elements (Semonin 1996: 71; Daston and Park 2001: chapter 9). Monsters increasingly became both figures of popular entertainment and the prime subject of curious inquiry during a century enthralled by 'forbidden topics' (Benedict 2001: 2). This was a century captivated by the natural world, once the prerogative of God but increasingly of interest to the rational inquiring mind, and with organizing it into discrete categories – as the work of natural philosophers such as Linnaeus indicates (see Thomas 1991). It was a period during which all people were fascinated by the wondrous, which meant that vulgar audiences were excited to see the Craws at the same time as 'distinguished Personages' of medicine and science satisfied their learned curiosity while asking 'questions that challenged the status quo' ('Advertisements and Notices', *Morning Herald*, 10 May 1787; Benedict 2001: 2).

The questions the Craws' peculiar bodies invited revolved around the nature of humanity and animality, and around the nature of acceptable sexuality. Because the Craws were 'deformed' and monstrous, by their very nature they were always liminally situated between the human and the animal. Fashionable throughout the early modern period into the nineteenth century, ethnological shows (the display of monstrous, wondrous and curious people) and exhibitions of animals coexisted alongside each other. Consistently blurring into one another, as Sadiah Qureshi argues, animal and human displays relied upon the 'alien' to create interest (2004: 237–8). While 'curious' humans and animals were exhibited, such as chimpanzees, polar bears, lions, kangaroo and other exotic beasts (Grigson 2016), those beings who deviated from the usual were especially popular. Indeed, those considered remarkably human, even devilish, for amazing abilities that fell outside of the customary 'dumb' and irrational 'brute' were a perennial favourite with audiences. The Learned Horse, the Learned Pig, various dancing dogs, the Learned Goose, singing cats, piano-playing mice and others thought remarkable, curious and wondrous often shared the stage with the Craws or were directly compared to them (Mattfeld 2015; 'News', *Gazetteer and New Daily Advertiser*, 24 January 1787). The Craws were consistently viewed alongside animal acts, and thus were frequently treated as animal themselves.

Indeed, the association of the Craws and other monstrous bodies with animal acts was well known by the Craws' handlers. Like many eighteenth-century owners or managers of the strange and wondrous, they consistently exaggerated the classification binaries inherent within their subjects. They were puffed (overpraised in paid newspaper advertisements) as 'Savage', 'wild born' and deformed monsters, while being irrefutably 'People', 'Human Beings' and 'of the same Species' ('Advertisements and Notices', *World*, 16 January 1787; 'Advertisements and Notices', *Public Advertiser*, 22 December 1786; 'News', *Morning Chronicle [1770]*, 16 April 1787). Such language indicates an awareness of and anxiety about the animal within them, the other animals on stage and their audience. However, this hybridity, as an inherent component of monstrosity, was amazing, and as such, desirable.

Dennis Todd argues that this desirability of the Other was intrinsic within 'monstrosity' itself. Although monsters were often greeted with fear, anxiety and disgust, not all were dangerous, and some might even be beautiful. The discourse of beautiful monstrosity was common during the eighteenth century. Many individuals who had a physical 'deformity' or 'defect' were described as monstrous, but then also affable, biddable or good looking (Todd 1995: 156–9). The mixed space between dangerous and even evil, and 'docile' and 'attractive', was for Todd one of the defining features of monstrosity and the clearest explanation for the ubiquitous popularity of the monstrous. 'Guardians' of the displayed were aware of the power that lay in the uncanny similarities between the monstrous and the 'normal', advertising their exhibition to the public by highlighting and exaggerating the blurry lines between object and audience, sameness and difference (Todd 1995: 157–8). Thus, with the Craws, monstrosity was both fearful and aesthetically pleasing.

In the eighteenth century, when anatomical difference was taken as an index of the mind within, the presence of monstrosity or defect was often interpreted as evidence of a depraved soul. William Hay, in his *Deformity: An Essay* (1754), among others, took to task this assumption (Pender 2000: 115), but the physiognomic argument of monstrosity's truthful body, the mark of a person lacking natural affection, remained a potential problem for the Craws' 'guardian'. Aware of monstrosity's latent negative aspects, especially its tendency to cause moral and social panic, he offset any potential 'alarm' or feelings of 'danger from them' (especially as may be felt by the visiting 'ladies') by exaggerating their docile affability ('News', 6 March 1787, *Morning Herald*). The negative monstrosity of the Craws was downplayed and their physical beauty and cordiality was embellished from the outset: 'These three truly surprising Beings', wrote the *Public Advertiser*, 'have attracted the most minute Attention and Great Admiration ... for their apparent and surprising Happiness and Content among themselves; most endearing Tractability, and respectful Demeanor towards all Strangers; as well as their unparalleled natural most cheerful, merry, and lively Disposition – Singing and Dancing at the Will and Pleasure of the Company' ('Advertisements and Notices', *Public Advertiser*, 22 December 1786). Indeed, they were 'docile, affable, entertaining' and even 'attractive' ('News', *Morning Herald*, 6 March 1787). They were astonishing creatures who drew audiences to them, while ensuring that once-stable categories of the self were continually in flux.

Monstrous attractiveness ensured their physical deviation from the natural body as a marker of absolute difference, while the rest of their bodies blurred the boundaries between 'deformity' and perfection, reviled and desirable, the animal Other and the human. Their 'endearing Tractability' and naturally happy disposition made them into ideal(ized) beings that encompassed desired (feminine) traits, but also situated them as biddable, domesticated, almost slavish, in their eagerness to please. Like the dancing dogs, they were reassuringly controlled within a clear hierarchy of species but also worryingly human/animal. Beings like the Craws questioned systems of power, the seemingly stable social hierarchy, the fabric of social make-up and the basic definitions of humanity.

Monstrosity on display also invites questioning of the nature of desire. The relationship between disability and desire is fraught. Most scholars and disabled people point to a long history of the disabled body as one that negates sexual attraction, where disability is isolating and often deemed 'disgusting'; it is a status that denies the eroticism of the disabled subject and the wider viewing public (Davis 1995; McRuer and Mollow 2012). As Davis argues, people with disabilities are 'by and large ... de-eroticized' (1995: 128) as part of the larger set of binaries between the able and disabled body. However, the experiences of those deemed 'monsters' undermines this overarching discourse and the 'immutable' nature of the constructed binaries of 'whole and incomplete, abled and disabled, normal and abnormal, functional and dysfunctional' (Davis 1995: 129), and desired and loathed. Eighteenth-century monstrosity invites the questioning of 'the contours of our sexuality' (Todd 1995: 156) alongside our humanity by acknowledging the often aesthetically pleasing and erotic nature of disability, while problematizing its social undesirability. Monsters are subject to a 'desire/disgust binary', to use Alison Kafer's phrase (2012: 336): reviled, dangerous, subversive, uncontrolled, but also beautiful, alluring and sexual.

For the Craws, this desire/disgust binary was typically associated with the women and had a profound impact on their lives as specimens of monstrosity. On 10 May 1787, the *Morning Herald* announced that the 'guardians' of the Craws were relaxing their stringent hours of operation, 10 am to 9 pm (*Collectanea*, f. 90v), to accommodate special requests. As the *Herald* stated: 'their guardians respectfully inform those distinguished Personages, who have from time to time applied to see them after nine o'clock at night, at which time they are stripped of their garments for public shew, that they may be waited on at their own houses with them, by giving previous notice before seven o'clock in the evening, at their exhibition place' ('Advertisements and Notices', *Morning Herald*, 10 May 1787). The Craws underwent a process of total dehumanization with the removal of any right to privacy and autonomy. Their bodies were objectified, as they were denied the human right to clothing and paraded as naked animals before the desiring gaze of London's elite.

Such displays were in keeping with the overt sexualization and erotic touching of the Craws (especially for the women). As the *World* on 17 March 1787 made clear, 'The old Female' Craw was 'not only admired for her attractiveness of extraordinary odd features and stature', but also for her 'most lively, prattling entertainment'. This entertainment was, of course, unintelligible, as the Craws did not discourse in recognizable language (probably a false performance). If she did speak as humans did in an intelligible language then, the paper titillated, 'many men have declared they would not more object to have a *close conversation* with her than they would with the naturally more engaging young jet-hair kissing one'. The male Craw's draw was his dancing – beautiful to observe but out of touch as decorum dictated for the female audience members ('News', *World*, 17 March 1787). However, the paper suggests that close sexual encounters between the female Craws and their (probably) male clientele were a usual occurrence – possibly as part of the later after-hours strip show as well.

Such interactions between audiences and the Craws (individuals worryingly of another species, or at least a sub-species, to humanity) invite questions of how desire, disgust, human, animal and speech interwove within the deformed body, and how they were negotiated by an admiring audience erotically aroused by monstrosity. A later puff from the Craws' time at Astley's Royal Grove can shed light on the complicated nature of eroticized eighteenth-century monstrosity on display and its implications for audience members acting on those feelings. On 6 November 1787, the *Morning Post* published 'A PARODY on a MODERN PUFF'. Intended as a political critique against the Duke of York and Prince of Wales, the puff took aim at those who sought out and believed the 'wonderful' and baffling performances of the older female Craw. In doing so, the puff made explicit the

Craw's dubious virtue, willingness to exceed the bounds of feminine decorum and absolute animal nature. The puff also argued that those men who invited her services, and believed them to be real, had slipped away from humanity and given in to the animal within that her monstrous body mirrored. Derogatorily labelling the two royals as '*imitatores!* [followers]' and '*servum pecus!!!* [slave cattle]' to the popular manipulations of the circuses and newspapers who consistently portrayed the Craws as unique, transgressive, exciting and morally pure, the puff argued that the Prince of Wales especially was like an unthinking animal – more animal even than the female Craw could ever be. Using oppositional and satirical language common to the era, the puff ran as follows:

> After the performance of this *extraordinary being* to a crowded audience at the ROYAL CIRCUS, a message was brought by *Mr. Hesse*, from their Royal Highnesses THE PRINCE OF WALES and DUKE OF YORK, signifying that they should think themselves *flattered* if the MONSTROUS FEMALE CRAW would favour them with a specimen of her performance.
>
> In consequence of this *request* the *Monstrous Female Craw* did not hold it *respectful* to refuse, and accordingly attended *Mr. Hesse* to Queensberry-House.
>
> Her performance consisted of the following *imitations*:
>
> The Learned Pig.
> The Singing Duck.
> Katterselto's Cat.
> The Drumming Hare.
> General Jackoo [the monkey].
> The Dancing Dogs.
> The Snorting [horse] Chillaby.
> And her own *natural* howl.
>
> During the exhibition, the most *flattering* attention was shewn by the PRINCE, who expressed high approbation at the *chastity* and [document damaged] powers of this *wonderful* being.
>
> The DUKE OF YORK took the *greater* part *upon trust*; but what he saw struck him as beyond conception *extravagantly great*.
>
> In tribute to the Female Craw, it seemed the universal opinion, that the ART OF IMITATION was, until *Thursday evening, totally unknown*; that *her's alone* was that which *baffled description*, and brought an absolute *identity* to the *animal it gave*; and high as the *public respect* has been in this subject, it did not equal the real.
>
> OURANG OUTANG.
>
> —*Collectanea*, Vol. 1, pt. 1

This parodic puff walks a fine line between truth and fiction, transparency and obfuscation, and the desire to harm and save. As a mock puff, it relies on the well-known advertising of the 'wondrous' acts of the Craws, especially their private shows and their hybrid animality. However, its diction, especially the italicized words, argues for their opposite. In keeping with period sentimentalized discourses around animal welfare and abolition, the puff humanizes the Craw (while remaining somewhat concerned about her animality) to illustrate the prince's complicit participation in ableist and anthropocentric systems of power that consistently dehumanize, objectify and commodify those with an atypical body – and by extension, harm the nation. The puff, in essence, and in keeping with period socio-political movements, is an abolitionist text that (somewhat) removes the animal within the victimized monstrous body to place it within the curious men who perpetuated morally corrupt backroom performances for their own erotic pleasure.

Indeed, as the puff implies, the *'respectful'* visit of the female Craw after the prince's *'request'* to join him was never something that she, or her proprietor, could refuse. He was a prince and she, as animal-human, was the slave-like property caught within a classed, gendered and ableist power imbalance. Her submission to his request was not about respect for his station, but simply because she could not decline. The prince's *'flattering* attention' was unwelcome, probably forced, and sexual in nature – as the reference to the Craw's dubious female reputation indicates. The female Craw was not known for her *'chastity'*, as previous puffs indicated, but resulted directly from a colonial society that enabled such behaviour on the part of her 'guardian' and 'audience'. For this anonymous author, her apparent animality, or non-human status as a result of her deformity, was used to harm and oppress her as a fallen woman. As a figure of failed femininity and a figure of common monstrosity because she was a woman, she certainly was not *'wonderful'*. As a victimized human fully capable of intelligible and rational speech, her *'imitations'* of animals, along with her own 'howl', did not bring 'an absolute *identity* to the *animal*' in question. Her performances of animal impressions in the Circus were anything but *'natural'*. Instead, her imitations were done by 'ART', or artifice learned as part of a well-known theatrical convention – something common to other human and animal acts that seemingly blurred species lines.

The puff pointed to the long history of charlatanism associated with monster displays (Pender 2000: 106–9) and was a part of the well-established tradition of satirizing learned individuals who were duped by them (Semonin 1996; Benedict 2001: chapter 1). As the 16 June 1787 edition of *Felix Farley's Bristol Journal* argued, the Craws were taught to imitate a lack of speech, the biggest defining feature of non-human status refuted by Sibscota. They were not 'wild born' but were 'taught a ludicrous gesture' and 'a more ridiculous unnatural gabble, without the least variety of sound or syllable' in addition to dressing in a 'grotesque manner'. The Craws' lack of intelligible, human-like speech (Green 1783: 59) came from careful training and acting and was not representative of truth or status as another species. The female Craw's animal imitations did not *'baffle... description'*, and they, along with the private nature of their performance, did not result in any *'public respect'* (original emphasis). What they did do, however, was illuminate the viewer's incapability of spotting a fake monster and their uncritical indulgence of desire for the Other (Pender 2000: 109).

Furthermore, the abolitionist mock puff was in keeping with late eighteenth-century discourses that, under the all-pervasive influence of sympathy, subverted the negative, animal nature of the different and disenfranchised. Just as Sibscota had claimed the animal to define the human, late-century authors rejected the animal in everyone, regardless of race or apparent monstrosity, to establish the human. Calling for the end of the slave trade and recognizing an affinity with those who were oppressed under slavery's yoke, abolitionists and animal welfare advocates demanded people's empathy. Images of tortured slaves, cruelly abused horses and the suffering deformed became stock in trade for social reformers (Abruzzo 2011; Boddice 2008; Perkins 2003; Preece 2002). Indicating a depraved soul and propensity to inflict similar destruction on those around them, harming an animal or an Othered human was increasingly understood as evidence of an immoral nature (Perkins 2003: 3). By the late eighteenth century, many claimed all humans and animals deserved love as creatures under God (Thomas 1983: 173). As a monstrous woman, then, caught somewhere between the human and the animal, the female Craw warranted better treatment. From an abolitionist and humanitarian stance, she deserved to preserve her modesty, freedom and autonomy. She and the other Craws should not have to publicly display themselves for the erotically hungry elite.

Philosophies that lumped the animal and the human together as equally deserving of care brought a swift end to the Craws' private shows – at least on the surface. Two weeks after the first advertisement invited wealthy patrons to indulge their desire for the monstrous bodies, the 28 May edition of the *World* stated that such 'repeated requests' to see the Craws after hours 'cannot possibly be complied with'. This was for two reasons. The first was because of 'the extreme fatigue they undergo, by being constantly exposed from ten in the morning til nine in the evening, demanding at that period an immediate rest for them' ('Advertisements and Notices', *World*, 28 May 1787). The Craws were suffering, exhausted, and as such required rest to maintain their health (and hence desirability).

These concerns were especially requisite for the youngest Craw. Of smaller stature, the young kissing Craw was ill for much of her time in London – the result, critics claimed (using overt animal discourse to describe her living situation), of 'her raw dinner' fed to her by her keepers. Her declining health should result in 'kindness', 'sympathy' or the meeting of the equally 'noble souls' ('News', *World*, 7 May 1787) possessed by the Craw and her sympathetic viewers. However, it seems even with the reduction in her hours and the removal of most private viewings that she remained ill over the next few months. Once the Craws were under the management of Philip Astley at the Royal Grove, the papers again expressed concern. Portraying her as an agentless 'creature' under the care of Astley, on 21 August 1787 *The Gazetteer and New Daily Advertiser* reported that the youngest Craw 'deserves the immediate attention of their proprietor'. Her 'food' was 'not congenial to her nature and constitution'; therefore, the correspondent implored, Astley should (as was 'proper') 'endeavour to find out what she has been accustomed to eat in her native soil'. Such philanthropic sentiment was not necessarily for the Craw's benefit, although she would 'be saved' through a changed diet, but so she could continue to serve as a money-generating commodity for her exhibitors and as spectacle for curious audiences 'desirous of gratifying their curiosity with seeing these astonishing living beings'. Such anthropocentric motivation for the alleviation of suffering was not unusual during the eighteenth century; however, regardless of such calls for the improved treatment of the youngest Craw, sometime around 5 September 1787 her presence in advertisements for the three 'monstrous Craws' disappears. The three silently and inexplicably became two.

With the youngest Craw's experience in mind, then, it becomes clear that humanitarian and abolitionist motivations were not the primary reasons for ending the Craws' private erotic shows. The youngest Craw continued to suffer, which was inconvenient for those who wished to continue profiting from her exhibition but was not necessarily grounds for ending the extra shows. What truly motivated the end of the private shows, I argue, was the second reason given for their cancellation: the transgression of the bounds of decency and human desire. The 28 May advertisement betrays an extreme fear about desiring, or acting on desire for, the monstrous Other to the extent that the author completely denied the existence of the original advertisement and the ongoing erotic interactions with the Craws. 'They also beg permission to give this public notice', the paper proclaimed, 'that they will ever tenaciously adhere ... to their first resolution, of not permitting any person whatever for any money that may be offered, to visit them in any parts commonly thought indecent, by either men or women, to be seen or exposed' ('Advertisements and Notices', *World*, 28 May 1787). It was 'their first resolution' to maintain the boundaries between decent and 'indecent' behaviour and of acceptable and unacceptable erotic interaction. Erotic desire for animalized monstrosity, and for the aberrant body, was simply intolerable. At least superficially. Of course, the presence of the 6 November mock puff targeting the princes indicates that the 28 May publication was done to assuage the sensibilities of the wider public, and that private 'conversations' continued in secret.

The anxious retraction of opportunities to indulge the audience's desire for the Craws, and insistence that such interactions never happened in the first place, raises serious questions about the nature of eighteenth-century taboo, sexuality and the position of the hybrid non-human within period constructs of curiosity's boundaries. Monstrosity's 'disgust/desire' binary stipulated that audiences were not to transgress on polite social decorum, nor were they to give in to their base desires to experience and even see the intimate parts of the deformed body. To do so introduced fears of the reproducing of monstrosity and, I suggest, of bestiality.

The perception of deformed or deficient individuals' sexuality as bestiality was a familiar construct in the eighteenth century, and it was a sexuality that had the potential to be the most 'outrageous' even in the most eyebrow-raising of centuries (Gabbard 2008: 377). As Carolyn Williams illustrates, the eighteenth century was remarkably full of implicit and explicit references to bestiality, with discussions of the subject appearing across the century and within obscure and canonical works of literature in equal measure. Designed for readers of all education levels, references to bestiality were 'fraught with anxiety, disgust, uncertainty and danger, and ... intimately concerned with human sexuality' (Williams 2006: 271). It is this concern, I suggest, that was at the heart of the quick retraction of the Craws' nightly shows and of the puffed attack primarily against the Duke of York. The prince was curious about and desirous of things he should not be and as a result placed his rational masculinity in jeopardy. Like the fops, rakes, mollies and hermaphrodites whose gendered and sexual performances, and physical bodies, made them monstrous and hence useless as civic men, the prince's desire painted him as someone who was incapable of fulfilling his duty to the nation during a time of social and political upheaval. To make matters worse, however, in the prince's case, his taboo desire also made him, like many others whose extreme curiosity made them 'monsters, 'queers' and curiosities, a traitor ... to ... his own species' (Benedict 2001: 2). His actions reversed the order of things, contravening all that was holy and natural in the world. Curiosity, then, made the prince equally animal to the Craw he so desired, and thus his hinted penchant for bestiality not only painted him as useless as a future ruler of the nation but also associated him with racialized miscegenation across the species line.

The association of disability with inheritable 'defects', and subsequent fear of such offspring, is well known (McRuer and Mollow 2012). However, because of monstrosity's animal nature, copulating with anyone or anything deemed animal could (many feared even during the Enlightened age) result in another monster (Todd 1995). Indeed, as Williams argues, with bestiality – and monstrous desire, I argue – 'The line between copulating like animals and with animals sometimes seemed perilously thin' (Williams 2006: 275). Therefore, because of his immoral desire, the betrayal of ideal masculinity and his own species, the prince was the one who was the true animal, the one who brought an 'absolute *identity* to the *animal*' (*Collectanea*, Vol. 1, pt. 1). Like the mercilessly satirized 'real connoisseurs of extraordinary beings, whether of the brutish or human creation' (Pender 2000: 109–10, 111–12; 'News', *Morning Chronicle [1770]*, 2 February 1787) who paid to attend the Craws privately, the prince was subject to his untamed curiosity and erotic desires forcefully fulfilled with a non-human/human animal. Thus, the prince was the 'real' animal, the true ape, or 'OURANG OUTANG' (*Collectanea*, Vol. 1, pt. 1), a species thought to be somewhat human or an evolutionary precursor to humanity (Thomas 1983: 132). The orangutan functioned here as an indicator of just how far man could fall if he insisted on irrational thought and brutish actions, and as a warning of what man would become if he gave in to his base desires. The prince allowed his unchecked enthusiasm for the monstrous body to override his civility, learned rationality and humanity. Such animalization of those who desired the monstrous, the non-human Other, was not confined to the 6 November puff, and was a common occurrence within critiques of audiences who enjoyed seeing the remarkable (human and animal) body on display (Mattfeld 2015). It was also well known by those who puffed the Craws, with Charles Hughes satirically claiming the female Craw had married the 'Black Prince, otherwise C – C – n' ('Arts and Culture', *World*, 15 October 1787). The fear of bestial miscegenation was potent and worrying, but also a prime motivator for audience curiosity.

ANIMALS, HUMANS, LEGACY

The Craws' time in London was short lived, and the last reference to them comes on 22 December 1787. Although they were not in London for long, the Craws left a legacy of monstrosity. Their name and image became standard referents for social and political excess, as James Gillray made clear in his 1787 *Monstrous Craws, at a New Coalition Feast* (Figure 4.3). Likewise, their defective form inspired a period fashion for enormous cravats, as appeared in Thomas Rowlandson's 1802 caricature. The wearers of the cravats, Rowlandson suggested, became monsters through their conspicuous display of fashionable excess, social ambition and questionable masculinity (Figure 4.4). They also became animals, as Rowlandson's caricature title hinted: *The Monstrous Craw; or a New Discovered Animal*. Monstrosity begets monstrosity, and monstrosity begets inhumanity; excess, lack, deformity, deficiency, oddity, Otherness and anything alien were at once human and always, mostly, animal.

This chapter has followed the defective and the monstrously deformed, thinking through the status of the Other as a lack, or lesser than, within an ableist society. In doing so, and by taking the presence of the animal as ubiquitous, it becomes evident that monstrosity, deformity and defectiveness

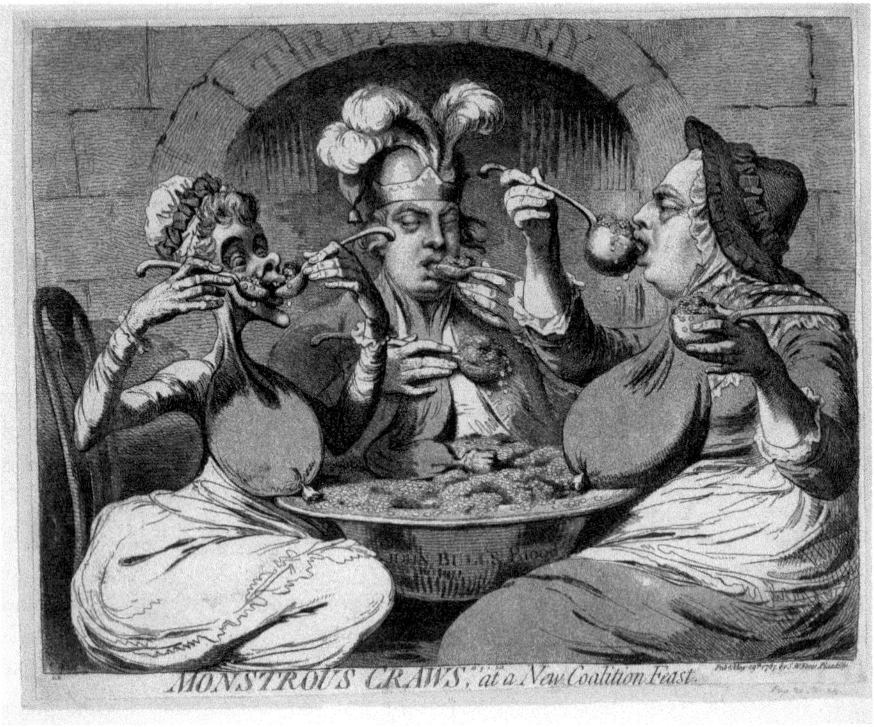

FIGURE 4.3: James Gillray, *Monstrous Craws, at a New Coalition Feast*, 1787. Credit: The Trustees of the British Museum, London.

were epistemological and ontological categories that ultimately destabilized the notion of 'human' while resisting or welcoming the animal in equal measure. Indeed, 'mixing distinct species together is at the crux of understandings of monstrosity' (Deutsch and Nussbaum 2000: 8), and the discomfort associated with that mixing was unique to the Age of Reason. During the eighteenth century, natural philosophers, such as Linnaeus, provided new classification systems that worked to clarify differences between human and animal (Wahrman 2004: 132–3), and medical advancements made with animals consistently tried to illustrate human uniqueness in the face of its apparent kinship with animal bodies. It was a period of urgency, as the very work that sought to ensure human distinctiveness in the natural world also definitively undermined it. The age's empirical advancements and global imperialism revealed that chimpanzees and orangutans were proto-humans, elephants could read and write, humans shared species characteristics with monkeys and bats, and human and animal bodies often functioned in the same manner. Within this consistently destabilizing narrative, and the anxious work to counteract it, the disabled and monstrous became living examples of just how thin the line between human and animal

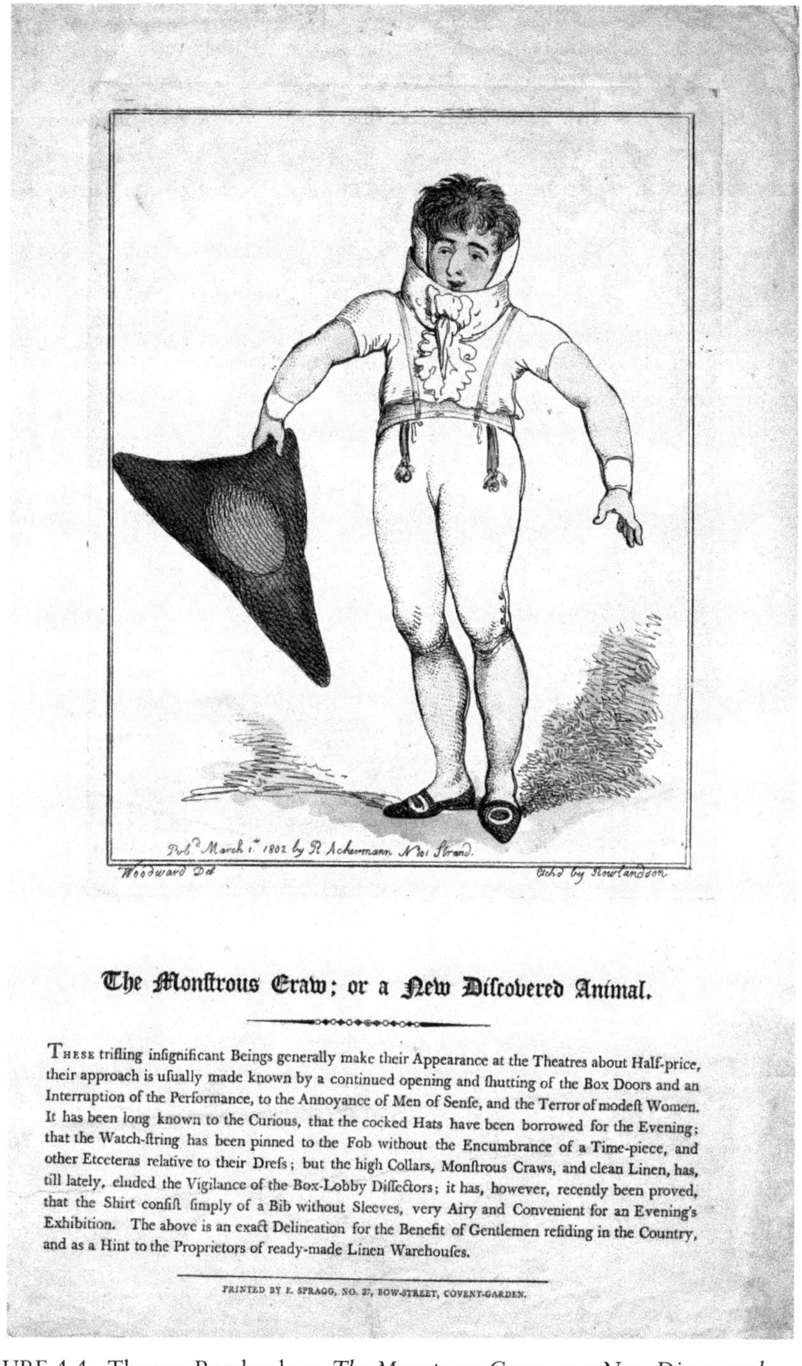

FIGURE 4.4: Thomas Rowlandson, *The Monstrous Craw; or a New Discovered Animal*, 1802. Credit: The Trustees of the British Museum, London.

actually was. Monsters and the disabled were prophetic beings who warned of a possible and (increasingly tangible) redefinition of humanity that erased all previous comforting delineations between species. Their deformed bodies demanded uneasy questions and created difficult answers. And no matter how hard naturalists, scientists and medical practitioners worked to ensure the stability of the human, and social commentators worked to police human morality, the presence of the defective and monstrous guaranteed the futility of their actions. As natural historian and taxonomist Georges-Louis Leclerc Compte de Buffon lamented, 'perhaps humiliating to humans: it is that we must classify ourselves as animals' (quoted in Guerrini 2010: 143). The animal was within everyone regardless of defect or deformity, whether people liked it or not, and regardless of how hard people worked to deny its presence.

CHAPTER FIVE

Objects

MARIEKE M.A. HENDRIKSEN

What do a drug jar in Poland, an English apothecary handbook, a skeleton carrying a scythe in Italy, four skulls from an Indonesian island, a wet anatomical preparation and an obstetric model in the Netherlands have in common? And what can they tell us about Enlightenment medicine? In this chapter I will argue that analysing the diverse but interconnected uses of one particular material, such as human bones, provides us with a more holistic, less linear understanding of the history of medicine. The history of medicine was long dominated by intellectual histories of ideas, and to a lesser extent by hagiographies of medical men. Over the past decades, the realization has grown that medicine was practised, used and developed by both men and women, by people from all levels of all societies, within and outside a variety of institutions, and that in the course of doing so, they created, exchanged, used, collected and destroyed a multitude of objects, texts and materials. Although people are undeniably important historical actors, in recent years it has become increasingly clear that objects play a significant role in how history is shaped and in our understanding of it – objects too, are actors.

This chapter explores the roles and meanings of a very peculiar category of objects in the history of Enlightenment medicine: those made partly or wholly of human bones. Such things possess a strange kind of agency; they are often simultaneously bone and the representation of bone, and possess a meaning that both stems from, and transcends, their materiality (Rheinberger 2012: 233–234; Brown 2001: 4–5). Before exploring the relationship between seemingly unconnected objects such as a human spine, a book and an obstetric doll, let us consider how objects came to take centre-stage in the history of medicine over recent decades.

It has been argued that speaking of 'turns' is a form of historiographical near-sightedness, but historians in many fields use the concept to signal shifting trends (Marr 2016: 1000). The 'material turn' in cultural history could be said to have started in the 1980s with a series of key works, such as those by art historians Michael Baxandall (1980) and Svetlana Alpers (1983), that drew attention to the circumstances and cultures in which works of art were produced and how these affected their production, meaning and materiality. In his edited volume *The Social Life of Things* (1986), Arjun Appadurai launched the idea that persons and things are not radically distinct categories, and that the transactions that surround things are invested with the properties of social relations. He argued that although it is formally true that things have no meanings other than those that humans and their actions endow them with, this does not illuminate the concrete, historical circulation of things, and that we thus need to study the thing-in-motion to illuminate its historical, human and social context. One of the more extreme approaches resulting from this material turn was philosopher and anthropologist Bruno Latour's Actor-Network-Theory (ANT, 2005), which put things at the centre of the study of existence. In the most radical form of ANT, nothing has special status; everything, whether human or object or phenomenon, exists equally and can equally influence other actors and events. These new approaches led to a raised awareness of the importance of materiality among humanities scholars.

Over the past decade, objects and their movements have been given an important role in the history of early modern science and medicine, too, with historians borrowing freely from methods and approaches originating in other fields, such as philosophy, material culture studies, anthropology and (technical) art history. Historians' turn towards the study of things stems partly from frustrations with history of science as intellectual history, based on ideas and texts (Hannan and Longair 2017: 15–42). By contrast, as Thatcher Ulrich et al. (2015) and Guerrini (2016b) have argued, a historiography of objects invokes a history of sensory involvement, a global history of movement across time, place and culture, and it is tied to a growing interest in social and cultural history more widely. It must be noted, however, that historians do not tend to focus on objects or artefacts and their physical qualities as such, but are instead interested in material culture: the myriad and changing contexts through which objects acquire, maintain and lose meaning (Harvey 2009: 3). Many now realize that objects can give us access to otherwise undetectable lives, such as those of the socially disadvantaged. Whereas text-based sources, which were created by a minority of people (usually elite and male), provide limited access to the everyday life of the many, material culture potentially gives us insight into such lives, for example by allowing us to trace and understand craft, domestic and trade practices that remained unrecorded in written sources (Thatcher Ulrich et al. 2015: 3–4).

However engaging and clarifying studies of the material culture of medicine can be, the benefits of the material turn need to be seen in perspective. First, although the material culture of Enlightenment medicine remaining today is rich and diverse, we have to keep in mind that when it comes to the material past, disappearance is the norm and preservation the exception, and these uneven survival rates can give a false picture of the past (Adamson 2009). Like any other kind of historical source, the objects that survive to this day represent only a fraction of the world of which they were once a part. Collectors, whether institutional or private, tend to favour certain objects over others – the exceptional, the perfectly preserved or cleaned and restored tend to be favoured, as do objects connected to the practices of learned white men, although this is slowly changing. To a researcher, an everyday, damaged, dirty object created by an illiterate woman of colour can tell a story that is at least as rich as, if not richer than, that of its exceptionally made, perfectly intact, cleaned and restored counterpart made by a university-educated white man. Unfortunately, the former will often have been lost altogether, while the latter is on display in a museum – an imbalance we should keep in mind.

Moreover, although we like to think that most of the things we still have are a collection of carefully curated and deliberately preserved objects, the reality is that they are often the remains of good or bad luck, individual preferences, serendipity and coincidence, rather than any intentional demarcation processes. This somewhat haphazard character of historical materiality should not prevent us from studying objects or from using them as the starting point for our research, but it is good to be aware of it, and to ask ourselves how we can use what remains to learn more about everything that has been lost, and why. We acknowledge that sometimes missing, destroyed or otherwise absent objects may be critically important for a nuanced understanding of the past.

Secondly, if there is anything that the past decades have taught us, it is that when studying the circulation of knowledge, not a single one of the core components – human actors, texts, material objects, networks, and immaterial objects or ideas – can be understood without the others. The material turn in the history of science has given us invaluable new insights into the importance of objects and sensory perception in the making and circulation of knowledge. However, to paraphrase Steven Shapin (2010), the historical study of science and medicine, and by proxy that of its objects, will never be 'pure'; it will always be a study of objects as collected or produced by people with bodies, situated in time, space, culture and society, and struggling for credibility and authority. Therefore it is important that when we study the material culture of medicine, we try to understand its changing relation to human actors over time. As Ludmilla Jordanova (2012: 157) points out, creators of objects – and the creators' nearest and dearest – are generally the first audiences for things, and understanding these audiences is integral to analysing artefacts.

These considerations have resulted in excellent historical studies that do not focus exclusively on objects and materials but pay attention to the role of people, ideas, texts and practices in early modern epistemic networks too. Many historians of science now successfully apply this integral approach and now have a fairly nuanced view about the agency of objects, reminiscent of Hacking's methods in *Historical Ontology* (2002: 17). Hacking did not, like Latour, advocate a parliament of things or strive to minimize the difference between the human and the non-human. Instead, he sees nature and objects as having limited agency, despite their role in the development of beliefs.

Bearing this in mind, I have chosen an object-driven rather than an object-centred approach (Prown 1982; Herman 1992: 3–14) for this chapter; I start from bones and objects (formerly) containing bones, but remain fully aware of the fact that they are little more than the lone coincidental survivors of historical demarcation processes. My aim is to gain a better understanding not only of this remaining material culture and its changes over time but also the many ways that bones were used and understood in Enlightenment medicine. Thus, human bones and objects, texts, and images related to human bones from this period are my starting point, but the bones themselves are far from my only source. For example, a rich collection of catalogues of anatomical collections from the long eighteenth century combined with documents created by anatomy professors and medical men provide insight into how the idea of anatomical collections changed in the eighteenth century. Moreover, I rely on a variety of written and visual sources, such as letters, diaries, drawings, prints and printed books, to explain the changing uses and understandings of human bones in Enlightenment medicine.

The main focus here is on bones and bone-related objects and sources created primarily in institutional, educational settings in seventeenth- and eighteenth-century Europe. There is simply too much to be said about human bone in other, related contexts, such as popular and non-European Enlightenment medicine, and contemporary supernatural beliefs and religion, to delve into here. For all the aforementioned reasons, this is by no means a full account, but analysis of these sources will show that bones were alternately destroyed, preserved, used and presented in a variety of ways in Enlightenment medicine, and that they were the subject of ongoing contention.

BONES DESTROYED

The apothecary jar shown in Figure 5.1 is part of the collections of the Apothecary Museum in Kraków, Poland (Bela 2013). Its exact provenance is not known, although the materiality of the jar itself can be studied for clues. It is made of white opaque glass, which was first produced in Venice in the sixteenth century. However, the jar's style – on a foot and heavily decorated –

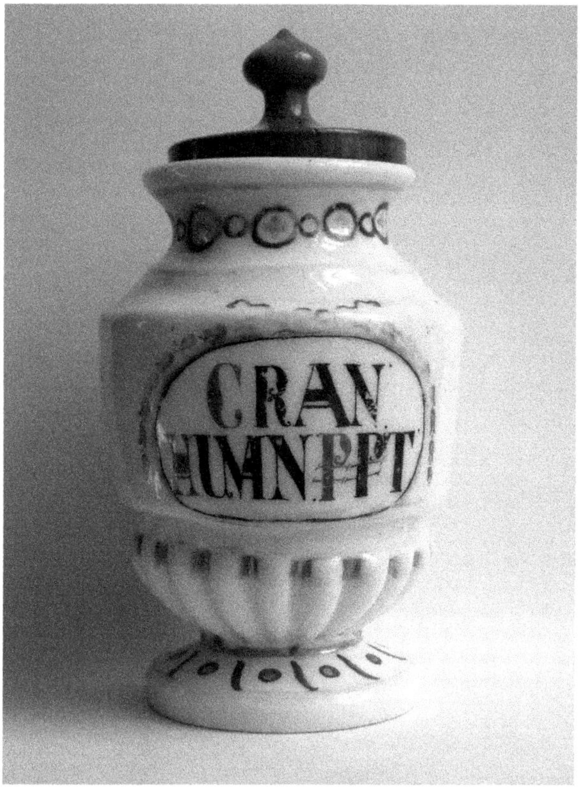

FIGURE 5.1: Opaque glass apothecary jar for preparation of the human skull. Credit: The Museum of Pharmacy at Jagiellonian University Medical College, Kraków, Poland.

was particularly popular in France in the seventeenth and eighteenth centuries (Drey 1978: 82–101). Part of a series of around fifty jars, it could also have been produced in north-eastern Europe or the Baltic region, home to a considerable glass industry in this period (Roosma 1969; Seela 1974). The wooden lid might be a later addition. Apothecary jars such as this one were widely used in apothecary shops throughout Europe to store *materia medica* or simples (the basic ingredients for drugs) in the eighteenth century. What is most interesting in this case is the ingredient this jar was supposed to contain: CRAN. HUMN. PPT is an abbreviation of *cranium humanium preparatorio*, preparation of human skull.

Among the many fascinating ways in which human bones were used in Enlightenment medicine, this one all but disappeared in the course of the eighteenth century. As recent research by Louise Noble (2011) and Richard Sugg (2015) has shown, 'corpse medicine', or the use of dead human bodies in

10. The finger of a mummy w. some of the leaves the body was wrap'd in. Un doigt d'une ancienne momie d'Egypte. Biron p. 277.

11. Hair an out of the ovarium?

12. Lapis o vesicula fellis humana — 0.2.6.

13. The monstrous head of a child.

14. The skeleton of a man made by Mr. Verier of the body of a Highwayman executed at Tiburn & bought by me — 3.4.6.

15. The skeleton of a youth made at Paris by Dr. Adair.

16. The arteries of the arm of a man injected with red wax given me by Mr. Bussiere.

17. The skull of an Irishman brought from Ireland for medicall use.

18. The skull of an Indian taken from one of the caves in Jamaica where they used to be interred.

19. A Jaw bone of the under side par of the same?

FIGURE 5.2: Page from Hans Sloane's catalogue of fossils, 'Fossils', Vol. 1, 'Coralls, Sponges, Crustaceae, Humana'. Entry 17 is a fragment of human skull intended for medicinal purposes. Other entries include various bone preservations. Credit: The Natural History Museum, London.

pharmaceutical preparations, was still fairly common by the late seventeenth century, though it had largely disappeared a century later. Early eighteenth-century apothecary handbooks still list ingredients like human blood, fat, mummified flesh, bones and skull as pharmaceutical ingredients. In the 1721 *Dispensatory of the Royal College of Physicians* of England by John Quincy (1721: 86), a recipe for a powder against epilepsy containing human skull is proudly described as 'a modern composition'. One of the reformers of the 1720 *London Pharmacopoeia*, the basis for this *Dispensatory*, was none other than Sir Hans Sloane. He kept a sample of pulv. Gutta., which is on display in the Enlightenment Gallery at the British Museum to this day.

Similarly, early eighteenth-century pharmaceutical handbooks published in mainland Europe, such as the Frankfurt *Dispensatorium* (Triller 1764: 538), also contain recipes calling for pulverised human skull. Cures calling for human bone are examples of sympathetic medicine: the historical medical practices in which a cure is 'sympathetically' related to the condition it treats. The cure relates to, involves, depends on, acts on or is effected by 'sympathy', a real or supposed affinity, correspondence or occult influence. The relationship between cure and disease in sympathetic medicine can take many different forms, and we can roughly distinguish between material and immaterial sympathetic medicine. The latter includes practices like pronouncing spells and incantations, while the former relies on a material relation between cure and disease. We can distinguish three different kinds of material sympathetic medicine (Hendriksen 2015b). The first type relates to similarity of colour, shape or substance, e.g. red materials such as rubies and iron oxides were thought to strengthen or cleanse the blood. The second type uses the cause as the cure. The third type is the 'pars pro toto treatment', in which bodily material of the patient (like excrement) or the object or substance that caused the ailment was treated, rather than the patient.

In the case of the use of human bones as ingredients for drugs, the underlying assumption was that the similarity of these materials to the affected human body or body part meant that the powers with which the material was imbued would permeate the diseased body or body part, thus healing it. That is why many such recipes called for bone and other body material from healthy young men who had died a violent death. The violent death was not the point; what mattered was that the source material remained healthy, containing the vital powers of the involuntary donor. It should not be spoiled by disease or accident (Sugg 2015: 184–8).

The word 'vital' in this context is to be understood more generally as the idea that matter within or outside a vegetable or animal body can have active, living properties that may influence the vital powers and thus the functioning of other vegetable and animal bodies. Although 'vitalism' is usually associated with the presence of a sensitive and inorganic soul and Romanticism, this is a narrow and somewhat anachronistic understanding of the term. Chang (2011) stresses the undeniable role vitalism played in alchemy, and in the work of 'mechanistic' philosophers and physicians. Ascribing active properties to matter after all suggests a certain vitalism: an understanding of life as generated and sustained through some form of non-mechanical force or power specific to and located in matter. However, by the end of the eighteenth century, these ingredients had all but disappeared from pharmaceutical handbooks.

It is too simplistic to argue that sympathetic medicine disappeared in the course of the eighteenth century because of the pervasiveness of the Baconian method or the rise of Enlightenment ideals of progress and methodological reductionism. As work by Israel (2006) and Vermij (2014) has shown, the period we now describe as the Enlightenment saw such a complex and continuously changing set of ideas and developments that the disappearance of particular phenomena cannot be explained simply by referring to 'the Enlightenment'. The fall of previously widely accepted ideas and practices is often caused by an interplay of many factors. There is not one straightforward explanation for these profound changes in the understanding of *materia medica*, such as the rise of chemistry as an academic discipline or even a chymical revolution; rather it was a complex interplay of epistemic, scientific and socio-economic factors that caused them (Hendriksen 2018a).

BONES PRESERVED

Whereas the use of bones as an ingredient for pharmaceutics almost disappeared in the eighteenth century, in another realm of medicine it changed profoundly, while in a sense it also remained remarkably stable. From the sixteenth century onwards, the practical study of anatomy was increasingly integrated in the academic study of medicine (Cunningham 2010: 8–16). This meant that professors of medicine gave lectures on human anatomy while a body was dissected by an assistant, a prosector, to illustrate their arguments. In the centuries that followed, it became increasingly common for the anatomy professor to dissect a body himself while lecturing, and for students to try and obtain bodies so they could dissect too. Moreover, medical men both within and outside the walls of the university attempted to preserve interesting specimens for their private and institutional collections, initially with limited success. Although human bones or a skeleton might seem fairly straightforward objects at first sight, they are almost always in a sense preparations, not some kind of *objets trouvées* (Santing 2008: 59). The obvious exception to this would be bones robbed from old graves, yet as these also needed to be cleaned and selected there appears to be a manufacturing and commodification aspect adhering even to these bones. Excavated bones were not very popular with anatomists, as they were frequently too badly damaged to be of any use. However, scarcity meant that anatomists often could not be too picky (Rosner 2010).

Bone constitutes a particularly interesting ontological problem here, as it initially appears to be just that: bare bone. Yet in the process of collecting, preparing, using, preserving and displaying bone, its materiality changes; it becomes an artefact and is invested with new meanings. As Hallam (2010) has pointed out, bones are relational entities, which emerge and take shape through the interactions that take place with them. Although the preservation of human bones, skulls and entire skeletons for the study of anatomy can be traced back at least to the Greek physician Galen (AD 129 – c. 216), the eighteenth century saw profound changes in both how and why bone material was preserved (Guerrini 2003; Hendriksen 2015a: 178–9).

As for the how, the very first bone preparations were either taken from graves or made using techniques that were based on natural processes of decay. Wet maceration, for example, was the cleaning of a skeleton of the last bits of soft tissue by lowering it into running water in a pierced case, or letting it decompose in water that is frequently refreshed. Andreas Vesalius (1514–1564), in his 1543 anatomical atlas, already recommended the repeated washing of a cadaver with slaked lime and water. Other tested methods of cleaning bones for preservation involved the removal of soft tissue with maggots and the boiling of bodies and body parts (Sturm 2007).

One of the first books to contain detailed instructions on how to clean and preserve human bones and entire skeletons that was also translated into the vernacular was written by Michael Lyser (or Leyser, 1624–1660). His hugely successful *Culter anatomicus* (The Anatomist's Knife) was first published in Latin in 1653, but saw numerous reprints as well as translations into German and English until 1740. As wet preservation methods were virtually non-existent in the mid-seventeenth century, the largest part of the book is devoted to the meticulous dissection of the human body. Only the fifth and final part (Lyser 1740: 225–76) focuses on 'the Method of making a Skeleton' and takes the reader through the steps of cleaning, separating and articulating (putting back together) the bones. Even though the skills of making a skeleton were quite possibly more often learned by doing and through one-on-one instruction than through using manuals (like Lyser's book), I will discuss this part of the book in detail, as its many reprints suggest a popularity among medical men and their students well into the eighteenth century. Moreover, it hints at the grimy details and hands-on nature of the process.

Lyser (1740: 227) advocates the use of a healthy, fully grown adult body, as he felt that the proportions of a child's skeleton were too different from those of an adult, and thus unsuitable for the study of anatomy. Moreover, he thought that young bones were softer and spoiled more easily than older bones. After a suitable specimen is selected, the bones have to be cleaned in five steps: first, the body needs to be divided into smaller sections to make it fit into a cauldron, then the marrow and medullary oil have to be extracted using pins, perforators and iron wire. Lyser (1740: 236) warns the reader not to throw away the marrow and medullary oil but 'to carefully put [it] up in a Glass, and set [it] in a warm Place to melt, till the Dregs subfide, and the clear Part afterward to be poured off'. For its 'many uses' he refers to 'Hilandus', by whom he probably means the German surgeon Wilhelm Fabry of Hilden (also known as Guilelmus Fabricius Hildanus, 1560–1634), who recommended the use of human medullary oil to treat burns (Jones 1960). This shows how the various parts of skeletons circulated between the realms of medicine – in this case, the production of *materia medica* was a direct result of anatomical dissection and preservation.

When the useful marrow and oil have been removed, Lyser continues, the bones have to be steeped in water for three or four days to remove blood and flesh. It is important that the water is refreshed once or twice a day, and the process works better in summer than in winter; if at all possible, the cauldron should be kept in a warm place. This would cause an interesting paradox for the anatomist, as public dissections were preferably held in winter to minimize the stink of the decomposing body. Moreover, boiling is not a good idea at this stage, as it will cause yellow discolouration. Lyser (1740: 227) credits his teacher Simon Paulli (1603–1680) with the invention of 'a Method of making the Bones as white as the finest Ivory'.

The whiteness of preserved human bones was very important to seventeenth- and eighteenth-century anatomists, as also suggested by other sources. For example, the Amsterdam anatomist Frederik Ruysch (1638–1731) (1744: 722) repeatedly mentioned whiteness as a desirable characteristic of bone preparations (as in his description of the preparation of a 'very white skeleton of a mole'), while the Scottish anatomist William Hunter (1718–1783) thought that boiling bones would give them a brownish tinge (Guerrini 2012b). Although bones are not at all white in situ, white is traditionally associated with purity, cleanliness and death (Gage 1993: 117–18, Zuffi 2012: 224–33). Moreover, as the whiteness was achieved by thorough removal of the medullary oil, it is likely that white bone kept longer and better than the yellowish variety.

According to Lyser, the bones need to be boiled to remove remaining flesh and ligaments, but not cartilaginous parts like the sternum, as these will discolour and dissolve. The author also warns that the bones of the hands and feet should be wrapped and tied in a piece of linen, as the cartilage will dissolve and the anatomist would thus end up with an almost impossible puzzle to reconstruct. Throughout the boiling process, the fat should be skimmed from the water, and when all the remaining flesh has become white, the bones are ready for their final cleaning. The appropriate cooking time depends on the age of the bones; Lyser (1740: 240) refers to the knowledge of common cooks, 'because they daily find that old Meat takes a longer Time in boiling than young'. As Guerrini (2016a) has shown, the drawing of parallels between the kitchen and the dissection room was fairly common in the early modern period.

The appeal to craft and even general knowledge is repeated in the final stage of cleaning the bones, when Lyser (1740: 234) writes:

> We now come to the cleaning of the Bones, upon which it would be trifling to spend many Words, Since this Exercise discharges the Office of a Preceptor, and everyone that can cut his Victuals, knows how to take the Flesh off from a Bone; wherefore I will say no more upon this Subject.

However simple Lyser deemed some of the skills involved, only a small number of seventeenth-century anatomists appears to have mastered the skill of preparing and preserving human skeletons. Moreover, although cleaned, dried and reassembled full adult skeletons would remain a popular mnemonic, the eighteenth century saw a number of new subdisciplines in medicine and anatomy that called for new ways of preserving human bones.

In the first half of the eighteenth century, for example, anatomists developed an interest in preserving the human skeleton in its various stages of development. Whereas infant and children's skeletons in Lyser's time were deemed imperfect, or perhaps no more than quirky decorative items, they became a valued part of anatomical collections during the eighteenth century. For example, Leiden anatomists interested in osteogenesis – the generation of bones – developed preparation techniques that made bones transparent, so as to clearly show the tendons and the structure of the bone. The interest in osteogenesis can be tied to shifts in the understanding of physiology in the eighteenth century, which changed the meanings of preserved bones.

In the course of the eighteenth century, the classical idea that disease was an imbalance in the humours that had to be corrected was more frequently dismissed in favour of the idea that disease was something that could just affect a particular organ or body part, and that could be treated by therapies that were aimed only at the affected part rather than the entire body (Hendriksen 2015a: 191–8). Given the more localized understanding of disease, pathology took on a new importance. Anatomists no longer focused on collecting bones that told a moral tale or that could serve as an illustration in anatomy lessons. Instead, they started to systematically collect bones affected by a particular disease or deformity, both human and animal. Moreover, anatomists became increasingly interested in the similarities and differences between people from different regions of the world, which led them to start ethnographic collections of human skulls and bone material (Hendriksen 2015a: 198–204).

These developments show, for example, in Thomas Pole's 1790 *The Anatomical Instructor*, a manual that provided methods for preparing and preserving different parts not only of the human body but also of quadrupeds more generally. Pole ranked his articles on the preparation of human bones and skeletons under a section on maceration techniques: in four sections, covering

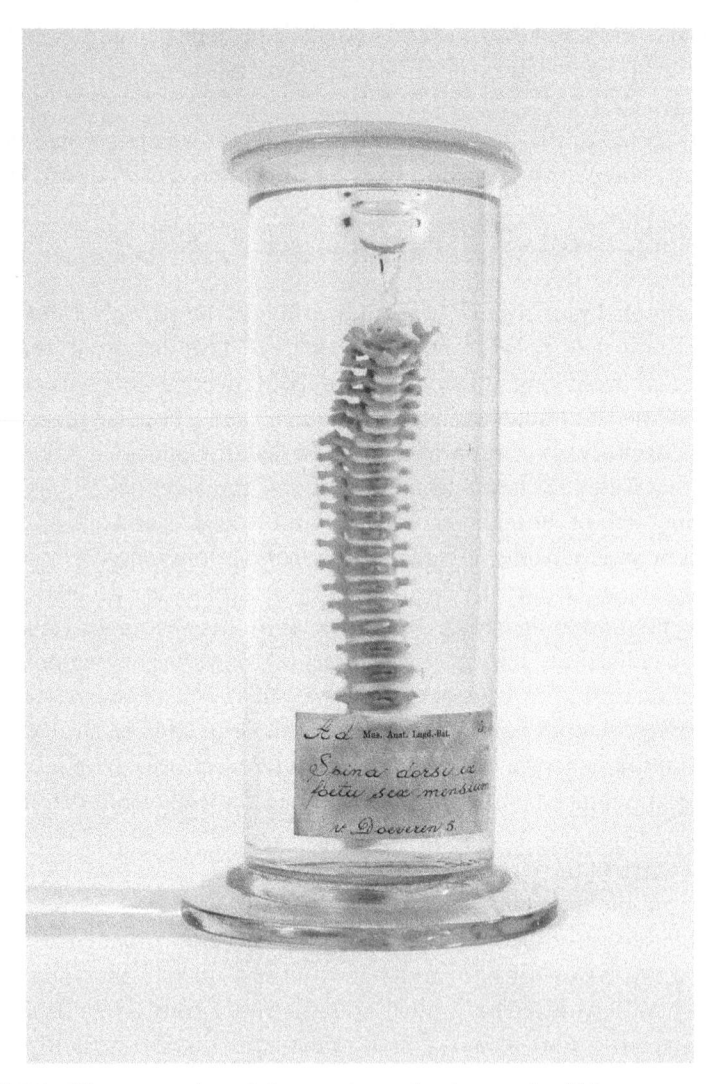

FIGURE 5.3: Wet preparation of the vertebrae of a six-month-old foetus, preserved to show the growth of the spine. Credit: Arno Massee/LUMC Anatomical Museum, 2012.

nine pages in total (Pole 1790: 148–57), he subsequently discussed the cleaning and preparing of bones in general, the making of the 'natural human skeleton', the cleaning and separating of the bones of the human head, and the cleaning and preparing of diseased bones. Another five pages (Pole 1790: 158–62) were devoted to the preparation of all other animal skeletons, including quadrupeds, fish and birds.

When we read Pole's text, it becomes at once apparent that human medullary oil and bone marrow were no longer sought-after commodities: without further ado, he tells the reader to remove as much of the fleshy parts as possible, and only to cut up the body as much as is necessary to put it in the maceration vessel. The body has to be submerged in clean water that has to be changed each day for at least a week, until no more blood discolours it. Then it should be left to macerate until all the flesh and ligaments are destroyed, which according Pole can take three up to six months, depending on the weather. At some unspecified moment during this period, holes the size of a swan's quill have to be bored in the larger bones, so the water can wash out 'the medullary substance' – but there is no mention of preserving it.

Once more, the whiteness of the bones is mentioned as an important aspect; it is the reason Pole (1790: 150) recommends that the bones be submerged in water throughout the maceration process, and the maceration vessels kept covered, especially in cities such as London, where the soot and other impurities in the air would otherwise pollute the water. When the soft parts are sufficiently macerated, they should be scraped off and the bones washed in clean water once more. Afterwards, the bones should be kept in a solution of water and lime or pearlash – a strong alkaline solution – for a week. Finally, the bones had to be rinsed with clean water once more, and then dried. Drying, however, should not be done in the sun or in front of a fire, as this would cause the remaining medullary oil to give them a 'disagreeable oily transparency' that 'spoils them of their Beauty'. Other ways to prevent this included boiling the bones in a pearlash solution to destroy the medullary oil, or bleaching them in pure air (especially on the sea shore, where they could be washed in salt water on a daily basis).

A new distinction made by Pole (1790: 151–7) was that between the natural and the artificial skeleton: the first was prepared in its own ligaments, whereas the latter was reassembled using materials such as hooks and wires. The method of making a natural skeleton was primarily suited to very young subjects, and was fairly impractical because the ligaments would become inflexible when dried, making the skeleton rigid. A separate section was devoted to preparing the bones of the human head, which Pole believed was particularly difficult to do well. As with the rest of the skeleton, the preparation process started with maceration and manual cleaning. When the skull was ready for drying, Pole advised filling it with dried peas and shaking it well, so the peas would absorb any remaining moisture. The resulting swelling would cause an even pressure on the inside of the skull, thus gently separating the main bones of the cranium. The head of a person of about twenty was recommended as a subject, as their skull would be whiter and their teeth generally better than those of elderly people, thus 'making a great ornament to the entire preparation'. Finally, diseased bones should be cleaned and prepared in much the same manner as normal bones, but extra care should be taken when handling them, as they could be shaped oddly and might crumble easily. When they were sufficiently prepared, they should be stored in glass containers to protect them from rough handling and dust.

Overall, Pole's work is more detailed than Lyser's, and the complete disappearance of the preservation of medullary oil is striking. Although there are some significant differences between the methods and goals described by Lyser and Pole, we can identify a number of commonalities and ongoing concerns, such as the visceral, hands-on nature of the entire process, which contrasts sharply with the desired clean, white, orderly results. These and other sources thus show that commodification of the human body, as either preparations or *materia medica*, as well as the discerning and preserving of order and even beauty in the repulsive and seemingly messy insides of cadavers, were important aspects in the self-fashioning of early modern anatomists (Hendriksen 2014, 2015a: 15–20). Moreover, the similarity to processes in the kitchen – the cutting, carving, boiling and drying – remains significant, and the influence of climate and surroundings is a concern in the late eighteenth century as much as it was almost a hundred and fifty years earlier. These aspects continued to link the anatomist's activities to those of other skilled practitioners such as cooks, and exemplified his dependence on and interaction with the material world around him.

Notwithstanding the frequent reprints of these books, which, as mentioned before, suggest a certain popularity, the question remains exactly how these texts were used in practice. Anatomists and their assistants working at universities most likely transmitted skills and knowledge about the preservation of bone material through one-on-one instruction, but given the multiple editions of both books, it is not unlikely that texts such as Lyser's and Pole's were used as mnemonics and handbooks by amateurs or less-skilled professionals, especially if they were far removed from those with specialist knowledge on the topic. Unlike some of the prestigious anatomical atlases of the time, which were printed on large folio pages, these books are pocket-sized octavos, confirming that they were made to be carried around and used rather than as status objects for book collectors. It is possible that they were also used by amateur natural philosophers, travellers and explorers in the field. For example, Jacob van der Steege (1746–1811), a physician of the VOC (Verenigde Oostindische Compagnie, the Dutch United East India Company), directing member of the Batavian Society and former student of the Groningen anatomist Petrus Camper (1722–1789), sent his old teacher a human skeleton, four human skulls, plus a tongue and a penis of a Javanese rhinoceros from Batavia in 1766 (Tulbagh, letter to Arnout Vosmaer, 1766). It is unclear whether van der Steege used Lyser's book or another, similar text, but Camper (1791) used the skeletons and skulls he was sent from abroad to develop his theories about local variations in human anatomy. Such donations show that preserved bones were also a commodity, used to maintain relationships with colleagues and acquaintances back home.

BONES DISPLAYED

The main aim of the sometimes unpleasant effort of preserving human bones was to study and display them, and presenting them as beautifully as possible was also a means to draw and retain the attention of the audience (Hendriksen 2015a: 20–2). The modes of displaying preserved bones give us insight into the changing ideals in anatomical study in the Enlightenment. In early modern Europe, there was a strong reciprocity between art and iconography on the one hand, and human anatomy in general and bones in particular on the other (Wallace and Kemp 2000; Hallam and Hockey 2001). Human bones, skulls and skeletons had served as symbols of *vanitas* – mortality and the futility and brevity of earthly existence – in funerary art since the Middle Ages, and this continued in early modern painting, especially in still lifes. The craftsmen making ivory memento mori (Buckley 2014), wax effigies (Messbarger 2010; Maerker 2011) and *vanitas* prints (Knoeff 2007) were often also the makers of anatomical ivory manikins, anatomical wax models and prints for anatomical atlases. The *vanitas* motives were echoed in public and private anatomical collections, which greatly increased in number from the seventeenth century onwards, not least because of the enhanced preparation and preservation methods discussed in the previous paragraph.

Although *vanitas* themes largely disappeared from both visual art and anatomical collections in the eighteenth century, at the beginning of the century human skulls and bones continued to be useful in explaining the world at large and telling moral narratives. Probably one of the most famous examples is the decoration of the Leiden anatomical theatre in the seventeenth and eighteenth centuries with a male and a female human skeleton adorned with an apple and a snake, representing original sin (Huisman 2009: 17, 48–54). Such biblical and moral references were widespread and widely used and understood, as also shows from the male and female skeletons carrying scythes created by Ercole Lelli in Bologna in the 1740s for the papal anatomy museum (Messbarger 2010: 40–6).

One researcher who has extensively studied and vividly described such practices is Rina Knoeff. She gives the example of the previously mentioned anatomist Ruysch, who had obtained the skull of a prostitute, Anna van Hoorne, which was visibly affected by venereal disease. Ruysch frequently took the skull out of its display case to explain to visitors the dangers of loose sexual morals, and would hold the skull near a candle to show that the corrosions of the disease had made it almost translucent in places. However, at some point the skull must have accidently broken as a result of being handled so frequently, because years later, Ruysch listed van Hoorne's skull, or rather the remains of it, again. However, by then only fragments of it remained, lying on the bottom of a phial, where they were 'trampled' by the foot of an innocent child. As

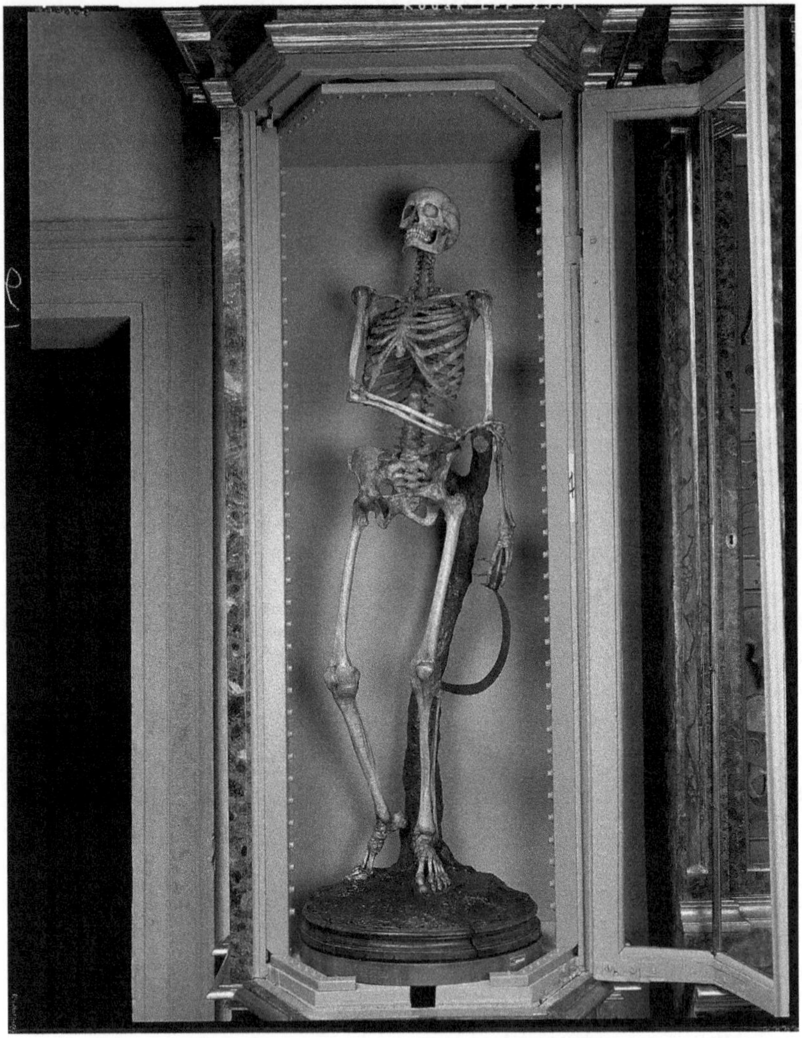

FIGURE 5.4: Ercole Lelli, female skeleton. Credit: Alma Mater Studiorum Università di Bologna – Sistema Museala di Ateneo – Museo di Palazzo Poggi. (Copyright: Università di Bologna/Fulvia Simoni).

Knoeff (2015) points out, this composition meant it was no longer possible to use the skull to explain the medical consequences of venereal disease, but the moral message remained and was even reinforced by the new composition.

In the second half of the eighteenth century, such use of anatomical preparations to teach moral lessons became increasingly rare. Instead, anatomical preparations became objects primarily used to study physiology, pathology and human variety. However, creating them remained a proof of skill for anatomists. Preparation served not only to illustrate certain medical ideas but also to demonstrate manual dexterity and elegance (Hendriksen 2015a: 210). These changing aims of preparations are reflected in the openness with which such collections were displayed. The Leiden anatomical collections, for example, had long been a great tourist attraction, but they became increasingly harder to access as the eighteenth century progressed. Initially, tourists would pay the custodian of the theatre, or his children, for a tour of the preparations and to hear the stories associated with the objects. However, around 1770, the refined preparations made by the admired professor Bernard Siegfried Albinus (1697–1770) were put in a separate room which could only be accessed under the supervision of the new professor of anatomy (Hendriksen 2017). Dániel Margócsy (2011) has convincingly argued that a successful preparation could long remain a valuable commodity. Yet at the other end of the spectrum, once-admired preparations were sometimes reused and cut up for new research (Hendriksen et al. 2013). Finally, around 1800, the old Leiden anatomical theatre was closed to the public and the collections moved to a purpose-built location consisting of research and teaching laboratories. The new building was further removed from the city centre, and access for the general public was limited (Huistra 2019: 57, 125).

HIDDEN BONES

Skeletons carrying scythes made by Ercole Lelli (for example, Figure 5.4) were part of a series of bone and wax models depicting the various tissue layers of the human body, and at the other end of the series were a wax Adam and Eve in which real human skeletons were used as a frame. Because of the serial nature of these wax works, there is little doubt that the full body models too contain human bones. Yet in some objects it is less clear that bones lie hidden beneath other materials.

An excellent example of human bones being used as the foundational structure for a medical model was recently discovered in the collection of the Leiden museum for the history of science, Rijksmuseum Boerhaave (van Calmthout 2016). Although it is not entirely certain whether this object is from the late eighteenth or early nineteenth century, it is too fascinating and relevant not to discuss it here. It is a so-called birthing phantom, which was a model used to help medical students practice difficult births; such models were a kind of doll in the shape of a woman's pelvis and abdomen with a baby doll and fabric placenta inside. Although using deceased pregnant women and their babies for such training was also common throughout the eighteenth century, the aspect of decay obviously made this an unpleasant and ad hoc activity (Schillace 2013). The birthing phantom, by contrast, could be used any time and lasted much longer.

The most well-known examples of early birthing models were probably those of Angélique Marguerite du Coudray (1712–1794), King Louis XV of

France's midwife. The only known remaining example of her work at the Musée Flaubert d'Histoire de la Médecine in Rouen, described by Carlyle (2018), contains a woman's pelvic bones and real vertebrae in the infant doll. The Parisian obstetrician Grégoire and one of his students, the Scottish surgeon-apothecary William Smellie (1697–1763), also used birthing models in their teaching (Owen 2016: 75–8, 95–101). Smellie (1876: 250–1) described Grégoire's 'simulator', which he witnessed around 1740, as follows: 'his machine was no other than a piece of basketwork, containing a real pelvis covered with black leather, upon which he could not clearly explain the difficulties that occur in turning children, proceeding from the contractions of the uterus, os internum, and os externum'.

Upon his return, therefore, Smellie started creating birthing machines himself, which also contained real human bones and mechanisms to make the simulated process more realistic (Owen 2016: 99). Although these sources show that the use of real human bones in birthing models was not unknown in the eighteenth century, very few models remain; with those that do, it is often hard to tell what is inside. When Rijksmuseum Boerhaave curators studied their particular phantom more closely, they saw material resembling bone sticking through the fabric. A CT scan at the Leiden University Medical Centre revealed that the phantom contained a human pelvis and a full baby skeleton.

It remains unclear how frequently and until when human bones were used in the creation of models such as this phantom. But in an 1804 article, the Leiden city obstetrician Gotllieb Salomon (1774–1864) still advocated it, saying that

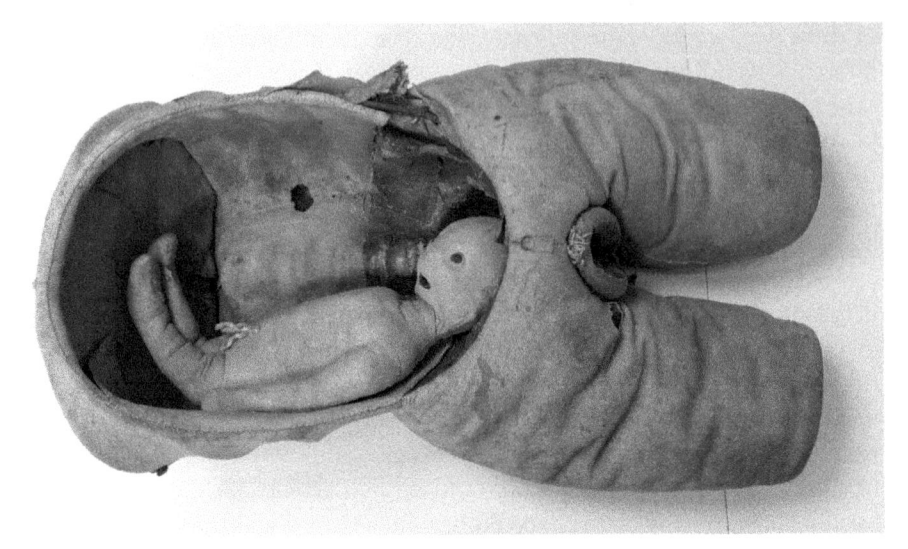

FIGURE 5.5: The birthing phantom at Rijksmuseum Boerhaave. Photographer: Tom Haartsen. Credit: The Rijksmuseum Boerhaave, Leiden.

he had first created such a phantom when he had to teach practical obstetrics to some students at the University of Danzig.

The case of the Leiden obstetric model suggests that the use of hidden human bones in medical models continued at least for some time into the nineteenth century, especially as they were also used in other models in this period. The French brothers Jules Pierre (1807–1837) and Jean Baptiste Édouard (1810–1868) Verreaux created taxidermy specimens of exotic animals for their father's Parisian shop selling natural historical objects, Maison Verreaux. They used human bones for models on at least two occasions, one of which was until recently believed to be a mannequin containing only human teeth. One specimen was known as 'el negro' or 'the negro of Banyoles' (Westerman 2004). The remains of a young African San man were stuffed by the Verreaux brothers in the 1830s, and remained on display in the local Darder Museum in Banyoles, Spain, until 1997. The remains were sent to Botswana in 2000 for burial. More recently, in 2016, a human skull was discovered in a mannequin that was part of an ensemble made by the Verreaux brothers (Gilligand 2017). Formerly known as 'Arab Courier Attacked by Lions', it was restored and returned to display at the Carnegie Museum of Natural History in Pittsburgh under the title 'Lion Attacking a Dromedary'.

These hidden human bones imply that the makers of these objects thought that the real thing would make for more convincing, if not more elegant, phantoms and models. After all, it would have been significantly easier to mount them around artificial skeletal structures, as happened in contemporary taxidermy (Hendriksen 2019). Strikingly, what remains largely hidden in all objects and materials discussed here are the lives and voices of the people whose bones were used and made into materials and objects in Enlightenment medicine. This includes both the bones hidden in objects and those clearly visible. Well into the nineteenth century, the idea of donating one's body to medicine after death was mostly unheard of, primarily because of widespread religious beliefs that required the intact burial of human remains in consecrated ground to ensure redemption and eventual resurrection (Bennett 2017). The bodies that formed the source for the materials and objects in this chapter disproportionally belonged to people on the periphery of early modern European society: convicted criminals for whom dissection formed part of their punishment, the poor, prostitutes, enslaved people and the Indigenous inhabitants of European colonies (Richardson 2001).

Although their stories remain largely hidden, even if we study the objects that were made from their bodies, the materiality of their remains does provide them with a certain agency. After all, they allow us to gain a better understanding of the time in which they lived and died, and continue to spark academic and social debate, about topics such as the preservation and display of historical human remains in museums (Knoeff and Zwijnenberg 2015; Devlin 2018). And while these and other uses of human bone discussed in this chapter may now strike us as strange, unusual, and even cruel or unethical, these objects and practices have to be understood in the context of the time in which they occurred and were created. It is our duty as historians to study them and reflect on them, so that we gain a better understanding of how something that seems as stable and solid as human bone can have such a fluid history.

CONCLUSION AND EPILOGUE

Whether human bones were destroyed for pharmaceutical preparations, preserved, decorated and arranged in wet or dry preparations in anatomical collections to study morals, anatomy, physiology, pathology or the exotic other, or merely used as a framework on which to sculpt a model made from another material, the examples in this chapter reveal two key issues.

First, and most importantly, there is the astounding variety of uses for human bones in Enlightenment medicine. In the case of the use of bone in pharmaceutical preparations, we see how the absence and destruction of the material can be as essential for understanding its importance as instances in which it has been preserved. This case also shows the clear, but thus far largely unexplained, change and eventual disappearance of a particular understanding of human bone as a medical material over the course of a century. A complex interplay of social, scientific and practical factors was at work, but even two well-researched books (Noble 2011; Sugg 2015) have not been able to provide a definite answer, which shows how hard it can be to grasp the factors contributing to such changes in hindsight. Moreover, apothecary jars and apothecary handbooks are the only material reminder of this use of bone; the actual bone preparation has gone in most cases, as has the medullary oil Lyser advised his readers to preserve.

The books by Lyser and Pole represent bones textually and as actual objects in their descriptions of how to preserve them. They provide insight into the very hands-on processes and practical skill required to preserve human bone successfully, as well as the challenges faced by Enlightenment medical men (and others) when it came to preserving bone. As texts and collected bone preparations show, the medicinal understanding and uses of bones changed during the eighteenth century; bone disappeared as an ingredient for drugs, while new anatomical interests – such as osteology, pathology and physiognomy – emerged. Despite these shifts, there were also continuities in how bone was preserved and used to study anatomy. As actual objects, the translation of Lyser's work and the multiple editions of both books, as well as their relatively small size, tells us that these books were in demand and made for practical use, rather than kept as prestigious objects.

The changing methods of displaying preserved bones in the eighteenth century suggests new relationships between science, art and religion. The decreasing accessibility of university anatomical collections, however, highlights a rift that developed between the professional preservation of bones and popular anatomy exhibitions, which became more common in the course of the nineteenth century. Human bones could also be hidden in objects such as the birthing phantom and later the Verreaux brothers' preparations, which indicates that the uses and understandings of human bones continued to change after the Enlightenment too.

What connects all the objects discussed in this chapter is human bone, a naturally occurring material. The stories and voices of the people whose bones were used to make them mostly remain silent, but we can still gain a better understanding of what the time they lived in must have been like because of the remaining material culture. However, the remains of these subjects were commodified and made into objects. All of them, including the ones that consist only of human bones or a part thereof – Lyser's medullary oil, Pole's natural skeletons preserved in their own ligaments – are artefacts. They were made intentionally by human hands, to serve a practical, scientific or ideological purpose – often all three at the same time. The history of objects and material culture is simultaneously art history, history of science, social history, economic and political history, and very much the history of making.

However understandable in their historical context, the objects that remain have become bones of contention (Sysling 2010). International ethical standards, such as the *ICOM* [International Council of Museums] *Code of Ethics for Museums* (2013), state that historical human remains in museum collections that have been obtained without consent from the subject or his or her descendants should be returned to where they came from, so they can be buried. However, the provenance of these objects is often unclear, and the thorough cleaning and preservation processes they underwent means that modern techniques are of little use in establishing provenance. Finally, it is good to realize that even today, human bones remain a commodity (Noble 2011: 161–4), and because of that, their meanings will remain multiple and instable. The meanings and uses of materials and objects have always been contextual and fluid, and will continue to be so.

CHAPTER SIX

Experiences

MICHELINE LOUIS-COURVOISIER[1]

Translated by Sylvia Smith

In a four-page letter sent to Dr Tissot in 1776, Madame Fol expresses a deep suffering, which involves her whole self. In a few lines she mentions her anxiety, horrible dreams, fears of nearly everything. In the main part of her narrative, she describes meticulously the interweaving of her bodily sensations with her anguish: quivering in the brain, 'astonishment to the brain', teeth cracklings, stomach palpitations, dizziness, kidney sweats. Her ears whistle and ring, and she feels 'beatings' along her kidneys and neck and within her head. She describes a sense of heaven and earth being upside down, and of the earth lifting her, making her feel like she is in a rocky boat.

Her text is written in a lyric language, hardly punctuated, unstructured, in a very approximate orthography. Her writing is vivid and makes her symptoms nearly contagious. But what does she even mean by 'astonishment' to the brain, and did she differentiate between brain and head? Her narrative calls on the senses of the physician, as well as his expertise. Even if we can no longer translate the term 'astonishment to the brain' into a contemporary bodily sensation, her account reaches out to the modern reader with its expressiveness (see Figure 6.1). Like many other written consultations, this letter demonstrates that the mind/body dichotomy is not relevant when investigating the experience of suffering in the eighteenth century. It also highlights sufferers' self-awareness of internal and external perceptions, and a flexible language precisely chosen to communicate specific sensations.

The cultural context of the doctor–patient relationship in the Enlightenment was focused on the modus operandi of the senses (Vila 2014: 12–20). As

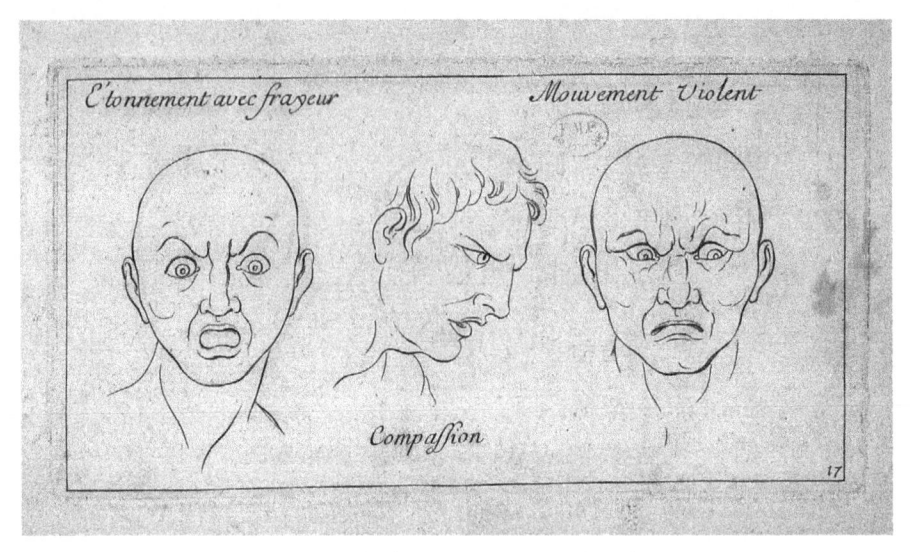

FIGURE 6.1: Astonishment with fright, compassion and violent movements. Movements could refer to the experience of internal passions and emotions as well as physical movement. From S. le Clerc, *Caractères des passions gravés sur les desseins de l'Illustre Mons. le Brun* (Paris: Chez N. Langlios, n. d. [eighteenth century]). Credit: BIU Santé, Paris.

Georges Vigarello notes, knowledge proceeds from senses before proceeding from thoughts (Vigarello 2014: 21). Any kind of disturbances *were part of* the experience of suffering in the eighteenth century and had to be transmitted to the doctor's senses. The internal and external sensations had to be communicated so that the physician could not only understand them but also *feel* them. That is why the context was also defined by a lyric language, at least in the parts of sufferers' narrative that described their symptoms. In these parts, patients used many comparisons and colourful images to activate the doctor's senses and experience. As we have seen with Mme Fol, the experience of suffering related most of the time to the flesh, mainly to movements that patients felt inside their body's fibres, humours and nerves.

At that time, three medical theories coexisted, theories which were well known even by laypeople. The first was the humoral theory that has been part of Western thought for centuries. In short, the four humours (the blood, the bile, the lymph and the black bile) were considered the principal components of the body. These humours were responsible for the organs' irrigation. To ensure good health, the humours had to be well distributed among them, their flow inside the body had to be unobstructed and a partial opening of the body's interior to the external environment had to be ensured, in particular by easy evacuations of all bodily fluids (Pilloud and Louis-Courvoisier 2003). The second was the animal spirits theory, which had been discussed not only by physicians but also by theologists and philosophers for centuries. Animal spirits were seen as tiny, invisible, subtle, and 'aerial' (made of air and very light) particles moving at high speed throughout the whole body. They were supposed to connect the body and the soul, conveying each internal and external sensation that was perceived, then transforming them into impressions in the brain/mind. Depending on the author, they were seen as circulating in the body through veins and arteries or through the nervous system. To ensure good health, they had to be very numerous, transparent, and to circulate quickly and together (Kleiman-Lafon and Louis-Courvoisier 2018; Smith et al. 2012; Sutton 1998). This theory fell into disuse at the beginning of the nineteenth century, but it was still common in French and English literature in the eighteenth century (Armand 2018; Bolens 2018). Third, the theory of nerves, widely debated during the eighteenth century, led to the distinction between irritability and sensibility (see Figure 6.2 for an anatomy of the nerves). Albrecht von Haller described the irritable fibre and the sensible fibre. The first acted on the muscles; the second transmitted the impressions to the brain. The key concept of sensibility was one, as Anne Vila notes, 'that bridged body, mind and milieu' (Vila 2015: 204). Sensibility could be a property related only to the nerves, or, as for the vitalist school, a vital principle that permitted a mind/body continuity. The sensible fibre was the place which connected together a sensory stimulus, an emotion, an idea. The sensible body was made up of innumerable nerve fibres, connected to each other, and traversed by micro-movements such as vibrations and oscillations (Wenger 2007: 39–49). To ensure good health, it was necessary to have a good distribution of vital energy through measured micro-movements. It is important to note here that these three theories were known and sometimes explicitly invoked by patients; depending on the symptoms they were suffering from, they could choose from among them which one(s) best suited their sensations and symptoms. There was a resonance between these theoretical medical models and the symptomatologic manifestation of the disease. This meant that the experience was quite easy to connect with the theory.

In this chapter, I will investigate the experience of illness and suffering in eighteenth-century French-speaking Europe, drawing on patients' written accounts. Writing letters was a common form of communication among the middling and upper classes. People used this means of communication to keep in touch with their friends, their relatives and their physician. For many authors, a blank page was not something to be dreaded but an invitation to record one's experience and to piece together fragments of one's daily life, either to share with others or to enhance self-awareness. Suffering was part of daily life and was recorded in detail – making personal narratives valuable material for historians today.

I will focus on the language that sufferers used. My analysis, based on a close and precise reading of these narratives, allows me to mark the historicity of the

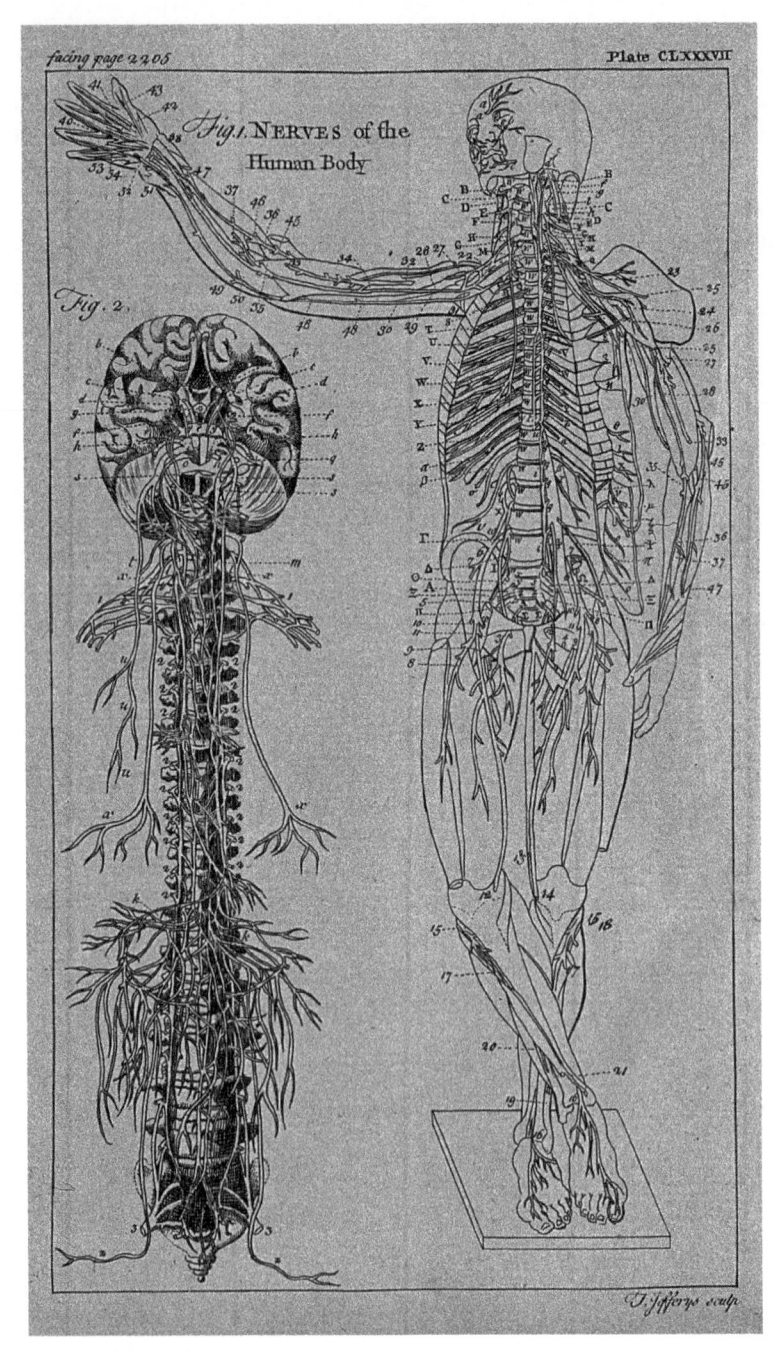

FIGURE 6.2: Two figures showing the brain, spine and nerves. Probably a plate for T. Jefferys, *A New and Complete Dictionary of Arts and Sciences: Comprehending All Branches of Useful Knowledge*, London: Printed for W. Owen, 1763–1764. Credit: Wellcome Collection, London/Public Domain.

body. Words are privileged data allowing us to get closer to past experiences. Yet a careful reading is important to investigate what those experiences really meant to the eighteenth-century writer. The difficulty for historians is to avoid an easy confusion with our own understandings, which could be quickly and unintentionally projected onto eighteenth-century patients' suffering. Some of these patients' descriptions seem to resonate with us today, but we should be careful to keep in mind the gap between our ways of perceiving ailments and explaining diseases, and those of eighteenth-century patients. Experiences are deeply shaped by the cultural context in which they take place.

We will see that the act of writing their narratives was an important one for the patients. It was not only a way to keep in touch with Dr Tissot but a moment in which to express a deep internal destabilization that they could no longer handle on their own. To get help, a sufferer needed to explore an experience in order to express it; the experience needed to be understood precisely. We will see, then, that the experience of suffering in the eighteenth century often affected patients' senses, particularly sight and hearing. But even the most common shared experiences of suffering were ultimately still qualified by the various tiny troubles of the flesh, manifested by numerous micro-movements and subtle changes in bodily consistency. Eighteenth-century people appeared to experience themselves as a fragile and disordered milieu that needed to be rebalanced and fortified.

READING BODILY EXPERIENCE

Using first-person narratives to study the experience of suffering in the eighteenth century is a challenge, and the first step must be to clarify exactly what is meant by the term 'experience'. Historian Séverine Pilloud has argued that experience of sickness is closely connected to narration and representation (Pilloud 2013: 4–6). I propose a different approach: an attempt to consider the relationship between the words on one hand, and the perceptions and sensations as they were experienced on the other hand. The *Oxford English Dictionary* defines experience as 'the fact of being consciously the subject of a state or condition, or of being consciously affected by an event. Also an instance of this; a state or condition viewed subjectively; an event by which one is affected.' Experience is therefore related to the idea of being conscious of oneself and of one's response to external events. In this chapter, I define the experience of suffering in the eighteenth century as the consciousness that sick people had of themselves, which they described through corporeal sensations; this entailed the physiopsychological condition of the whole subjectivity. The concept of aesthesis as proposed by historian Joanna Bourke is useful in thinking in *one-word* perceptions, feelings and emotions (Bourke 2003). Aesthesis also helps us to avoid the mind/body dichotomy when considering eighteenth-century experience.

Therefore, the notion of suffering should be used in the broadest sense and should be related to a disruption of the aesthesis as an individual experienced it. According to Bourke, drawing a distinction between pain and suffering can contribute to outlining the mind/body distinction (Bourke 2014: 21). Javier Moscoso links the history of pain to the history of experience, again without recognizing the mind/body dichotomy, and therefore uses 'pain' and 'suffering' indifferently (Moscoso 2012: 2). In this chapter, I intentionally choose the word 'suffering' to make sure that it covers the numerous sensations (and not only physical pains) and discomforts, of highly varying degrees, that eighteenth-century patients were aware of and that they described in detail to Dr Tissot.

A historical study of such self-consciousness requires the analysis of patients' written accounts of physical and psychological events that indicated changes in the physical and mental conditions they felt were significant enough to be recorded and relevant to be shared. Although one has access only to written fragments frozen in time, these fragments remain vibrant through the language patients employed. Several categories of sources are available to historians interested in the experience of suffering as defined above. These include personal diaries, correspondence and consultation letters (Digby 1994; Lyon-Caen 2016; Lane 1985; Rieder 2010). This chapter focuses on the latter form of written account for several reasons. First, such letters are comparable to laboratory notes of self-observation and constitute a summary of the arduous things patients experienced, as we will see later. Second, they were written to a specific person: the words were carefully chosen and sentences precisely written so as to be understood adequately. And third, they are a concentrated record of the sensations that patients felt in their bodies and translated into words.

Drawing on Linda Pollock's method for reading sources to consider the lived experience of emotions (Pollock 2004), I will treat patients' words as an expression, or even an aesthetic, of what they really experienced – instead of viewing their letters primarily as vehicles for transmitting content or explaining their suffering. Written consultations were a form of cultural script in that they aimed to communicate *and to share* patients' experiences with Dr Tissot. They called on the physician's senses as well as on his scientific expertise to interpret their suffering. Sufferers' need to share their experiences offers historians today an opportunity to get closer to the 'heart of the matter' (to borrow from Jacot Grapa's 2009 title); consultation letters reveal patients' attempts to make sense of their suffering as they experienced it – in their minds and bodies, and in relation to their environment.

It is important to note here that this 'heart of the matter' concerns a specific category of the eighteenth-century European population: those wealthy enough to be able to afford a consultation with a famous physician. Such patients had time to focus on their symptomatology, as well as the cultural and economic means to communicate it and seek relief. This does not mean, however, that the remaining population did not experience a similar kind of suffering, but it is difficult to locate because of a lack of sources. The experiences described by letter-writers *made explicit* a deep unease present in wider society. For example, in her analysis of late eighteenth-century hospital files, Heather Beatty observes that nervous diseases did not affect only the elite (Beatty 2012: 91). Similarly, in her book on suicide in eighteenth-century France, Dominique Godineau notes that workers, too, experienced and expressed a deep suffering that pushed them to take their own lives (Godineau 2012: 157–8). The notion of aesthesis suggested by Bourke, as well as its possible disruption, affected everyone. Although we must be aware that the status of letter-writer and recipient could shape the way that patients put their suffering into words, these narratives could represent more than the European elite. Elite or non-elite, the eighteenth-century letters point to a gap between the letter-writers' cognitive, mental and sensorial worlds and ours.

Written consultations were frequent in Europe at the time. Such consultation letters were a common way of making contact with a doctor (Brockliss 1994; Wild 2006; Stolberg 2011; Smith 2008; Coste 2014). Sir Hans Sloane (Smith 2003; *The Sloane Letters Project*), William Cullen (Risse 1974; Shuttleton n. d.) and many other physicians in Europe dealt with patients by letter. Between 1750 and 1797, Swiss doctor Samuel Tissot received over 1,300 consultation letters and essays from patients across Europe, documents which are now archived and on which this work is based. Most of them came from middle- and upper-class individuals who had already tried several treatments unsuccessfully (Pilloud 2013: 52–7). Their letters ranged from a brief page of notes to a thirty-page epistle and contained all the details that patients felt necessary and relevant for the doctor to understand the unique nature of their illnesses. Some patients identified the presumed cause of their suffering, described their personal circumstances and explained the consequences of their affliction on their lives. Others were very to the point. As noted by several historians, letters are 'messy documents' (Boon 2016: 37–9). There was no 'typical' letter; the content of each depended on what the writer believed was important to communicate at that point in time. There are multiple possible ways to read these archives. In order to approach the experience of suffering, I examine letters that concern patients' descriptions of symptoms that they were experiencing and their language for sharing their experiences.

LANGUAGE AND THE HISTORICITY OF EXPERIENCE

Words are the only data historians have for gaining insight into a patient's experience. As Jean Starobinski notes, historians have access only to what patients describe in their narratives when it comes to examining affective experience (Starobinski 2012: 257). Joan Scott goes further by reducing experience to language; 'subjects', she states, 'are constituted discursively and experience is a linguistic event' (Scott 1991: 793). Without deciding whether a chasm exists between experience and language, it is obvious that language remains the surest means to attempt to understand the realities experienced by patients in the past. Patients' narratives remain the most faithful transcription to be found of their experience, due to the kind of language they use. The choice of expressions or figures of speech to describe their experiences are traces of the universe that sufferers lived in, felt and perceived.

Influenced by the theory of close reading, this chapter therefore takes a close look at the language used by patients to recount their experience. At that time, knowledge obtained from experience and theoretical knowledge were not mutually exclusive (Cook 2000). Doctors placed a great deal of importance on experience both in their practice and, as Sophie Vasset points out, in their scholarship, where they included discussions of their own experience and sensations (Vasset 2013: 115–17, 124). For eighteenth-century people, personal experience was an essential part of medical and lay culture that was included, alongside reasoning, analysis, classification and deduction, in the construction of knowledge. The languages of experience and theory went hand in hand in medical journals. The history of the epistemological value of the experience is still to be done, but a quick look at its definition in the dictionary reveals that the definitive opposition between reason and reasoning on one hand, and experience on the other hand, was only introduced in 1932 in the *Dictionnaire de l'Académie française*.

Both doctors and patients accepted personal narratives as a valid medium for communicating information on which medical practice was based. Eighteenth-century diagnoses and treatments were based on patients' translations of their symptoms into words (Fissell 1995). We can also consider, as does Philip Rieder, that the subjective feelings that patients put into words were perceived as objective facts by their friends, family and physicians (Rieder 2010: 361). Language was unanimously viewed as the fundamental essence of the relationship between doctor and patient. Patients often used metaphors and comparisons to describe the physical and mental manifestations of their illnesses, so that their descriptions may be seen as reflecting their actual conditions as accurately as possible, even if misunderstandings did occur and were reported (Louis-Courvoisier and Mauron: 2002). Eighteenth-century doctors believed figures of speech to be valid, as they were not yet looking for – either in patients' words or despite them – the 'silent truth' hidden in a patient's body (Foucault 2011: 33). It was not until the nineteenth century that doctors viewed such figures of speech with scepticism – or even as signs of pathological deviance (Rigoli 2001: 91–244).

Owing to the semantic ambiguity inherent in several words used both in the eighteenth century and today (humour, emotion, sensitivity, embarrass, beaten, etc.), it is necessary to look beyond our own mental paradigms and modern-day classifications. This ambiguity reflects the close and even confused relationship among thoughts, emotions and physical sensations (Sugg 2013: 316); it should not be taken as an incomplete expression of patients' thoughts and experience but rather as a flexible means of accommodating the complexities of their experience. As Julie Neveux indicated in her research on John Donne's work, monism (or the absence of distinction between the mind and the body) is located in the feeling and in the language of the feelings (Neveux 2013:15). The same monism is present in some patients' words in the eighteenth century. Experience was still closely tied up with physiology, emotions, circumstances and language; it is ambiguous in our eyes, but it fitted with the rationality of the Enlightenment.

The historicity of the body can be seen as a relationship between individuals' flesh and words, as described by Barbara Duden (Duden 1992; Rieder 2010: 300). Nobody knows what the authors of the eighteenth-century letters were 'actually' experiencing. But we do know what expressions they thoughtfully chose to relate what they were feeling. And we know that in their eyes, those words were the best way to depict what they were going through. As Richard Sugg states, we must accept that their experience was real, despite the fact that it has since 'vanished' (his term) and even if it seems strange to us today (Sugg 2013: 20). Anthropologist Laurence Kirmayer sees this as a dialectic between a patient's body and written narrative (Kirmayer 1992: 324). It is only by identifying the nature of such a dialectic that the historian can move beyond a patient's body image (as Kirmayer calls it) to access the patient's embodied experience. By studying the expressions and lexical associations of patients in the eighteenth century (or by deconstructing patients' narratives), I will connect patients' words to their experience of suffering.

HISTORIANS AND THE STUDY OF THE EXPERIENCE OF SUFFERING IN THE PAST

The process of deconstructing patients' narratives and attempting to discern their experience through the connections between their words and bodies also involves reviewing research already undertaken on consultation letters. The research of Séverine Pilloud (2013; Pilloud and Louis-Courvoisier 2003), Philip Rieder (2010), Michael Stolberg (2011), Robert Weston (2013), Sonja Boon (2016), Joel Coste (2014), Nahema Hanafi (2017), Patrick Singy (2014), Daniel Teysseire (1993, 1995), Wayne Wild (2000) and Lisa Smith (2008) offers a solid framework for the experience of illness and suffering. Their work clarifies the prevalence of some diseases in the eighteenth century and representations of those diseases, illustrates the importance of friends and family in helping patients to cope, highlights representations of suffering, focuses on gender conditions, depicts the sexual behaviour of men and women, and underscores the impact of certain diagnoses within the context of eighteenth-century medicine, incidentally telling stories of individual patients and identifying narrative frameworks. The historical study of illness and the experience of suffering is a lengthy undertaking and should be taken step by step, since it is a mix of so many components.

The danger of confusion

A superficial reading can lead historians to identify patients' narratives with their own experience and induce them to project their own experience onto past patients' words – after all, who hasn't suffered at some point? Over-simplistic identifications with eighteenth-century patients, however, are misleading and ignore the divide between historical and modern experiences. Even when the events a patient describes are vastly different, there is always a risk that historians project modern-day classifications onto the patient's narrative.

Unless we set aside our own experience and modern-day mental paradigms when reading consultation letters, interpretation can be contaminated by projections of our own emotions, experience and classifications. In his chapter on 'the travel of the historian', Siegfried Kracauer suggests a process of self-effacement; he recommends that scholars adopt an 'active passivity' when reading archives, which assists in widening one's vision and resisting one's mental habits (Kracauer 2005: 131–66; Ginzburg 2013). This recommendation is particularly relevant for topics related to bodies, suffering and everyday experiences. According to Kracauer, historians belong to two ages: the one they live in, and the one they work on. Even when looking at something that appears to fit modern experiences, deliberate 'estrangement' through close reading can enable the scholar to better connect language and thoughts with historical experience (Herrstein Smith 2016: 70).

Accepting this estrangement, however, requires that we also recognize a kind of scholarly experience that goes beyond the rational and cognitive, and is not entirely controlled. At the first step, estrangement is more a feeling than the result of an analysis. In that sense, the researcher's subjectivity is at stake and influences their research. Although we do not need to go as far as Andrew Johnston and Russell West-Pavlov, who assert that 'scholarly neutrality and objectivity are more rhetorical façade than genuine fact' (Johnston and West-Pavlov 2015: 4), researchers' own experiences shape their historical analyses in multiple ways, starting with their choice of archives and interpretation of sources.

The active passivity recommended by Kracauer is the first step in a process of reading these letters that progressively makes the scholar aware of the feeling of estrangement. The identification of the components of this feeling and their analysis comes as a second step. A close reading enables the scholar to move on from feeling to analysing the sources, and to reconstruct as far as possible the mental and perceptual structure of the eighteenth-century patients' experience.

Finding the right distance

Paradoxically, close reading helps to maintain a minimal distance between our own experience and that of eighteenth-century patients. The process begins with the transcribing of the patients' letters, then reading them several times in order to identify the relevant passages. This slow, methodical approach has enabled me to assimilate the letters' language word by word and to spot unusual lexical and grammatical structures that might have been overlooked if they had been read too quickly. My research on experience was initially an analysis of 100 letters sent to Dr Tissot between 1750 and 1798, which I selected specifically to study the experience of melancholy (Louis-Courvoisier 2015; 2017). I then compared my findings on melancholic patients with 370 other letters written to Dr Tissot by sufferers.

As the letters do not follow rigid codes and vary considerably in length and structure, it is impossible to identify a fixed set of criteria to analyse them. Moreover, each letter reflects a patient's particular circumstances, which makes comparisons tricky and generalizations unsuitable (Grassi 1998: 5–6). What is more, each sentence and expression within a letter raises several questions that, instead of leading us to a descriptive or explicative summary, result in even more bewilderment. With so much variation, it was essential to identify some form of firm ground. I identified two common elements: the act of writing and patients' language. In the first section below, I will show that patients wrote letters to describe a destabilization within their bodies that had become unbearable, and that the person to whom they wrote influenced the way in which they recounted their experience. The subsequent section will deal with the components of the sensible/sensitive experience. I will show that the experience of suffering was defined by many patients by external troubles affecting the writer's senses, mainly problems of sight and hearing. But the most commonly shared experience of suffering was characterized by a cenesthesic chaos (or subtle internal sensations), such as deep changes to their bodily consistency or violent micro-movements affecting each part of the body.

THE ACT OF WRITING

For some patients, writing to Tissot was comparable to calling a doctor today, a moment when a person decided to become a patient (Zola 1973: 679). Something critical happened which led an individual to seek medical help. What pushed them to write at that precise moment? Which details did they chose to express the singularity of their experience? To focus our attention on these questions means to concentrate on a specific moment of the experience and on its context. It helps to catch it as a concrete reality perceived and communicated by patients while they were writing.

Signs of disarray in patients' 'animal economy'

Writing is an act triggered by one or more experienced events that prompt an individual to put their observations, thoughts and reactions on paper. In eighteenth-century consultation letters, the act of writing was sometimes motivated by a desire to send an update to a doctor following a face-to-face consultation, to inform a doctor of the effects of the treatment he had prescribed, to express thanks once an illness was cured or to solicit a reply. In these cases, the letters typically followed well-established letter-writing conventions, and the act of writing was prompted not by disturbing symptoms but by the social conventions of the time, especially in high society.

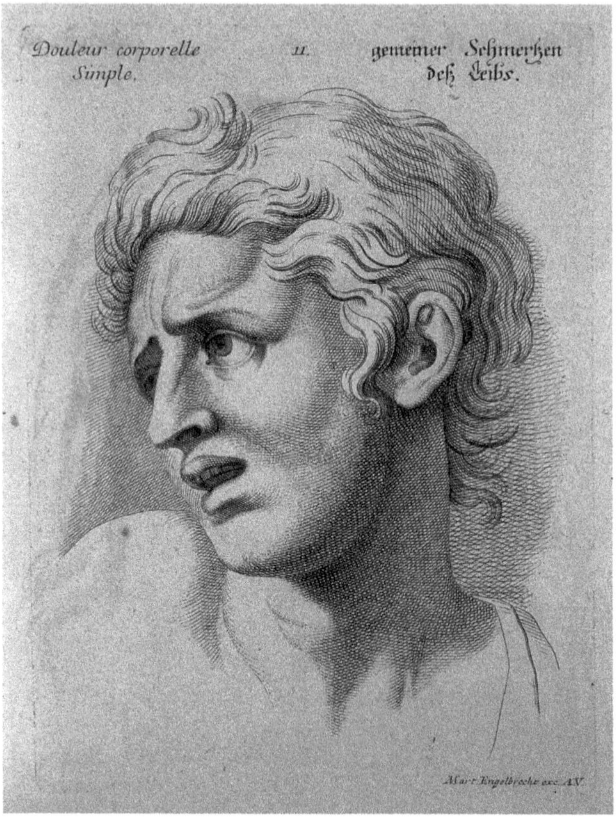

FIGURE 6.3: The face of a man expressing simple bodily pain. Engraving by M. Engelbrecht(?), 1732, after C. Le Brun. Credit: Wellcome Collection, London/Public Domain.

In other cases, letter writing was prompted by excessive pain or discomfort, as if a patient's tolerance limit had been reached for an identified or supposed illness, or more often for a group of disparate symptoms which had lasted long enough to become unbearable. They felt like a disturbance of the patient's bodily functions and internal movement, or in other words, of their animal economy. On 2 April 1774, La Comtesse de Vury de Remiremont consulted Dr Tissot about 'an infinite number of small pains, the sum of which are making my life miserable'.[2] (Figure 6.3 depicts the facial expression of simple bodily pains, which seems to fit this case.) She also said that she felt 'delicate' but not necessarily ill. Although some patients used medical terms and discussed their symptoms and diagnoses, in general they did not write to say they 'had' dry patches or rheumatism, for example; such statements would have had at most an explicative value. Lisa Smith is right to consider that such narratives are not the result of a fully interpreted experience (Smith 2008: 460). Instead sufferers wrote to present to Tissot (rather than to represent) how they felt: the disarray of their 'animal economies', the changes in their moods, their worries, their ill ease, their torments. On 17 November 1776, Le Comte d'Halgouet, who blamed a variety of symptoms on his obstructed spleen, said that his disease worried him more than it pained him, because it made him 'think dark thoughts, as I am naturally melancholic'.[3] It was often an accumulation of different symptoms, the chronic nature of their symptoms or an increase in their symptoms' intensity that pushed patients beyond a threshold and prompted them to write to the doctor, seeking relief, consolation and sometimes a cure.

Occasionally pain was the main reason for consulting the doctor, but not always. 'It's not exactly a pain, but something mute that's bothering me under my ribs', wrote Le Chevalier de Rotalier. He continued, 'It feels like there is a weight or a lack of elasticity in the muscles and nerves under my ribs; however, when I press on the area with my hand, I don't feel any pain'.[4] Patients experienced a wide variety of unpleasant sensations in their bodies – and the word 'pain' was far from sufficient to cover them all.

Despite claiming to be in good health, some patients wrote to Tisssot for advice. Mr Desbordes spelled out a host of symptoms but nevertheless said in the same letter on 10 August (n. d.), 'Otherwise, I feel fine, I eat well, sleep well, and don't do anything to excess; I have good colour, like a man in perfect health'.[5] For Ms De Chastenay on 8 November, 1784, the contrast between her good health and her state of anxiety was striking: 'I'm almost always in a state of agony, and convinced that my health is good, I'm never sure of even the next quarter of an hour of my existence, because I always fear that my ideas, my thoughts, or a conversation will make me experience a revolution that will kill me'.[6] Ms De Chastenay used the terms 'agony' and 'health' in the same sentence, as if the word pair of suffering/wellbeing did not coincide with sickness/health. It was possible for some letter-writers to suffer and yet to consider themselves to be in good health.

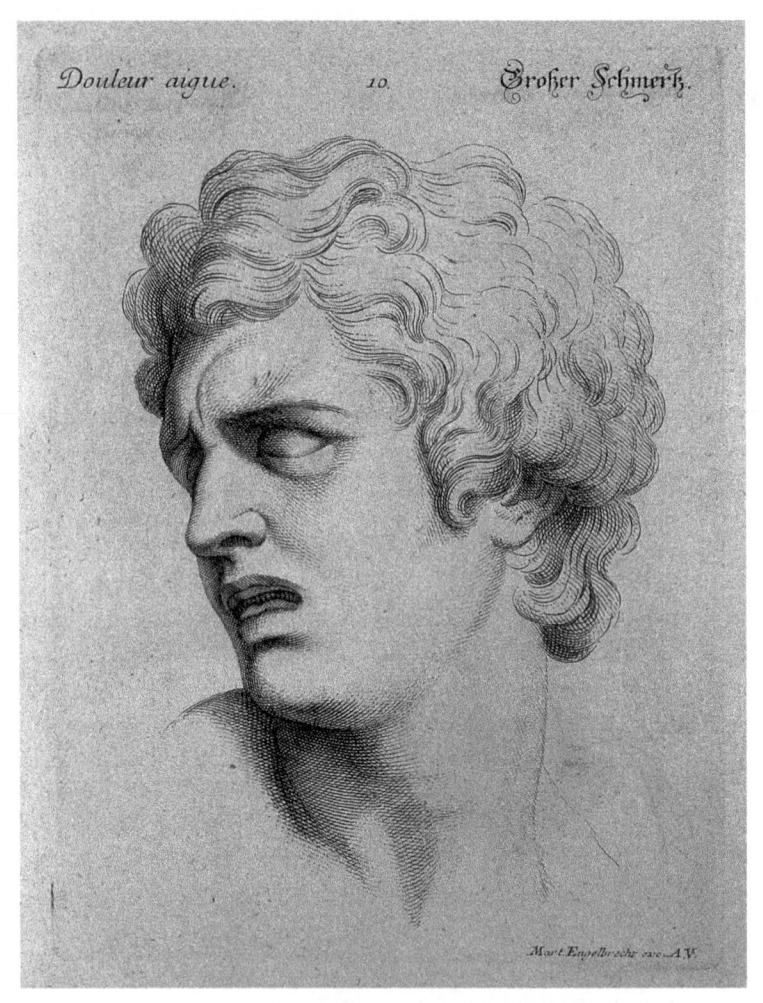

FIGURE 6.4: A man suffering acute pain. Engraving by M. Engelbrecht (?), 1732, after C. Le Brun. Credit: Wellcome Collection, London/Public Domain.

For many patients who consulted Dr Tissot by letter, but who were not already part of a social or therapeutic relationship, the decision to write was prompted by the fact that daily life had become unbearable. Even if they suffered a chronic disease, it appears that they were experiencing, at the moment of writing, an acute suffering that drove them to write down their ailments.

The importance of detail

Generally, details were important to characterize the uniqueness of an experience. In the eighteenth century, the word 'detail' was sometimes used to qualify a narrative; it referred also to 'anything related to circumstances and particularities in the matter at question' (*Dictionnaire de l'Académie française* 1762).⁷ Some patients used 'detail' when writing to Tissot. For instance, on 24 January 1772, Colonel Jungkenn asked the doctor, 'May I take the risk of displeasing you, Sir, with such a circumstantial detail?'⁸ He sent Dr Tissot a consultation letter and a memoir that together made up around a dozen pages, providing all sorts of specifics about his symptoms. Patients' letters were filled with 'circumstances' and 'particularities', all of which they felt were important to include because they revealed different aspects of an illness they believed to be 'singular' or 'unique'. They therefore wanted to paint as complete a picture as possible for the doctor.

The details in patients' letters covered their assessments of their conditions and antecedents, as well as the consequences of their illness for their daily lives and for their friends and family. Patients also elaborated on any domestic treatments and opinions or prescriptions from previously consulted healers. They provided their own thoughts on the diagnosis and possible causes of their illness. But the most striking details, especially for a study of the patient experience, were the minutiae of their sensitive reality (*réalité sensible*) and their physical and psychic conditions.

Such details were not intended for Dr Tissot to only read and analyse. Some patients explicitly called on the doctor's senses. 'Deign to listen to me, Sir, lend a favourable ear to the account of a despairing man's pain', wrote Mr Muros de Laborde on 15 February 1772, before continuing his narrative on seven pages, as if he were channelling oral discourse through written discourse.⁹ Some attempted to 'paint a picture' (*tracer un tableau*) of their ailments, explicitly soliciting the doctor's eyes, as did Mr De Lavau, on 14 July 1793, and the Abbot Tinseau (no date, 144.03.03.25). On 17 November 1776, Le Comte d'Halgouet asked the doctor to perform a specific movement to help him localize the area where he had pain: *'Please take care to note that my pain is centred on my left side, at the lower section of my ribs; bend your left arm while you are standing up, as if you were going to put on your coat, that's where the pain is, and it extends pretty much down to my kidneys'* (original emphasis).¹⁰ Although patients related their experience in writing, beyond the act of putting pen to paper, when they reached out to the doctor, they explicitly invoked his body and senses so that their words activated his whole self. The patients needed to be 'heard', 'seen' and understood by all the doctor's capacities.

THE SUFFERING EXPERIENCE AS A COLLECTION OF PERTURBED AND AGITATED SENSATIONS

The patients' experience of suffering was made up of a collection of sensations – sometimes concurrent and often fleeting, complicated and volatile. By writing them down in detail, patients were attempting to break down the sensitive components their experience and to recompose it through the process of wording. This process could be therapeutic in itself, as noted by Smith (2008: 466) and Rieder (2010: 54–7). The quantity of details patients needed to write down suggests that the temporality of writing helped them to find the precise connection between experience and language, in order to give a form to their suffering and then to communicate it to their reader.

Disturbances of the senses

The experience of suffering was sometimes caused by external factors that provoked dis-ease in the senses. The senses most often mentioned in patients' descriptions of their symptoms were hearing and sight. The eyes were the organs most commonly afflicted, either causally or pursuant to other symptoms – or because of the eyes' sensitivity. Patients found vision-related disturbances particularly worrying. For instance, Ms Doxat de Champvent (1790), who suffered from headaches, completely lost her visual references: 'My vision suddenly becomes obscured, to the point that objects in front of me fade away and my eyes seem to be constantly covered by a dark veil' (no date, 144.05.02.23).[11] Another patient, Ms Dubois (29 January 1792), felt that her eyesight would sometimes be obscured by a 'violent attack of grief'. She saw black flies in front of her and felt as though a veil covered her eyes.[12] Le Comte de la Porte (27 May 1782) believed he was falling ill because his vision was blurred, as if he was looking at objects 'through flashes of light'.[13] Ms Fol reported on 26 August 1766 that she could no longer stand 'the light of dusk, this fallacious day, which gives me agitations as if I was having convulsions'. Worse yet, she found that 'when I hold my head up with my hand, it seems as if the earth and the sky switch places, the same topsy-turvy feeling I have in my body'.[14] Patients experienced an altered sense of vision: blurred, shadowed, interrupted by flashes of light or obscured by flies.

Some patients heard occasional buzzing or ringing in their ears. A few simply mentioned it, but others sought to make the doctor understand what they were experiencing. On 10 October 1774, the Abbot Debonne heard a sound 'similar, but not as loud, to the one a river makes when it crosses a dam by a mill'.[15] La Comtesse de Werthern heard 'snapping sounds, like the crackling of a twig in a fireplace' (3 May 1793)[16]. Ms Fol heard such a racket that her entire body was affected: 'I hear explosions in my head, whistling, and horrible buzzing sounds, which cause all my limbs to agitate' (26 August 1766).[17] Mr Le Meilleur wrote on 26 March 1770 that he heard sounds originating in his brain: 'but having woken up around midnight, I was surprised to hear an extraordinary sound in my brain, somewhat like the sound a taut fishnet makes when it is torn; in addition, I heard a murmuring that can best be compared to the sound of earth dried by the beating sun, and that has just been watered'.[18] And Mr Hartman noted on 22 May 1792 that he heard a constant 'croaking' in his abdomen every morning that was accompanied by a bothersome, but not painful, feeling in his intestines'.[19]

Since these sounds were hard to describe, patients often compared them to familiar sounds they knew the doctor would have heard, such as the crackling of a burning twig or dried earth, the gurgling of a river or the cawing of a crow. They believed that since the doctor was familiar with these sounds, he could 'hear' them. At the same time, these examples reveal the 'operative machinery' (Herrstein Smith 2016: 60); the authors were also trying to activate perceptive simulations (Bolens 2014) in order to share experience. The number of metaphors or comparisons included in the consultations suggests that the authors used them as a driving force that could improve Tissot's judgement through his imagination.

Troubles of the flesh

Patients who wrote to the doctor themselves did so because they knew better than anyone else what they were suffering from (Pilloud 2013: 94–6). Reflecting the popular Enlightenment concept of sensitivity, the words 'feel' and 'feeling' were used constantly, such as in 'I feel', 'it feels like' or 'a feeling of'. According to some linguists, the term 'feeling' can relate to a 'synthetic event' (Neveux 2013: 11–12) and includes both a physical and a psychical state (Polguère 2013). This double understanding of the term is important to keep in mind when reading such letters, as it enables us to recognize and to accept the sometimes strange bodily sensations that eighteenth-century patients described.

A 'fibrillar' suffering   Medical theories in the eighteenth century focused on fluids' circulation and nerves' routes which organized the inside the body. Consultation letters show more sophisticated internal sensations, that could occur in any solid, aerial or fluid part of a patient's body. Some, like Mr Le Meilleur and Ms Fol, suffered from various sensations *inside* their brain; others complained of drafts between their skin and flesh, winds in their bowels, vapours in their hypochondrium, beating or sweating in their kidneys, and heart and stomach palpitations. Their sensations did not always follow set trajectories of human anatomy, and the organs they mentioned were not necessarily organs defined by science; as historian Jackie Pigeaud argues in his discussion of anatomy in antiquity, 'forms' would be a better description (Pigeaud 1985: 56). Patients' experiences reveal more sophisticated sensations than those indicated by medical theories of the time. The fibres of Mr Godet du Peret (3 June 1789) were 'dry, sensitive and irritable beyond expression'.[20] Ms Nomis, on 16 April 1785, hoped to find something to strengthen her nerves and to convey strength to the fibre.[21] Some authors explicitly mention the fibre, but the sophistication of the sensations is also revealed through other discursive technics.

Mr Torchon Defourchet (who had 'sluggish and flaccid' fibre) added that he felt 'in his shoulders a shivering as if my skin became unstuck and as if somebody had blown air between skin and flesh' (no date, 144.03.06.19).[22] Mr Bertolot had worryings all around his navel; he felt hot vapours rushing towards his neck (no date, 144.04.04.02). On 10 June 1771, Mr Charier had a 'beaten stomach and a sort of twisting in his throat'.[23] The internal upheavals he felt led to others, and Mr Charier made his reader understand that his internal geography was in disorder, his bodily integrity was impaired, and some of his bodily trajectories were distorted and causing strange sensations.

The letters contain many and repeated examples of cenesthesic chaos. Patients could feel pain and discomfort in any part of their body, and these feelings accumulated, propagated to other areas and affected their physical beings. Patients experienced their body and their selves in the thickness of their flesh, through the sensitiveness of each fibre. If their bodily model can be related to a body shell enveloping humoral and nervous systems, as shown by Pilloud (2013: 177), the description of their experience seems also close to the 'fibre body' as described by Hisao Ishizuka (2012). According to Ishizuka, historians of medical theories have neglected the concept of fibre, which was the minimal unit of the body until the mid-eighteenth century, in favour of the nerves. Elasticity was the essential property of the fibre, involving features such as movement, resistance and restoration. The cenesthesic chaos, and its internal geography that does not follow only the nervous and humoral paths, is in line with the rehabilitation of the fibre (Wenger 2007: 39–42; Vila 2014: 4).

The violence of internal movements A variety of movements participated in the patients' cenesthesic sensitivity. Although several historians have noted that patients felt pain move within their bodies (Rey 2000: 145–9), the movements felt by patients did not concern only pain. Patients used a variety of motion-related words to describe their disturbing, or even unbearable, symptoms: agitation, trembling, vibrating, stirring, quivering, twisting, emotion, transporting, revolution, shuddering, trembling, palpitations and beating (Louis-Courvoisier 2018a).

The way patients described such internal movements, and how they experienced them, enables several observations. First, these were sensations shared by many people. Second, in addition to movements of the nerves (mentioned by both patients and doctors), the movements involved many other body parts. Patients suffered from 'revolving bile' (Mrs Vibraye de Roncée, 15 February 1773), 'stirring bile' (Mr Cherot du Marois, 16 January 1786), stirrings in the fibres and frontal blood vessels (Mr de Corsier, 20 August 1793), blood agitations (Mrs Wilmsdorff, 8 April 1783), emotion in the blood (Baronne de Portzig, 16 August 1776), 'a painful movement or labour in my nerves *as well as my flesh*' (my emphasis, Chevalier de Soran, 17–23 October 1771), transporting within the brain (Mr Pollet, 20 April 1772), and boiling between the skin and flesh (no name, no date, 144.05.04.19).[24] Winds were also non-negligible sources of discomfort: 'I am tremendously bothered by winds, which travel along my hypochondrium and go up my chest', complained Mr Pollet on 20 April 1772.[25]

Patients often described the intensity, or even the violence, of the movements they felt: 'Far from it, my blood rushes to my head even more violently than ever', described Mrs De Brackel on 9 May 1790.[26] For Mr Reichert, 'my blood is thick and flows impetuously', while Mr Walmöden reported that 'with the heat flashes that are somewhat intense, the flowing and agitation in my brain increase to an alarming point' (no date, 144.05.02.40).[27] On 10 December 1789, Ms De Diesbach felt 'pain throwing around in my stomach'.[28] Ms Fol, by contrast, described on 26 August, 1766 the fact that she did not have a single body part that was serene: 'I was in a state of anxiety, a delirium, I couldn't sleep without having horrible dreams, melancholy, dizziness, shaking, fright, trembling in my entire body, heart and stomach palpitations, and beating in my kidneys.'[29] The word 'revolution' was frequently used to describe the violence of the movement.

As Rieder contends, body and mind coincide in a shared reality (Rieder 2010: 103). This coincidence was not only in a shared reality, in a moment of experience, but was enclosed in some of the words themselves (Smith 2008: 463–5). The emphasis on bodily movements reveals the ambiguity of these terms. Among them, 'emotion' and 'uneasiness' could refer to either a mental state or a fleshy or humoral movement (Louis-Courvoisier 2019). Beside the emotions in the blood mentioned above, we can find also expressions, difficult to understand today, such as 'A kidney is giving me emotion that makes me tremble all over' (Mr Snell, 19 March 1793).[30] Mr Buyrette suffered from 'a uneasiness' in his palate, anus, and ear (27 February 1770), just as Mr Walmöden had a 'uneasiness' on the skin (no date, 144.05.02.40).[31] On 24 July 1776, Le Chevalier de Valpergue reported experiencing a 'uneasiness, especially in my legs, which seems to come from an overly taut fibre'.[32] Abbot Bertolot had the same kind of uneasiness 'all around my navel' (no date, 144.04.04.02).[33] In each of these instances, the uneasiness related to a localized fibrillar agitation that caused the pain.

A close reading of these letters shows that the suffering experience of illness in the eighteenth century was linked not only to pain that moved about but also to a body in which every element was continuously in a state of disorder. These painful internal moving sensations were not only related to the humoral and nervous systems; rather, they can be seen as the pneumatic and fibrillar 'pulsing body-machines' (Sutton 1998: 39).

The sensations can also be understood within the context of the theory of animal spirits. As philosopher John Sutton observes, 'wriggling spirits, then, were phenomenologically felt' (Sutton 1998: 39–42). Some vitalists still used the term in their medical writings in the middle of the eighteenth century, as well as the word 'fluid', which is sometimes considered synonymous with animal spirits (Carnicero de Castro 2014). Unlike English-speaking letter-writers (Beatty 2012: 89–98), French-speaking letter-writers sometimes used the term 'fluid' – though they rarely mentioned animal spirits explicitly in their narratives. The description of uncontrolled and messy movements, linked to vapours, blowing air, wind and more generally to pneumatics, led to similar descriptions of the moving and sensing animal spirits and their functions in the body. It is as if these writers had embodied the properties of the movements of animal spirits but left aside the theory (Louis-Courvoisier 2018b: 92).

Changes in bodily consistency The changes that patients felt inside their bodies also involved a sense that their bodily consistency was being altered. Patients often used the French term '*fonte*' ('melting') to indicate an improvement in their condition. Ms Bonville d'Achy, on 7 April 1793, wrote that she twice experienced 'a considerable melting of bile' that made her feel better.[34] On 14 May 1774, Mr Vauvilliers also said he experienced a 'considerable melting', noting in the margin of his letter that it involved 'fifty-two evacuations in one night' (no date, 144.02.04.26).[35] These 'meltings' should be considered alongside the importance given at the time to evacuating humours and relieving the plethora (Pilloud and Louis-Courvoisier 2003: 461–2). 'Meltings' were usually helpful for patients since they alleviated obstructions, feelings of fullness or a poor composition of humours.

However, other feelings of a changing bodily consistency were markers of suffering. Sometimes, humours changed consistency, as was the case for Mr Gaspary on 18 May 1773: he felt air mixing with his fluids 'whenever I hear distressing news, or if I'm expecting some occurrence that will bring me grief. My phlegm acts as if my breath has a soufflé effect, and it feels like air can't enter into my lungs.'[36] Sometimes, as for Mr Bournouville on 7 October 1768, the writer's humours got thicker: 'The fourth day I felt a heavy weight and considerable thickening of my humours and in all my fluids, to the point where I didn't have the strength to move or accomplish even the smallest task.'[37] Note the link that Mr Gaspary makes between the feeling of thickening humours and his subsequent sense of inertia. What might be called today a 'lack of energy' was then associated with the consistency of a person's humours. Figure 6.5, for example, depicts '*abattement*', a term that referred to loss of spirits and/or energy in the eighteenth century (*Dictionnaires d'Autrefois*). The image captures a sense of wilting and weakening that was as much emotional as physical; physical disturbances were intertwined with psychological phenomena.

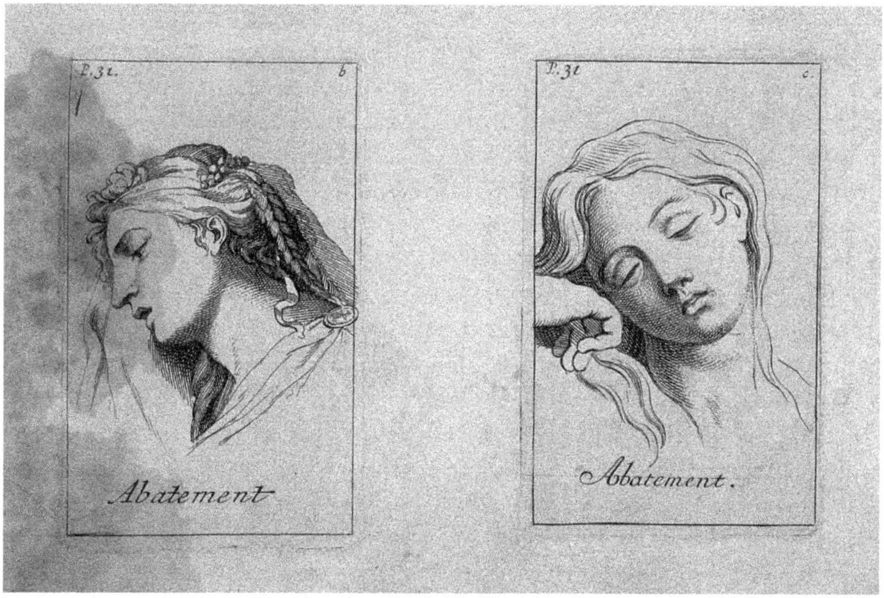

FIGURE 6.5: Abatement, described in the Wellcome catalogue as 'Two faces expressing dejection'. Etching by B. Picart, 1713, after C. Le Brun. Credit: Wellcome Collection, London/Public Domain.

Mr Dorc's blood, on 5 December 1773, was 'full of phlegm and humour, or too thick, or worn out'.[38] In other cases, patients experienced a feeling of emptiness, crushing, decomposition or dryness that was bothersome: 'sometimes it feels like my brain is dry and empty' wrote Mr Claret on 7 April 1790.[39] La Comtesse de la Rivière (4 January 1792) felt a 'decomposition' that made it hard for her to speak.[40] Another patient said his pain felt 'like someone was crushing the entrails on my right side' (no name, no date, 144.03.06.28).[41]

Floating entrails, a dry and empty brain, vapours that become tears, blocked kidneys and brain, dry fibres, a stomach that is stuck to the kidneys, a vaporous body and soul, dried humours, thick blood – all these expressions depict painful experiences that were real for the patients who wrote them.

CONCLUSION

A study of the experience of illness and suffering in the eighteenth century as described by patients in consultation letters carries with it two significant biases: that of condensation and that of intensification. By condensation, I mean that patients concentrated the elements of their experience into a single document that was intended to help the doctor understand their case and find relief. For some, the document was written at a breaking point when their experience, until then bearable, had become unbearable. By intensification (Veyne 1996), I am referring to the nature of the source. The letters were written within the context of a daily life that involved not only what the writers experienced in their bodies, but also other events in their lives, whether professional, economic, political, societal, or related to their friends and family: everyday events that we would have found in a diary. In their consultations, however, patients left these events out to focus on their suffering, thereby providing or strengthening the intensity effect.

It is important to highlight and take into account both of these biases, although it is precisely these biases that give us a better comprehension of the letter-writers' experience. Even though the patients' illnesses were generally chronic and had been affecting them for a long time, several patients decided to write Dr Tissot when they could no longer stand the symptoms. The factors leading up to the writing of their letters imply that they went through a process of reconstituting and concentrating their experience. This, in turn, enables modern-day historians to identify and analyse the elements most commonly chosen by eighteenth-century patients to express their suffering.

As we have seen, the experience of suffering is embedded in its cultural context. The eighteenth-century context entails various components which shape this experience. Among them was an 'easy writing' context: upper- and middle-class people were used to writing about their everyday life. This practice had encouraged the development of written consultations all around Europe. This frame of consultation involved time for self-observation and to bring numerous symptoms to consciousness. It thus allowed the connection between subtle and intimate sensations and a precise, detailed and creative language. This language was necessary for the physician not only to understand but also to feel the patients' symptoms. In the eighteen-century doctor–patient relationship, the experience of suffering had to be contagious and not only explained. Furthermore, eighteen-century patients were able to reclaim the different medical theories and to integrate them with what they were feeling when suffering. 'Revolving bile', 'blood agitation', 'dry and irritable fibres' or 'blowed air between skin and flesh' were all symptoms 'borrowed' from the nerves, humoral or animal spirits theories and embodied by patients.

These letters reveal a suffering experience that was characterized by a cocktail of internal and external sensations, and by self-awareness that includes each kind of bodily matter. It meant changes in the bodily consistency, which consisted of various gases, liquids and solids in a state of flux – making patients feel liquefied, 'scattered with holes' or even disintegrated. Violent and subtle internal movements that could involve each fibre of their body also affected patients.

A close reading is necessary to be aware of the gap between our contemporary categories which shape our experience and those of the eighteenth century. Of course, we would not say to our physician today that we were suffering from a blood revolution or from vapours rushing towards our neck. Here, the historicity of the experience is quite clear. Nevertheless, there is a less visible blurred area enclosed notably in the 'flexible' words; research is still to be done on these words to detect them. If we have been aware for some time of the semantic ambiguity of some of these words, such as 'humour' or 'transport', for example (Pigeaud 1985; Nahoum-Grappe 1994), numerous others, such as 'astonishments' or 'uneasiness', are more difficult to identify. It takes time and requires a repeated and precise reading, as well as a willingness to feel the 'estrangement' they induce, in order to recognize that these words refer to both a mental state and a bodily condition. But these steps are necessary. A hasty reading can lead to a misinterpretation, or at best to a partial understanding, conditioned by our mental patterns, and that would miss the complexity that shaped the eighteenth-century experience.

NOTES

1. I am very grateful to Philip Rieder and to Lisa Smith for their fruitful comments.
2. 'infinité de petis meaux dont la somme totale font de ma vie un etat facheux'. All the original documents quoted in this paper are easily searchable by name in the Fonds Tissot: Archives du corps et la santé au 18e siècle database, http://tissot.unil.ch/fmi/webd/Tissot.
3. 'occasionne du noir, etant naturellement melancolique'.
4. 'Ce n'etoit point precisement une douleur, mais quelque chose de sourd, qui me genoit sous les côtes . . . C'est comme un poids ou un manque d'elasticité dans les muscles ou nerfs qui sont sous les côtes; cependant, lorsque j'appuye la main dessus, je n'eprouve aucune sensation douloureuse.'
5. 'Du reste, je me porte bien, mange bien, dort bien, ne fais aucun excés; j'ai bonne couleur, comme un homme en parfaite santé.'
6. 'Je suis presque toujours dans un état d'agonie, et persuadé que ma santé est bonne, je ne suis jamais assuré d'un quart d'heure d'existence, parce que je crains toujours que mes idées, mes réfléxions, une conversation ne me fasse éprouvé une révolution qui me tue.'
7. 'signifie tout ce qu'il y a de circonstances et de particularités dans l'affaire dont il est question'.
8. 'Pourrois-je craindre à vous déplaire, Monsieur, par un detail si circonstancié?'
9. 'Daignez donc, Monsieur, m'ecouter, daignez preter une oreille favorable au recit des maux d'un infortuné.'
10. 'Je vous prie de faire grand attention que le siege de mon mal est au costé gauche, à la chute des costes; pliéz le bras gauche, lorsque vous seréz debout, comme si vous vouliéz le passer dans vôtre veste, c'est là qu'est mon mal, et qui s'etend plus ou moins au reins.'
11. 'tout à coup, ma vüe s'obscurcit à tel point, que les objets fuyoit de devant moi, une toile noir passoit continuëlement devant mes yeux'.

12. 'un chagrin violent ... des mouches noires, un voile devant les yeux'.
13. 'comme à travers des éclairs'.
14. 'la lumiere du crespuscule, ce faux jour, me donne une agitation dans mon corp semblable à des convultion ... soutenant ma tête de ma main, il me semble que le ciel et la terre se renverse, de même que mon corps'.
15. 'approchant celluy que fait une riviere, mais pas si fort, en franchissant la digue qui la traverse près d'un moulin'.
16. 'cracs, semblables aux petillemens d'un fagot dans une cheminée'.
17. 'Il se fait des éclats dans ma tête, des siflements, des bourdonnements afreux, toutes ces choses me donnent de l'agitation dans tous mes members.'
18. 'mais m'étant réveillé vers la minuit, je fus étonné d'entendre, dans mon cerveau, un bruit extraordinaire, à peu près comme si c'eut été de petits filets fortement tendus qui se feraient rompre; de plus, un murmure que je ne scaurais mieux comparer qu'à celui que rend une terre desséchée par les ardeurs du soleil, qu'on viendrait à abbreuver'.
19. 'un croacement continuel'.
20. 'mes fibres sont sèches, sensibles et irritables au-delà de toute expression'.
21. 's'il ne se trouve pas un moyen, de fortifier mes nerfs, et de donner plus de force à la fibre'.
22. 'j'ai ressenti dans les epaules un frissonnement comme si ma peau se décolloit et comme si l'on m'avoit soufflé entre cuir et chair'.
23. 'j'ay l'estomac abbatu, je veux dire delogé, c'est ce qui me cause des tiraillements au coup et un certain tortillement dans le gosier. Voilà la source de mon mal.'
24. 'revolutions de bile', 'remüements de bile', 'remuement dans les fibres ou les vaisseaux du front', 'agitations de sang', 'emotions de sang', 'mouvement ou travail avec douleur tant dans les nerfs que dans les chaires', 'transports au cerveau', 'ébullitions entre cuir et chair'.
25. 'je suis prodigieusement incommodé des vents, qui le long des hypocondres montent dans la poitrine'.
26. 'Bien loin de ça, mon sang ce porte à la tête avec plus de violence que jamais.'
27. 'mon sang est épais et court avec impétuosité'; 'dans les chaleurs un peu vives, l'ecoulement et les agitations du cerveau augmentoient à un point allarmant'.
28. 'les douleurs se jettent dans l'estomac'.
29. 'je fus dans l'angoisse, le délire, ne dormant qu'avec des rèves afreux, la melancholie, des vertiges, des tressauts, des frayeurs, un tremblement dans tout mon corps, des palpitations de coeur et d'estomac, un batement dans les reins'.
30. 'Un rein me donne de l'émotion et me rend tout tremblant.'
31. 'inquiétude au palais, au fondement ou à l'oreille'; 'inquiétudes sur la peau'.
32. 'une inquiétude et surtout aux jambes, qui me semble venir de la fibre trop tendue'.
33. 'tout autour du nombril'.
34. 'une fonte de bile considerable'.
35. 'une fonte considerable ... cinquante-deux évacuations en une nuit'.
36. 'lorsque je viens de recevoir quelque nouvelle affligeante, ou que je prevois avoir quelque occasion de me chagriner. Dans ce cas, ma pituite fait l'effet d'un soufflé, et il me semble que l'air ne peut entrer dans mes poumons.'

37. 'Le quatrième jour j'ai senti beaucoup de pesanteur et un épaississement considerable dans les humeurs et dans toutes les liqueurs, au point de n'avoir pas le courage d'agir et de m'occuper en la moindre chose.'
38. 'plein de glaire et d'humeur, ou trop espay ou trop usé'.
39. 'on diroit quelquefois que mon cerveau est vuide et desseché'.
40. 'sentiment de décomposition'.
41. 'comme si lui écrasoit les boÿaux du coté droit'.

CHAPTER SEVEN

Mind/Brain

CLAUDIA STEIN AND ROGER COOTER[1]

Culturally speaking, the brain didn't exist in the Age of Enlightenment. Unlike in today's 'Age of the Brain', no one reduced behaviour, emotions and feelings to cerebral states. Of course, the brain had long been known among anatomists, who often observed the porridge-like stuff under the cranium. But that had no cachet, no cultural significance; it didn't touch, move or inspire any public. What mattered in the Age of Enlightenment was not brain but mind and thinking. Only at the very end of the eighteenth century did the brain surface as the 'organ of the mind'. It was a breathtaking biologization; it literally blew minds – blew them out of the window along with everything that accompanied considerations of mind and soul. In retrospect, it demolished mind, secularizing it away from its moorings in the realms of metaphysics and spirituality. No longer would rational man need to refer to philosophy and/or God in relation to thinking. From now on, 'Nature' would suffice.

The distinction between mind and brain would have puzzled many eighteenth-century physicians. It was an impossible distinction for them to make. Dualisms they were comfortable with, but it was mind/matter or mind/body (more precisely, soul/mind and soul/body) that they worried over. The distinction between mind and brain rests on the idea that our minds reside somehow outside of nature, or at least beyond any technique which the natural sciences may develop to study it (casting into stark relief the need for 'psychosomatics' to investigate the inexplicable). But that was a nineteenth-century puzzle. Eighteenth-century medical practitioners knew that the mind influenced the body – they would wonder why the brain had been singled out – and they knew that the body influenced the mind. That was not the problem. The problem was what the mind actually was, how it was involved in the regulation of health and resistance to disease, and how one could maintain the former and alleviate the latter – all the while maintaining the epistemological standards which dominated the Age of Enlightenment.

This chapter is divided into two parts. The first discusses central ideas about mind that emerged in the eighteenth century and that guided thinking about the mind all over Europe. The focus is on Britain and its celebration of the idea of sensationalism, a radical idea about human knowledge production and the mind that found many enthusiasts throughout the eighteenth century. Invented by the British physician and moral philosopher John Locke (1632–1704), sensationalism fitted well the new aspiring Age of Enlightenment and its central idea of rational 'man' ('man' being used then in the sense of 'humankind'). The chapter's second section moves on to a cultural understanding of these ideas and how they garnered new social hierarchies particularly in relation to women.

Through a new sort of reasoning in the eighteenth century, the 'scientists of man' aimed to define a new human. 'Rationality' meant objective thinking without passion, prejudice and superstition and without reference to non-verifiable statements such as those of religious revelation. The new human was no longer the miserable sinner of old but an autonomous being, one that took delight in man himself as the apex of creation, guided by reason and above all with an investigating nature, including investigation of humankind. Society was the product of free humans, it came to be believed – persons who came together to set up a political society to protect fundamental rights, liberty and property. 'Man' became the master of nature (Outram 2013).

John Locke provided the eighteenth century with its conception of mind and a vision of humans as natural and social beings. Indeed, for him the principles of both metaphysics and medicine should be the same. After all, he was a physician, educated at Oxford and Leiden, who provided medical care for his patron – Lord Anthony Ashley Cooper, Earl of Shaftesbury. To modern eyes, Locke's ideas can look remarkably familiar. In his 1689 [1694] masterwork, *An Essay Concerning Human Understanding*, he successfully laid out what would be the model of the new human for the new Age of Enlightenment. He had been inspired by the moral philosopher Thomas Hobbes' *Leviathan* (1651), a book that famously laid out a theory of society that was grounded in a mechanistic understanding of human beings and their passions. While Locke agreed with Hobbes in principle, he dissented from his negative view of human nature as eternally sinful and brutish (and therefore in need of strict governmental control). Locke believed that humans were not born with eternal moral characteristics, basic principles and ideas, but rather that they acquired them throughout their lives through the capacity of reasoning. He therefore decided to ground his research on a radical analysis of how humans think. Unlocking the possibilities and limitations of human reasoning, he thought, would get him closer to revealing what humans really were and would offer insight into their morals and sociability.

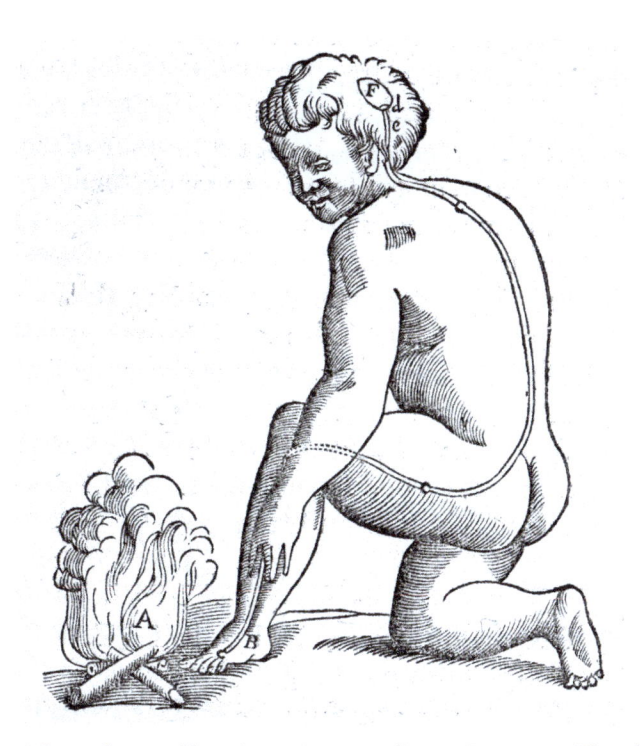

FIGURE 7.1: The pathway of burning pain, according to Descartes. The physical sensation was sent through the body to the pineal gland. In this way, pain was a physical sensation above all. Credit: Wellcome Collection, London/Public Domain.

To know 'man' was to know human reasoning, its possibilities and limitations. Locke's method of investigation was empiricism, a way of exploring nature first championed by the English natural philosopher and statesman Francis Bacon (1561–1626) and so popular in Britain that it was taken up by the Royal Society after its founding in 1660. Locke's choice of method and his belief that all human ideas come from sensation and reflection (i.e. that all human knowledge is founded on experience) set him firmly against another philosopher fashionable at the time, the Frenchman René Descartes. Descartes' dual and mechanistic view of the human body was based on the belief – not unlike Hobbes' – that humans are born with a set of innate ideas and general principles of logic. Locke's idea that humans acquired ideas and knowledge through the combination of sensations and reason was foreign to Descartes' philosophical system.

Initially, Descartes had aimed to establish principles of truth that humans could not doubt (Porter 2005: 65). Having questioned everything deemed 'truthful' in human knowledge, he arrived at the one thing so self-evidently true that it could not possibly be questioned: his own consciousness – *cogito, ergo sum*, or 'I am thinking, therefore I exist'. Descartes deprecated the idea of sensory knowledge, later praised by Locke, as the basis for all reasoning. In his view, subjective judgements were too uncertain. Instead, he ennobled reason above the senses; they were ontologically distinct for him. Because the notion of thought precedes that of all corporeal things, he claimed, it must be the conscious mind (*res cogitans*) which forms the essential I. Man was essentially dual, according to Descartes; he consisted of matter independent of mind, with the rational soul (situated, he believed, in the pineal gland) controlling a body-machine. The rational soul he suggested operated, via its pineal gland anchorage, throughout the body by means of animal spirits in the nerves and blood. The rational soul, the animal spirits and other faculties by which the body channelled sense impressions were themselves attributes of the flesh (Porter 2005: 68). What was novel to Descartes was the view that there was only one soul; the body was a machine, pure and simple, with no subaltern souls of its own, as the ancient Galenic theories, still prevalent at the time, suggested. In his view, the animal spirits and other faculties by which the body channelled all its sense impressions were themselves attributes of the flesh.

The importance of Descartes lay in his bold designation of the soul as a philosophical rather than a religious principle, an immaterial thinking thing (Porter 2005: 68). While upholding the Christian soul, he transformed its status into *cogito*, rendering it independent of divines and ministrations of the Church. Crucially, Descartes understood 'thought' as the awareness of our actions and the moral standards against which we measure them. In short, natural philosophy was founded on moral philosophy (Hennig 2010). Only in later works, such as the *Passion of the Soul* (1649), did Descartes confront a key problem of this mechanical dualism, namely the fact that it did not account for the multiple interactions between mind and body. What about human passions of the mind such as blushing in shame, feeling hot in anger or cold in fear? Didn't they arise by or with the help of the bodily senses? Descartes provided no answers.

Descartes' lack of answers bothered many intellectuals at the time, not least John Locke. For him, Descartes' mechanical system provided no answers to the body/mind problem: the problem of thinking and action and the question what the 'I', or the self, really was. Far from affirming Descartes' idea that the mind possessed an intuitive knowledge of the indivisible soul, Locke even doubted that we could know anything of its nature – hence, he believed that personal identity or self was the problem that needed to be addressed (Porter 2005: 72). For Locke, man's mind was a blank slate, a *tabula rasa*: there were no lingering *a priori* innate truths or ideas, as Descartes suggested. Knowledge, he claimed, was partial and acquired passively by humans only by the incessant and uncontrollable accumulation of experience through the five senses.

> Methinks, the *Understanding* is not much unlike a Closet wholly shut from light, with only some little openings left, to let in external visible Resemblances, or *Ideas* of things without; would the pictures coming into such a dark room but stay there, and lie so orderly as to be found upon occasion, it would very much resemble the Understanding of Man.
>
> —quoted in Porter 2005: 73

The mind was an empty 'slate' at birth that only came to be filled subsequently by ideas impressed, like wax on a seal, through sense perceptions. For Locke, the experience of the senses led to the accumulation and consolidation of probable empirical truths sufficient for God's purpose for man. No moral absolutes were engraved upon man's heart or head, only the psychological mechanisms of pleasure and pain or desire and aversion could bring about a sound practical grasp of good and bad, vice and virtue, in society.

> Self is that conscious thinking thing, whatever substance made up of (whether spiritual or material, simple of compounded, it matters not) which is sensible or conscious of pleasure and pain, capable of happiness or misery, and so is concerned for itself, as far as that consciousness extends.
>
> —Locke 1694: 185

This thinking provoked criticism. Where did Locke's empiricist critique of Descartes leave the very concept of integrity and moral agency, his critics asked? If everyone was an empty void at birth, was there any stable, constant individual self? Locke's thoughts on consciousness, particularly his reasoning on the unity of the self through consciousness and memory, drew praise and blame throughout the eighteenth century. Metaphysicians pressed further into how ideas were the source of our knowledge, but worried about what exactly the knowledge was that this gave us, and if it gave us as much as Locke wanted to believe (Dyde 2015). Most notably, the Scottish moral philosopher David Hume believed that ideas gave us no idea outside of those ideas themselves: no material worlds, no selves. In *A Treatise of Human Nature* (1739), Hume took Locke's epistemology of human understanding and the self a step further – something that seemed to many of his critics to be a dangerous and cynical relativism. Far from being unitarian creatures who are 'every moment intimately conscious of what we call our SELF', Hume argued, we are instead 'nothing but a bundle or collection of different perceptions, which succeed each other with an inconceivable rapidity, and are in flux and movement' (Hume 1739: T14.6.1, T1.4.6.4). The unified self was a fiction or artifice – a notion that attracted the outrage of more religiously inclined moral philosophers of the time.

That our sensual experiences are the only key to human reasoning and knowledge became a key tenet for historians, moral philosophers and political theorists at the time, from Montesquieu in *De l'esprit des lois* (The Spirit of the Laws, 1748) to Adam Smith in his *The Wealth of Nations* (1776). Here a new discipline – called the 'Science of Man' in Britain, 'anthropology' everywhere else – took for granted that we have minds. Instead, the focus was on what spurs our passions, what thoughts we think in different environments, what new selves we may become, and what personal and social relations we commerce in; these were humanity's endeavours to perfect the social and political world around it. Locke's empirical epistemology that limited experience of knowledge to the processing of sense perception was a success across Europe, everywhere spurring investigations into what mind and human thinking was, what was the self, what were sensations, and which was the most important. The more practical-minded among the medical men, such as the Swiss anatomist Albrecht von Haller (1708–1777), began to focus on the anatomical investigation of the nervous system in animals and humans, hoping to identify the channels of sensation and, ultimately, the seat of mind (Boury 2008). Other scholars were more interested in a hierarchy of the senses, hoping to identify the most important ones. The French Abbé de Condillac, for example, opted for touch, which he thoroughly investigated in his famous study *Traité des sensations* (1754). He also proposed famously not only that sensations were given, but that they could be trained in every single human. Locke's sensationalism was successful because it offered the possibility of change and betterment in individual humans and society as a whole.

Locke's legacy to the eighteenth century was a cautious confidence in the educability of man's mind and, thus, in humans as transformable and progressive social creatures. If man's mind was malleable, he could change it for the better. Locke's 'malleable mind' reflected a key belief and the greatest hope of the eighteenth-century Enlightened elites: that we can become better, more peaceful people, that human society would be governed by rational human beings training and using their sensibilities to bring happiness to all. However, the discussion on human mind and its malleability among Enlightened thinkers also pointed to one of the starkest problems in the Age of Enlightenment, at least from today's perspective. Although the Enlightenment project had the happiness of all in mind on paper, in the realities of daily life certain social groups were excluded. Non-European ethnic groups were certainly among these. After all, enslaved people were considered 'property' of white men, their work being the backbone of many eighteenth-century economies as in Britain (Curran 2011; Schiebinger 1993). But also among the white population in Europe, the aims of universal human nature, reason, progress, freedom, equality and brotherhood were 'lived' and 'experienced' differently. Historians have drawn attention to the fact that Europe's poor were hardly included in the Enlightened elites' thinking. Nor were women.

Women were assigned a specific place in European Enlightened society based on what was increasingly implied: their different 'natures'. Some women, particularly from the elites, came to participate in intellectual debate, particularly as hostesses of a new intellectual and social institution that emerged from the seventeenth century: the salon. More generally, however, women were denied full human status as individuals at precisely the time that men were increasingly defining themselves as autonomous individual actors in the legal and economic spheres. Between men and women, a gap opened in regard to the rights and autonomy increasingly demanded by men and the dependence still demanded from women (Outram 2013: 85). Some women, such as the early feminist Mary Wollstonecraft, became fully aware of these inconsistencies arising from the new liberal Enlightenment ideals of a universal human nature and a society and daily life that was still organized on patriarchal structures.

Specifically, Enlightenment thinkers made great efforts to define femininity and to assign women to the domestic sphere. In moral, philosophical, medical and scientific advice literature, which became popular at the time, it was implied that women were virtually a separate species within the human race. Increasingly, their anatomy – their minds and bodies – were put forward to cement their separation from men. Women were characterized by their innate inferior capacity for rational reasoning due to their small anatomical build and skulls, their reproductive functions and their nerves. Rational reasoning was simply not for them, as much medical advice literature drummed home. In other words, women were not capable of thinking without passion, prejudice and superstition, or without reference to non-identifiable statements (such as religious revelation) in ways that would keep incoming sensual perceptions in check and ordered, according to sensationalists such as Locke or Hume (Outram 2013: 100). Women, it was implied, were 'different' human beings from men by their very nature. To paraphrase Mary Wollstonecraft's *Vindication of the Rights of Women*: the male is male at certain moments, but – forever denied education – the female is female her whole life. Men had 'at least an opportunity of exerting themselves with dignity, and of rising by the exertions which really improve a rational creature', but women's 'moral character may be estimated by their manner of fulfilling those simple duties [as daughters, wives and mothers]' (Wollstonecraft 1792: 48, 122).

These contradictions about gender clustered around the ambiguous concept of 'nature' (Outram 2013: 87). Nature, the very subject matter of political, legal, and philosophical as well as medical and scientific thinking, became something like the ethical norm and authority of Enlightened eighteenth-century society. What was natural must be 'good', was the motto. Jean-Jacques Rousseau, in his widely read educational work *Émile, or On Education* (1763), was to define femininity as 'natural' and hence both right and ineluctable. In doing so, he and his many followers attached the debate on femininity and rational reasoning to one of the central concerns of the Enlightenment: the nature of 'nature'. 'Natural' could mean many things, as Dorinda Outram has made clear. It could mean 'not socially defined', 'not artificial' or 'based on the external physical world' (Outram 2013: 87).

Overwhelmingly, 'the natural' was used (often in a mixture of all these meanings) to legitimate and control arrangements that in the twenty-first century we would see as socially created. But 'naturalness' was also often used to legitimate arguments aimed at bringing into being a state of affairs which did not yet fully exist. 'Natural', in other words, was an excellent way to argue for points of view that were in fact often novel and always highly prescriptive. Social arrangements could be given additional validation by being presented as natural. And nature and its laws were usually considered above politics. Arguments for the naturalness of feminine roles could thus, because of the ambiguity of the term, gain force simultaneously from biological arguments about created nature and from repeated Enlightenment polemics against 'artificiality' in society. By artificiality, Enlightenment thinkers meant social practices that were held to be at odds with the true structures of 'human nature'.

The extreme ambiguity of the term 'nature' could thus be used in multiple ways to define femininity in this period. As Outram explains, women were increasingly defined as closer to nature than were men, as well as being more determined by 'nature', meaning, increasingly, their anatomy and physiology. The notion that women were closer to nature than men included both the claim that because of their physical nature they were prone to sensations, emotional, credulous and incapable of rational reasoning and, at the same time, that due to their reproductive organs and 'finer nerves' women were the carriers within the family of a new morality through which the 'unnaturalness' of civilization, its artificiality, could be transcended and a society created which was natural, polite and modern (Outram 2013: 87). Despite all the ambiguities, one point stands out clearly. In spite of the Enlightenment tendency to define the 'natural' as good, women's equation with nature did not operate in such a way as to give them equality with or superiority over men; rather, on the contrary, it operated to define women as 'the Other'. The 'Other', moreover, was to be defined, unlike men, whose nature was obvious and right.

From the seventeenth century on, all sorts of moral, philosophical and educational texts, together with sermons, poetry, novels, conduct literature and pedagogical writings, discussed the natural role of women as part of 'the betterment' of society. Originating in court culture and in the polite salon society of France during the seventeenth century, and reaching the British Isles in the later seventeenth century, these writings advanced the then novel idea that women's inherent moral and intellectual differences embodied all the good and beautiful in the 'new' society. Women were born to keep the 'unruly' male in check, it was claimed. In a world in which liberal and democratic tendencies were increasingly discussed, women, with their innate 'chastity' and 'delicate timidity of mind', were assigned a key role in upholding the social order and preventing potential anarchy. Central to this Europe-wide discussion about the natural rights of the sexes was Rousseau's *Émile*. It opened the flood-gates to modern prescriptive literature on the proper character and education of the sexes by emphasizing the development of the soul not through cultivating the mind but through improving mind and body in concert with one another.

For Rousseau, it was the purpose of natural philosophy to read in the book of nature 'everything which suits the constitution of her [woman's] species and her sex in order to fulfil her place in the physical and moral order' (quoted in Schiebinger 1986: 67). Thus was initiated the view that women's inherent physical, moral and intellectual differences from men suited them for roles in society vastly different from those of men (Schiebinger 1986: 91). *Émile* presented woman as being naturally fitted to domestic duties, particularly to providing warm maternal care for her children and loving companionship for her spouse. Woman's natural role, Rousseau argued, was that of a mother, an ideal considered to be natural and therefore both 'right' and inescapable. This notion was even propagated in the fine arts, where it was fashionable to paint

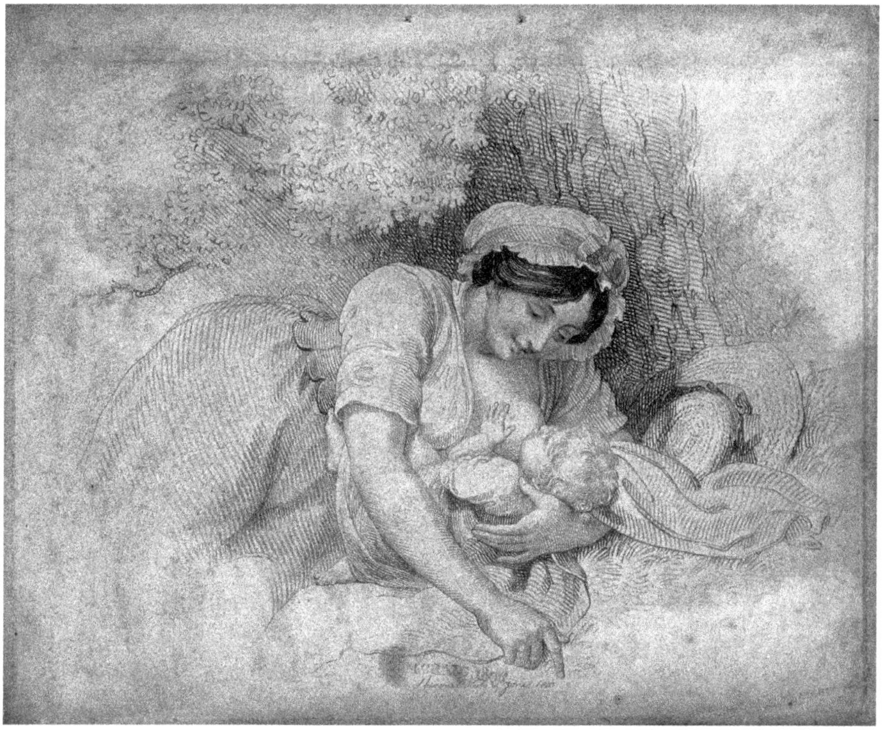

FIGURE 7.2: A woman breastfeeding her child, 1810 (after W. M. Craig, 1806). Credit: Wellcome Collection, London/Public Domain.

pictures of mothers holding their children – often breastfeeding. The breastfeeding simultaneously demonstrated women's closeness to 'nature' and emphasized the unnaturalness of wet-nursing, which was typically practised by well-to-do European families (Schiebinger 1993: 66–70).

The home was the realm of the female 'Other', Enlightened opinion-makers agreed. But so too was the world of polite sociability, for which certain traits ideally fitted women: namely, love of peace, natural refinement of manner and, most crucially, instinctive tenderness or sympathy for others – attributes characteristic of all good Christians but present in women to an exceptional degree. Women, British Enlightenment thinkers agreed, were primary bearers of the 'affections', meaning not just love of family and other intimates but the 'social sympathies' on which civilized progress depended, since it was through feminine influence that bellicose men and their uncivil sex were 'softened' into social beings (Taylor 2005: 42). What 'better school for manners' could there be, it was rhetorically asked by the moral philosopher and champion of sensibility, David Hume:

> than the company of virtuous women, where the mutual endeavour to please must insensibly polish the mind, where the example of female softness and modesty must communicate itself to their admirers, and where the delicacy of that sex puts every one on his guard, lest he give offence by any breach of decency?
>
> —quoted in Taylor 2005: 42

Hume also backed up his view on the natural place of women in Enlightened society through history. Together with other Scottish thinkers, such as Adam Smith, Adam Ferguson or the more controversial Lord Monboddo, Hume was significant in popularizing a linear 'conjectural history' or 'stadial history' of humankind which traced the progressive story of human civilization from stages of savagery – passing societies of hunting, pasture and agriculture – to the Enlightened European society of commerce. Such thinking became widespread and gained great credence. And women were central to it – to the stories of civilization that traced progress from 'savagery' and 'slavery' to 'civilized' members of advanced societies of 'commerce'. (Indeed, the word 'commerce' incorporated the essence of all that Enlightenment writers considered 'modern'. Formerly it had referred only to relations between the sexes, but the Scots broadened it to include financial and intellectual exchange [Sebastiani 2013; Hirschmann 1997]). Most Scottish writers within the tradition of conjectural history saw human history as being marked by a process of 'feminization', while the condition of women was taken as a benchmark. However, as historian Silvia Sebastiani has aptly remarked, this also marked the limit to the progress of civilization. Monogamic marriage was considered by Hume and fellow historians to be the natural locus of the relationship between the sexes, thereby confining the horizon of women to the private sphere and family relations. Women's minds had a narrow space in which to dwell (Sebastiani 2013: 134).

Such underlying presumptions about the natural role of women in society became so deeply engrained that they were imbibed even by early feminists, such as Wollstonecraft – one of the fiercest critics of Rousseau's views on women in *Émile*. While on the one hand she aimed to achieve a character as a human being, regardless of the distinctions of sex, on the other, she took for granted that women were *naturally* more modest. She believed that 'all the causes of female weakness' resulted from the 'want of chastity in men' (Dabhoiwala 2012: 190). Most feminists followed her in this. Her friend Mary Hays, for example, an equally bold philosophical and political thinker fighting for women's intellectual equality and rationality, thought it obvious that

> modesty is innate to a much a greater degree in women than in men. The history of all nations, – of the human races, wild and tame, social and savage – all, all agree in this great truth; and would delicacy permit, a thousand and a thousand arguments might be adducted to support a fact, so undeniably, so sacredly true; – so dear to the happiness of individuals and society; – so essential to domestic bliss. And, at the same time a truth, the most honorable and flattering to the female sex; enslaved and mortified as they are, in so many other cases.
>
> —quoted in Dabhoiwala 2012: 190

For Wollstonecraft and Hays, and many other feminists of the eighteenth century, women were more chaste than men, and it was important to them that it should remain so, for the laws of reason and nature alike. This idea continued to gain strength, being accepted as virtually a self-evident fact by the twentieth century. This was ironic, since it strengthened a sexual double standard. The idea that women's moral superiority would improve men's manners could not easily be decoupled from their assumed intellectual inferiority (Dabhoiwala 2012: 190).

Medical men were prominent among the writers on women's physical and intellectual capacities. The knowledge of their profession, so they claimed, bestowed on them the special authority to speak and write on the laws of human nature. It placed them at the forefront of discussions about women's capacities and the relation of the sexes in polite society. Although medical theories on women's weaker minds and bodies originated in antiquity, what changed in the Enlightenment was the increasing reliance on medical 'evidence' to back up these ideas. Medical treaties were heavily quoted in moral philosophical, historical and pedagogical texts on the origins and development of mankind and the differences between the sexes. The eighteenth century, Dorinda Outram reminds us, did not make our modern distinction between nurture (the role of education, training and social expectations in the making of human character) and nature (the role of human biology). Rather, many thinkers believed that physical differences directly generated the social roles assigned to each sex. Based on the implications of contemporary medical texts, Rousseau in *Émile*, for example, authoritatively claimed that women's occupations 'were taken to be rooted in, restricted to, and a necessary consequence of their reproductive functions' (Jordanova 1989: 29). Of course, it must be said that the deep divide between 'nature' and 'nurture' is essentially a nineteenth-century one, as is the idea that the scientific medical 'gaze' is objective, neutral and devoid of any social and cultural implications (Daston and Galison 2007).

Among those who promoted the differences between the sexes was the Aberdeen doctor John Gregory (1724–1773). He had moved to Edinburgh in 1764 when he was appointed to the chair in medicine and became royal physician (Lawrence 2004). Gregory was the author of one of the most renowned and bestselling books on feminine conduct of the second half of the eighteenth century: *A Father's Legacy to His Daughters* (1774), 'a study not merely fitted to amuse and gratify curiosity, but a study subservient to the noblest views, to the cultivation and improvement of the Human Species'. Gregory drew not only on conjectural history as evidence for his claims but also on the findings from a new field in medicine that gained prominence during the eighteenth century: comparative anatomy. Indeed, it has recently been argued that the new progressive conception of history actually emerged from a systematic use of the comparative approach in medicine (Sebastiani 2013: 136–7).

Comparison with animal bodies and behaviour, Gregory argued in one of his earlier works (*A Comparative View of the State and Faculties of Man with Those of the Animal World,* 1765) made it possible to assert man's peculiarity and to place his social characteristics in a natural hierarchical order. To Gregory and many others, comparative anatomy thus offered 'to the bone' evidence as to the debates on the different mental, bodily and social capacities of men and women. The female skeleton, including the skull, became of interest to anatomists only during the eighteenth century, as Londa Schiebinger (1986) has shown. Early anatomical drawings, by contrast, such as the famous ones by Andreas Vesalius, had depicted an idealized male body only – the default body according to classical medical theory. Earlier images showed two major differences between men and women: those of the external bodily form and the reproductive organs. But the first drawings of female skeletons that appeared in England, France and Germany between 1730 and 1790 reflected a growing interest in the finer delineation of sex differences; the goal was to discover, describe and define sex differences in every bone, muscle, nerve and vein. The *Encyclopédie* article of 1765 on the 'skeleton' devoted half of its text to a comparison of the male and female skeleton. Differences were laid out in detail, including the male and female spine, clavicle, sternum, coccyx, pelvis and skull. The article concluded: 'All of these facts prove that the destiny of women was to have children and to nourish them' (quoted in Schiebinger 1986: 68). Interest grew. By 1750, Edmond Thomas Moreau published a slim book in Paris entitled *A Medical Question: Whether Apart from Genitalia There Is a Difference Between the Sexes?* His answer was 'yes'. In 1775, the French physician Pierre Roussel reproached his colleagues for considering woman similar to man except in sexual organs: 'The essence of sex', he explained, 'is not confined to a single organ but extends, through more or less perceptible nuances, into every part' (quoted in Schiebinger 1986: 51). This belief was also expressed in contemporary writings on disease, especially those of the nerves.

In *The English Malady or, a Treatise of Nervous Diseases of all Kinds; as Spleen, Vapours, Lowness of Spirits, Hypochondriacal, and Hysterical Distempers, Etc.* (1733), George Cheyne diagnosed eighteenth-century England as suffering from a chronic condition that was the flip-side of Enlightenment reason: hypochondria (in men) and hysteria (in women). Heavy diet, comfortable and sedentary lifestyles, and urban living had resulted in nervous disorders running rampant. The historian George Rousseau notes that hysteria was reframed as a nervous problem over the course of the century and increasingly was seen as the same problem as hypochondria. The popularity of the nervous body, he argues, was closely connected to the Enlightenment insistence on formal behaviour and the demonstration of reason; the opposite was the abnormality and pathology of the uncontrolled and uncontrollable body. Nervous illness had its own language, which could be learned: fainting, weeping, blushing. The public sociable personality of daytime might, at home in private, suddenly become subject to the dark fears of night-time, dreams of incubi and succubi, sleepwalking – moments when unreason might re-emerge (Rousseau 1993: 158–62).

Indeed, nerves and reason went together. Popular medical practitioners such as Sir John Hill and other Enlightenment thinkers recognized that learned men were most subject to hypochondria; intellectual work was fatiguing. It provided insufficient exercise to keep the fibres of mind and body in tip-top condition. For women, however, the diagnosis of hysteria was a sign of their irrationality and weaker nature. Not all of them were content to accept this diagnosis, however, as some contemporary medical consultation letters suggest (Beatty 2012). For example, between 1722 and 1734, Lady Catherine Sondes wrote to the eminent London physician Sir Hans Sloane to ask advice on her bodily twitching, drooping on one side of the face, rising nerves, fast heartbeat, flatulence, strange frights, bad dreams, gnawing pain and memory loss. Initially, her personal physician Dr Colby diagnosed her as hysterical, which Lady Sondes rejected. She was satisfied with Dr Colby only when he changed his diagnosis to a blood disorder. For Lady Sondes, who discussed her satisfaction at being busy and physically active, a diagnosis of a nervous disease that came with the stigma of sedentariness and weakness was wholly unacceptable (Smith 2008: 468–71).

Women also became potentially subject to their embodied passions in another way: lustfulness. George Rousseau suggests that diagnoses of hysteria throughout history were often linked to a concern with women's raging sexual appetites and were sometimes related to lovesickness. Although hysteria was subsumed under the nerves and made parallel to men's hypochondria, this did not make women's bodies any less animal (1993: 105, 112, 180). It merely shifted the problem to masturbation fears, which can be situated within the wider social changes that prioritized penetrative and reproductive sex (Laqueur 2003; Hitchcock 2012). The anonymous author of *The Ladies Dispensatory* (1739), a popular advice manual, recounted two cautionary tales of masturbating women. One young woman abused herself between the ages of fourteen and nineteen, resulting in a *furor uterinus* (nymphomania). During increasingly violent fits, the woman undressed and violently attacked any man nearby. She died soon after, at which point doctors and surgeons anatomized her. They found that her clitoris had swollen abnormally and that her blood appeared especially sharp and corrosive. In the other story, a young woman discovered masturbation at the age of eleven with her mother's chambermaid. Seven years later, she had developed a clitoris so large that she appeared to be a hermaphrodite. The doctors attributed this to clitoral relaxation. Through masturbation, both young women became masculine and sexually aggressive, with uncontrollable bodies (*Ladies Dispensatory*, 1739: 8, 10). Taking this to its logical conclusion, the body of a female masturbator might even create its own offspring, independent of human action. Thus, physician G. A. Douglas argued in his book *The Nature and Causes of Impotence in Men, and Barrenness in Women* (1758) that false conceptions could be caused by self-abuse. He suggested that women needed vaginal stimulation in order to make an egg descend. If a woman used 'those shameful implements' to stimulate herself, she would produce an egg that would remain unfertilized and grow so that it resembled a pregnancy. Women, he warned, 'should know this and tremble' (Douglas 1758: 16–17). Given the loss of bodily control, it is no wonder that female masturbation was seen as dangerous. Masturbation resulted in inverted social and sexual hierarchies: men became womanly and women became manly. Worse yet, the uncontrolled female body, devoid of any reason and unthinkingly following lust, made a mockery of the ends of marriage.

If women's bodies were not to be trusted, neither were their minds; women did not need to be hysterical to have excessive imaginations and fears. Women (and servants) were blamed for instilling unreason in their children. In *Some Thoughts Concerning Education* (1745 [1693]), Locke described the bogeyman Raw-head and Bloody-bones, a story told by nursemaids and mothers that was allegedly as pernicious as a disease in its effects on their minds:

> [their] usual Method is to awe Children, and keep them in subjection, by telling them of Raw-head and Bloody-bones, and such other Names as carry with them the Ideas of something terrible and hurtful, which they have Reason to be afraid of when alone, especially in the Dark. This must be carefully prevented: For though by this foolish way, they may keep them from little Faults, yet the Remedy is much worse than the Disease.
>
> —Locke, 1745 [1693]: 200

The real problem was the long-term damage of such tales in the education of young *men*. Locke noted that the minds of the young were impressionable and that such fancies 'frequently haunt them with strange Visions, making Children Dastards when alone, and afraid of their Shadows and Darkness all their Lives after' (201). He provided a cautionary account: 'There was in a Town in the West a Man of a disturbed Brain, whom the Boys used to teaze when he came in their way.' One day, the man seized a sword from a nearby cutler's shop and chased a boy. The boy escaped to his house, but chanced to look behind 'to see how near his Pursuer was, who was at the Entrance of the Porch, with his Sword up ready to strike; and he had just Time to get in, and clap to the Door to avoid the Blow, which, though his Body escaped, his Mind did not' (202). The boy was haunted into adulthood by the memory, always having to check behind him when going in that door.

Others, such as James Forrester in his *Dialogues on the Passions, Habits, and Affections Peculiar to Children* (1748), amplified and elaborated such stories, casting blame specifically on nurses, mothers and grandmothers. Forrester mused that 'something of Raw-head and Bloody-bones occurs to you as often as you look into a dark unfrequented Corner of a Church', which came from 'some Remains of the Nursery, some Remnants of Fear, and that Idea of Dread, which, Thanks to our Mothers and Grandmothers, is constantly connected with Churches, Church-years, and Charnel-houses' (Forrester 1748: 27). Once again women were painted into a corner, accused of emasculating males, virtually denaturing them. 'If the Spirit is kept long in this Subjection', argued Forrester:

> Timidity becomes a Habit, and nothing afterwards can persuade it to look at the most visible Terror, and all he Marks of Cowardice, which is the lowest and most abject State, to which a rational Creature can be reduced.
>
> —37

The reasons behind Raw-head and Bloody-bones' punishment apparently needed no explanation, since the real terror of the nursery – for the Enlightened male – was the long-term effects on masculine rationality, perpetuated by the wild imaginations of women and servants.

From a modern perspective, what is most interesting about all this writing on nerves, passions, hypochondria, child terrorization and so on is that the brain is never the central link between these discussions in medicine, pedagogy, or moral and natural philosophy. Its place in the debates about humanity was wholly inferior. It was only at the end of the eighteenth century that this changed, and forever. This was largely due to one man, Franz Joseph Gall (1758–1828), along with his German physician colleague, Johann Spurzheim (1776–1832), who was to be responsible for disseminating Gall's ideas in Britain. Gall was something of a showman who gallivanted around Europe entertaining popular audiences with an impressive collection of skulls. But he was also a serious physiologist and what we would call today a neuroanatomist. He lectured on his ideas to august medical audiences. After graduating from the Vienna school of medicine in 1785, he set up in private practice in a fashionable part of the capital. But he aspired to more. He wanted to make a name for himself in science and medicine, specifically to contribute to the Enlightenment project of a science of humankind. In the best spirit of the Enlightenment, he rejected classical interpretations of the soul. Becoming obsessed with the observation of individual personality traits and differences in behaviours, he eventually arrived as his theory of *cranioscopie* or *organologie* (later popularized, by Spurzheim, as phrenology, the theory of brain and science of character based on reading from bumps on the skull).

Through *cranioscopie*, Gall, 'the naturalist of the mind' (as he has been called), posited not only that the brain was the organ of the mind but that individual character traits could be localized in different compartments or 'faculties' of the brain. Moreover – and this was what made phrenology anathema to upright philosophers and intellectuals, but at the same time made it especially popular in early nineteenth-century Britain – Gall claimed that the inside contours of the brain could be read from the outside of the skull as a result of its early ossification. Initially, he identified some twenty-six separate mental faculties, such as those for 'wit', 'religion' and 'love of offspring'. These were organized according to a conventional hierarchy, with the morally superior faculties such as those of 'language' and 'religion' at the top and front of the brain, while those more 'primitive', such as the 'conjugal', were relegated to a lower and more posterior position.

The idea of 'mental faculties' was not new; it was well-worn in contemporary metaphysics and moral philosophy as well as in medicine, as in John Gregory's *A Comparative View of the State and Faculties of Man* (1765). But in those writings, 'faculties' were conceptual entities, not material things. Gall's immortal claim to fame was to transform the conceptual into the material, reifying mind into matter through biology (Young 1970). In so doing, he undermined the *tabula rasa* idea of mind promoted by John Locke, the line of thought that ascribed more to nurture than to nature (van Wyhe 2002). For Gall, 'brain

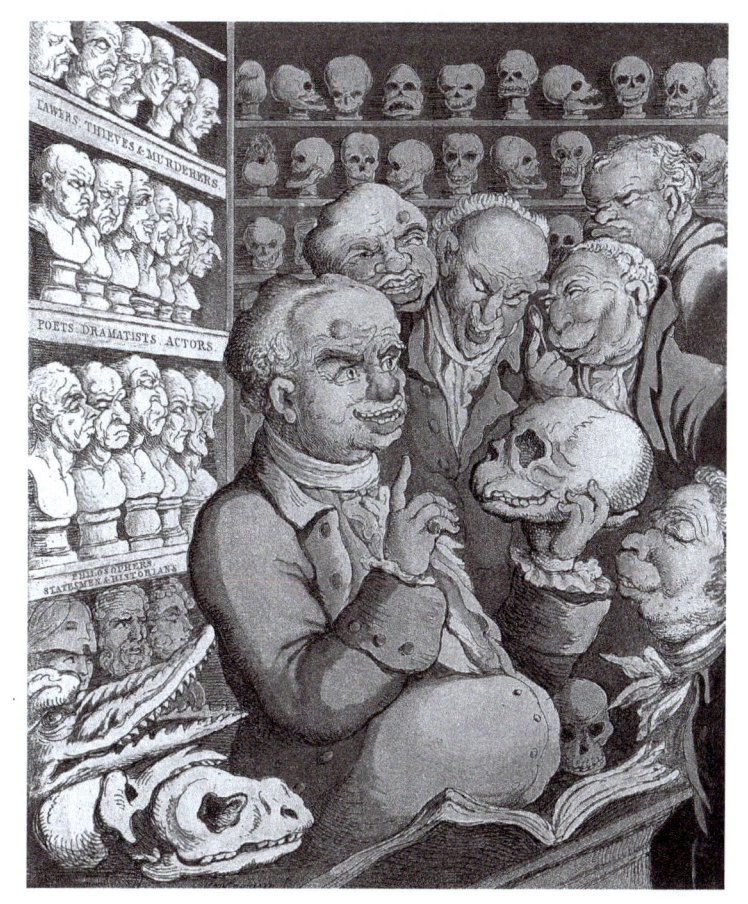

FIGURE 7.3: Franz Joseph Gall leading a discussion on phrenology with five colleagues, among his extensive collection of skulls and model heads, by Thomas Rowlandson (1808). Credit: Wellcome Collection, London/Public Domain.

organization' pointed to individual differences that could be passed down in families and remain stable over a lifetime. In 1791 he published the first volume of his findings, which were later extended into what was posthumously published, in English, as *On the Functions of the Brain and Each of its Parts: with observations on the possibility of determining the instincts, propensities and talents, or the moral and intellectual dispositions of man and animals by the configuration of the brain and head* (1835). It was a work that, along with Gall's lecturing on the subject, lead Francis II to banish him from Austria in 1801 on grounds of being a heretical materialist. Gall then took up residence in Paris, spending most of his time examining the skulls of inmates of prisons and mental asylums, especially murderers and sexual 'deviants' (Young 1990).

The materialization of man through brain biology was something difficult to resist except though religious argument. Nor were the racial and gender implications of Gall's theory of brain easily contested, or desired to be. By then, as we have seen, these social hierarchies were well established; Gall simply biologized them in the brain. Understanding and explaining individual differences was, in fact, a major aim of his research programme. And of course, within this programme, women's brains were deemed to be smaller and more delicate.

With this biologization of mind into brain, the inherent contradictions of the Enlightenment disappeared. The new theory of brain (as a fixed, non-malleable thing) trashed the old Enlightenment ambiguities. What was now to be legitimated through biology was straightforward double standards, about which no one had to be guilty; they were solidly legitimized in the brain with its hierarchy of functions. Character was no longer infinitely malleable (van Wyhe 2004). Gall and Spurzheim had introduced a biological predestination: you were what you were by birth, 'nature'. And 'nature' now was unambiguous; the facts of brain science wouldn't allow ambiguity. Nature had been made limited and finite, caged in the skull. Ironically, the only place left for the *inherent contradiction* of the Enlightenment was in the mind – in minds like that of Mary Wollstonecraft that were torn between what they believed was the 'nature' of women and their legitimate arguments for change and rights. With the biologization of the brain, so ended the Enlightenment's preoccupation with the dualism of mind and matter, reason and thinking, and sensationalism and imagination; the Enlightenment's inherent contradictions were smoothed away.

NOTE

1. This chapter was originally composed by Sean Dyde, who, through illness, was unable to complete it. We have used some of his material in the first section. We are grateful to Lisa Smith for helping us with the final version and allowing us to include sections on pages 162–3, sometimes verbatim, from her blog posts at *Wonders & Marvels* on 'Nursery Terrors' and 'Masturbation & the Dangerous Woman'.

CHAPTER EIGHT

Authority

ANGELA HAAS

When Marie-Anne Pigalle began to cough up blood in November 1758, her physicians and surgeons did everything in their power to heal her.[1] According to her own deposition, she endured three bleedings over the course of January 1759. As her condition worsened, her doctor prescribed broths of red cabbage, veal and frogs, and the following month he prescribed her cows' and asses' milk to ease the stomach pains these broths had caused. She then developed a fever. After bathing in various concoctions of the doctor's invention, her fever continued to worsen. On 25 March, her doctor decided to try each of these remedies a second time, only to conclude that she had incurable tubercles in her lungs. She saw another doctor, who bled her twice more and prescribed her a broth of frogs and snails, which complicated her condition further; he eventually concluded, too, that she was incurable. At last, Marie-Anne decided to decline all further treatment, placing her faith in the divine power of the Eucharist, by which she was reportedly healed on 14 June (de L'Épée 1759: 1–22).

In the eighteenth century, licensed medical practitioners commonly presented their art as the surest source of better health. Church and state authorities turned to those educated in Europe's most elite institutions as the official judges of novel remedies, extraordinary cures, and various legal matters related to health and the human body. Despite these duties, many people – ranging from religious polemicists to humble practitioners to mesmerists – argued that this authority was undeserved. For example, published narratives of extraordinary sicknesses and cures sometimes subtly (and often overtly) showcased the incompetence of medical practitioners. These accounts included detailed narratives of sicknesses and medical treatments, usually from the perspective of female patients and their familiars, and commonly expressed their frustration with ineffective remedies. A demonstrated inability to cure patients meant that the formal medical authority of elite practitioners could be easily contested in the printed debates of the Enlightenment, as authors asserted that perhaps patients, rather than practitioners, were most qualified to judge matters of health and sickness.

Historians have long overlooked the failures and limitations of medicine, focusing instead on success stories of medical breakthroughs and developments. Before the late twentieth century, scholarship on pre-1800 Europe sought to identify the origins of the modern medical profession, crafting a teleological story of the triumph of scientifically minded male practitioners in the wake of the Scientific Revolution. Scholarship focused principally on famous medical men like Andreas Vesalius and William Harvey (O'Malley 1964; Whitteridge 1971). Their authority, it was generally thought, eclipsed that of laypeople and practitioners whose approach to health and healing appeared less scientific – and thus less familiar to modern eyes. By the 1970s, historians were challenging such triumphalist narratives of professionalization, questioning whether the groups that so closely related to modern medical practitioners (licensed physicians and surgeons) had been uniquely skilled or readily granted authority in the past. Thomas McKeown, for example, considered whether medicine had even contributed significantly to the general decline of mortality rates in Europe from the eighteenth century (McKeown 1979). Even the rise of clinical medicine, often seen as the most important medical development of the eighteenth century, had its drawbacks. Michel Foucault famously argued that the rise of teaching hospitals had deeply negative consequences, including the dehumanizing process of separating the patient's body from their self (Foucault 1973).

By the 1980s, scholars had shifted their focus to the social history of medicine, with its 'bottom-up' view of the pre-modern medical world. Following the lead of historians in the Annales school, who had incorporated discussions of the popular experience of medicine and disease into their 'total histories', scholars of France began to consider medical authority from the perspective of patients and the various factors that limited the power of elite practitioners (Forster and Ranum 1980). For example, François Lebrun's detailed study of popular views of medicine revealed that French people had recourse to a wide range of healers – from physicians and surgeons to empirics and healing saints – all of whom possessed medical authority. While earlier professional histories traced the rise of the professional and the fall of the charlatan, Lebrun (1983) argued that the divide between the 'official' medical profession (which focused on natural healing) and other medical practitioners (who relied on magical and religious healing) was artificial. Using a social history approach, Matthew Ramsey (1988) suggested that there was a sharper divide between popular and learned medicine but found negative popular attitudes towards elite practitioners. As scholars began to study the perspectives of laypeople, it became clear that a wider range of practitioners enjoyed some degree of medical authority and, significantly, that the skill of 'professionals' was disputed.

Considerations of lay perspectives also led to a breakthrough in understandings of patients' power over their own health and medical services. For example, rather than being pushed out of the medical world by the monolithic power of professionals, it became clear that patients played an important role in shaping medical services and practices in their capacity as consumers. Studies on the 'medical marketplace' revealed that practitioners of all types competed for patients' approval. Indeed, elite practitioners often had difficulty keeping up with those who were more skilled in the art of self-promotion. In the English context, scholars such as Harold Cook, Roy Porter and Mary Fissell showed that the early modern medical world was unregulated, with few signs of a distinct, scientific medical culture before 1800 (Cook 1986; Porter 1989; Fissell 1991). Scholars such as Colin Jones (1996), David Gentilcore (2006), Isabelle Coquillard (2018) and Philip Rieder (2018) have identified similar trends in France and Italy. The 'medical marketplace' has become a staple concept in histories of early modern medicine. Not only does it allow scholars to consider the choices of laypeople, it also provides a framework for discussing interactions and conflicts between different types of practitioners.

Historians now know that medical authority was shared by a much wider range of practitioners and lay healers than previously thought, and that medical knowledge, commonly associated with the European male, was shaped by contemporary views of gender and race. Since the 1990s, scholars have considered medical practitioners who had been marginalized in teleological histories of the emergence of modern medicine. For example, the histories of medical professions had typically treated them as masculine domains, overlooking the authority of female practitioners. The medical practices of women, even midwives, were treated as inferior, and thus were destined to be supplanted by those of professional, male practitioners. Susan Broomhall's work on female practitioners in early modern France (2004), by contrast, shows that women enjoyed a considerable degree of medical authority, providing the majority of medical care to rich and poor alike – and using dynamic medical practices. Contributors to Hilary Marland's edited volume *The Art of Midwifery* (1993) revealed the great range of skills, functions and statuses of female midwives across Europe. Lianne McTavish's study of midwifery in France (2005) shows that male and female midwives alike embodied both feminine and masculine characteristics in their treatises and that their authority was challenged in similar ways. Scholarship on female midwives has further suggested that they were not supplanted by male practitioners in all parts of Europe, and that where they were, the process had less to do with the inferiority of their practice and more to do with a growing tendency to associate rationality and scientific medicine with men (Kosmin 2020; Cody 2005). Histories of female practitioners reveal that medical authority in

Europe was not exclusively male or masculine. Recent studies in the colonial context have shown similarly that medical authority was not exclusively European, as historians have begun to reveal the medical authority of Indigenous and enslaved people, who helped to shape European medical theories and practices (Chakrabarti 2010; Schiebinger 2017).

While scholars have identified common trends across regions, in all cases local structures affected power dynamics in ways that can only be fully understood within specific cultural, social and political contexts. When studying a single region, it is easier to see how unique factors, including political disputes, social hierarchies and religious structures, shaped medical authority within a specific time and place. This chapter uses eighteenth-century France as a case study for examining the shifting boundaries between formal medical authority, granted by law, and informal medical authority, granted by popular consent. Those who practised medicine legally within the kingdom did so with royal or local permission. The basic structure of the corporative medical community emerged in the sixteenth century as a tripartite system of guilds, which granted licences to physicians, surgeons and apothecaries. Traditionally, those trained in the prestigious medical faculties, such as the Faculty of Medicine in Paris, enjoyed the highest social status and the greatest legal authority, and surgeons and apothecaries were legally subordinate to physicians. However, by the middle of the eighteenth century many of these traditional boundaries were blurred – the prestige of graduate master surgeons was comparable to that of physicians; critics characterized the Faculty of Medicine in Paris as backward; and the roles of physicians, surgeons and apothecaries increasingly overlapped, leading to conflicts over jurisdiction (Gelfand 1980; Rabier 2007). Many outside the tripartite system also practised legally, including expert oculists, herniotomists, dentists, midwives and bone-setters, while others enjoyed de facto legal status. To further complicate matters, most actually practised within what Lawrence Brockliss and Colin Jones call the 'medical penumbra', which included a wide array of unlicensed empirics and drug peddlers (Brockliss and Jones 1997). Even the most elite physicians found themselves competing on a relatively open market with those who were legally at the bottom of the hierarchy and technically breaking the law, a testament to the fact that legal status and prestigious training did not always translate to medical authority from the perspective of patients.

Within the context of the Enlightenment, the expansion of literacy and print further undermined traditional medical authority as established by law. Using discourse analysis, this chapter examines the polemical strategies authors employed to bolster or undermine the reputation of certain groups and individuals and thus their authority to judge matters of sickness and health. The work of Lindsay Wilson and Cathy McClive on medical debates during the French Enlightenment has shown that medical and legal debates often accentuated the uncertainty of medical judgement (Wilson 1993; McClive 2008, 2012).

Print could be a useful tool for medical practitioners looking to gain the support of the reading public, but it was an equally useful tool for their opponents. This chapter addresses the use of printed media to reinforce practitioners' authority as judges. However, I focus especially on opposition to the practitioners and the various polemical devices used to exploit their weaknesses and undermine their authority, while simultaneously bolstering the authority of lay witnesses to interpret events.

While the authority of the medical community was already dispersed among a wide range of practitioners, medical controversies threatened to further dilute that authority as those without medical training claimed the ability to judge medical matters. This was especially the case in the printed debates that form the basis of this study: publicized medical controversies over reported marvellous or miraculous cures and illnesses. Historians long ignored such controversies, which were eclipsed by discussions of the secularization and naturalization of medicine, or 'the desacralization of sickness' (Lebrun 1983: 8). Viewing the Enlightenment as a rationalizing and secularizing force, traditional histories of the Enlightenment largely ignored religious currents and sympathetic discussions of the supernatural, or pitted reason (physicians and anatomists) against superstition (folk medicine) (Cunningham and Grell 2007: 1). Historians of medicine have overlooked debates about supernatural phenomena during the Enlightenment, seeing them as irrelevant aberrations in an age of reason and scientific progress. This chapter elucidates those discussions, building on recent historiographical shifts towards the cultural history of ideas and examining debates beyond the elite circles of the philosophes and their patrons.

To understand Enlightenment medical authority, it is crucial to pay attention to reports and discussions of the preternatural (beyond what is usual in nature) or supernatural (beyond the laws of nature) phenomena; indeed, most 'triumphant' stories of bodily healing during this period had little to do with medicine. Eighteenth-century medicine failed the most basic function of being able to heal people, which left a chasm for other sources of healing. Cures were attributed to unofficial saints and magnetizers, who professed to heal people through the use of iron filings, rather than to physicians, surgeons and apothecaries. Famous philosophes may have launched a full-scale attack on the supernatural, but it proved resilient. The eighteenth century saw some of the most widely attested and debated miracles in French history, and publications containing stories of marvellous events abounded. Lorraine Daston and Katherine Park remind us that even those Enlightenment philosophers who rejected the supernatural did little to debunk marvels or miracles, preferring to ignore them as something associated with the 'vulgar' masses (Daston and Park 1998). Even so, people from all walks of life were fascinated by controversies over the supernatural (Darnton 1968; Fleming 2013). Authors even appealed to their broad readership by carefully laying out the evidence for or against the authenticity of these cures and illnesses. As such, printed debates over supernatural and liminal phenomena can be especially useful for examining medical authority, as they enabled a large segment of the population to judge for themselves which medical authorities – whether elite physicians, local oculists or patients – they found most reliable. Medical controversies reveal competing views of the authority of medical professionals, the reliability of witness testimony and the prerogatives of patients.

There were two antagonistic trends at work in eighteenth-century France. On the one hand, scholars like Lindsay Wilson have shown that medical practitioners, supported by church and state, sought to take medicine 'out of the hands of local empirics and of the people themselves' (Wilson 1993: 114). On the other hand, partly in response to this first trend, people sought to recapture this control through alternative means such as medical self-help literature, the medical marketplace and mesmerism. Ramsey argues that distrust of professional medicine gave rise to 'medical republicanism' in late eighteenth-century France – that is, 'the view that medicine belonged, not to the doctors, but to the people' (1988: 69). A 'publicist' vision for medicine emerged during this period, championing the public as the best judge of the viability and scientific authority of medical cures (Brockliss and Jones 1997: 31). The examination of debates over miracles, medical marvels and mesmerism presented below provides further evidence of these trends. It was through these debates that the authority of elite practitioners was both challenged and reinforced, and patient voices were simultaneously defended and trivialized. Reports of miracles and medical marvels were difficult to verify but also, if one trusted witness testimony, difficult to debunk. Elite physicians and surgeons bolstered their authority through print and championed their art as a reliable science to compete with other authorities – patients attesting to their sicknesses and cures, witnesses of sudden healings, mesmerists claiming the power to heal all ailments, and irregular practitioners. By the eve of the French Revolution, medical authority was clearly divided. Some placed their faith in the hands of the medical elite, while others rejected this formal authority and placed their trust in the untrained eye, unhindered by pride, jealousy or antiquated medical theories.

MIRACLES AND THE TRANSFER OF MEDICAL AUTHORITY

In Catholic tradition, miraculous cures were verified through extensive testimony from doctors, clerics and laypeople who had witnessed the persistence of and sudden recovery from ailments. Although medical experts had traditionally played some role in the process, in 1678 the Congregation of Rites made medical testimony a requirement to verify miracles in order to counter accusations of superstition; Pope Benedict XIV (1675–1758) further medicalized the process. Despite the rising standards of the Church and the philosophes' mockery, Catholic traditions of miracles and saints carried on relatively unchanged during the Enlightenment (Santing 2007; Duffin 2009; Pomata 2016). Even Protestant England saw a surge in reports of healing miracles, though there were no formal mechanisms in place to authenticate them (Shaw 2006: 69). In France, the Roman Catholic Church officially remained the arbiter of miracles, but in practice, the publicity surrounding miracles during this period meant that readers were also in a position to act as judges. Most miracles reported in eighteenth-century France were embroiled in controversy, most famously those associated with the convulsionaries of Saint-Médard. By mid-century, many medical practitioners declined to provide testimony to authenticate miracles, owing to scepticism or a fear of reprimand and mockery. Without formal medical judgement, supporters of reported miracles could not obtain the official approval of the Church – but by transferring the authority to assess the medical aspects of miracles to laypeople, they might obtain the approval of the reading public. Although lay witnesses, especially women, were increasingly disparaged, controversies over miracles in eighteenth-century France fostered a novel discourse that criticized elite medical experts and championed the medical judgement of laypeople.

Most reported miracles during this period were controversial because they were linked to figures condemned by many members of the clergy (including the pope) for their ties to Jansenism. Jansenism was a catch-all term for supporters of various unorthodox political, ecclesiastical and theological ideas. Louis XIV, for example, had condemned the Jansenists as republicans in both church and state. In 1713, Pope Clement XI (1649–1721) promulgated the bull *Unigenitus*, denouncing various doctrines associated with Jansenism, such as predestination and lay reading of the bible. It also confirmed the hierarchy of the Church: the pope over regional bishops, bishops over the lower clergy and spiritual authority over temporal. Opponents of the bull, called *anticonstitutionnaires*, were commonly associated with Jansenism; the group included lawyers, several bishops and nearly three-quarters of the lower clergy in France, as well as their loyal congregants. Thus, although 'Jansenist' was once a term most commonly applied to erudite theologians, from the 1720s the term applied to anyone who opposed *Unigenitus* on legal, political, theological or devotional grounds. Popular opposition to the bull grew as Jansenists began to publicize reported miracles as proof that God approved of their cause.

The most famous of these miracles occurred in the cemetery of Saint-Médard in Paris where the Jansenist deacon François de Pâris was buried. Soon after his death on 1 May 1727, crowds of pilgrims flocked to his tomb, reporting miraculous cures from blindness, deafness, paralysis and other afflictions, often following bodily convulsions. Reports of these miracles spread across France, causing one of the century's most heated debates. Between 1731 and mid-century, supporters of the miracles published at least 300 works in defence of the miracles and convulsions (Maire 1985: 24). Between 2,000 and 6,000 copies of the illegal Jansenist newspaper the *Nouvelles ecclésiastiques* were distributed each week, publicizing hundreds of reported miracles from across the kingdom (Maire 1998: 115–62). Opponents of the miracles published hundreds of other works, mocking the miracles and convulsions and condemning the Jansenists as heretical frauds.

From the outset, doctors and surgeons played a central role in verifying or disproving these miracles. Supporters of the popular cult that had developed at Saint-Médard created a *bureau de vérification* in which medical experts, lay officials and priests worked together to examine those who sought cures at the cemetery (Kreiser 1978: 151–2). Jansenist polemicists used the authority of medical practitioners to validate the miracles' authenticity. When reports of miracles worked by the popularly acclaimed (although officially condemned) saint's intercession arose in the diocese of Auxerre, the *anticonstitutionnaire* bishop wrote a pastoral letter to the faithful of his diocese, reminding them that the doctors and surgeons who testified to these miracles were among 'the most

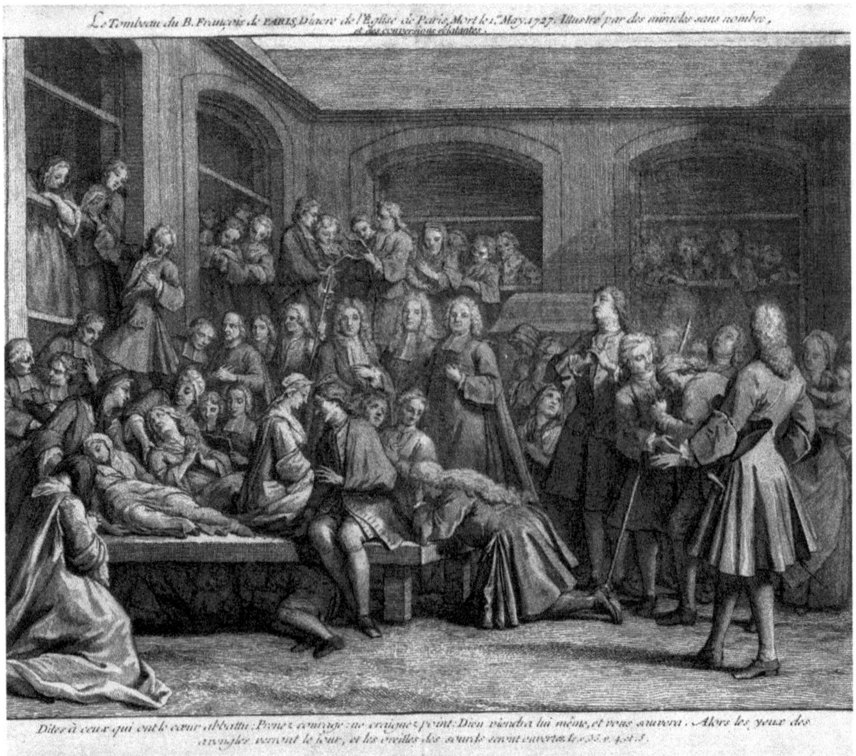

FIGURE 8.1: The tomb of M. de Pâris, from *The Truth of the Miracles worked by M. de Paris' Intercession (La verité des miracles opérés a l'intercession de M. de Paris)*. Credit: BIU Santé, Paris.

qualified and trustworthy people of the city' (Caylus 1735: 18). For this bishop and other supporters of these miracles, the testimony of licensed medical practitioners proved that these miracles were authentic and the Jansenist cause was righteous.

However, most authorities, whether church or state, held that the miracles were hoaxes, feigned by a heretical cabal in hopes of misleading the simple-minded, and they had medical consultants of their own. One of the most widely publicized and criticized miraculous cures was that of Anne Le Franc, which occurred shortly after the dismissal of her Jansenist-leaning priest from his post in 1730. After suffering from blindness in one eye and partial paralysis for almost thirty years, she was reportedly cured at the tomb of François de Pâris. The archbishop of Paris, Charles Galpard Guillaume de Vintimille (1655–1746), assembled a commission of two physicians and three surgeons to examine the miracle. Upon questioning forty of the original 120 witnesses, the commission decided the miracle was a hoax. Physicians maintained her affliction was the result of a 'hysterical illness' produced by menstrual irregularity (Vintimille 1731: 31). Surgeons concluded that she had a 'hysterical affliction' and that only 'those who are not versed in the art of healing could have found something extraordinary in the sickness and healing of Anne Le Franc'. As experienced practitioners, they had seen similarly afflicted patients 'healed by ordinary means' and, furthermore, her recovery was not sudden (Vintimille 1731: 33). The commission attacked Anne's ability to trace her own sickness and recovery, reinforcing the superior judgement of elite physicians and surgeons. This, then, was the archbishop's principal evidence against the miracles at Saint-Médard; he attached medical reports at the end of a pastoral letter, forbidding any forms of devotion to the Jansenist deacon, as well as the publication of miracle reports without his approval.

The pastoral letter was read in the parishes of Saint-Médard and Saint-Barthelemy on 22 July 1731 and throughout Paris soon after. Vintimille did not stifle the cult, but instead publicized it. The number of reported miracles increased, with the cemetery becoming so popular that police officers were needed to keep order. The development of a religious cult linked to Jansenism alarmed the authorities, who feared its potential for social, political and ecclesiastical disorder. However, it was the convulsions that often accompanied the physical and spiritual healings which most worried the authorities and tainted the cult's reputation. While many considered these convulsions miraculous, others described them as 'diabolical' and 'obscene' (Strayer 2008: 245). When convulsions occurred, one could hear 'weeping, moans, and frightening cries' from some parts of the cemetery and, in others, people laughing 'at such a comedy' (AB 10196). Those healed were of all ages, sexes and social backgrounds, but opponents insisted that only children, women and the poor were 'miraculously' healed, strengthening the idea that the cemetery was a haven for the superstitious and ignorant (Maire 1985: 87–8). The predominance of women at Saint-Médard led many commentators to argue that convulsions and miracles resulted from feminine imaginations and humoral imbalances.

Royal authorities saw the burgeoning devotional cult as a threat to social stability and ordered the arrest of anyone convulsing in public. In January 1732, the first minister of France – and fierce anti-Jansenist – Cardinal de Fleury (1653–1743) aimed to discredit claims that the convulsions had divine origins. He placed René Hérault, Paris's lieutenant general of police, in charge of interrogating convulsionaries held in the Bastille. After one convulsionary recanted his avowal that he had faked convulsions, Hérault invited twenty-four surgeons and physicians to examine the convulsionaries again as a precaution. Some had considerable ailments, showing that they had not been miraculously cured at the tomb of M. de Pâris; others had been relieved of such minor ailments that the medical examiners refused to consider them miracles. For example, Guillaume-Antoine Maupoint declared that after his convulsions he could suddenly pronounce the letter 's', which he had been unable to do before (*Procès Verbaux de plusieurs médecins et chirurgiens* 1732: 6–7). Still others admitted that their convulsions were voluntary. Medical experts unanimously agreed that the miraculous events were contrived. Hérault published the medical reports hoping to turn the public against the Jansenists, who printed reports of new miracles on a weekly basis in the popular *Nouvelles ecclésiastiques*. The medical reports also justified Louis XV's closure of the cemetery on 27 January, with his ordinance referring to the unanimous declaration 'that the said movements were not convulsive or supernatural, and that they are entirely voluntary'. Crucially, the king pronounced that 'they obviously sought to work illusions' to take advantage of credulous people. Closing the cemetery would stop the crowds and the 'opportunity for licentious speech, theft, and libertinage' (Louis XV 1732: 2).

The controversy surrounding this particular series of miracles fundamentally altered how defenders of miracle reports authenticated them throughout the rest of the century in France. The miracle verification process became less focused on formal medical judgement and more focused on the testimony of lay witnesses. Although authors on both sides of the debate had sought medical experts to justify their interpretation of the events at Saint-Médard, as the controversy intensified many practitioners refused to provide their testimony. One anonymous defender of the miracles accused these practitioners of being jealous of God and resenting 'this competitor' who came 'to meddle in their art, or rather to embarrass it' and its 'useless remedies' (*Lettre à un confesseur* 1733: 3–7). Those who were willing to provide testimony that might authenticate the miracles ran the risk of having their authority publicly challenged. For example, when, in 1735, the archbishop of Paris ordered Nigon de Berty, his inspector general, to conduct another inquiry into the miracles, the report concluded that the medical judgement which Jansenist polemicists presented to authenticate them was faulty and biased. In the case of Marie Massaron (reportedly miraculously cured of apoplexy and paralysis), de Berty accused her surgeon of being a Jansenist partisan and declared that her physician had inadequate experience; neither had paid sufficient attention to the progression of her ailments and the timing of her recovery. Under pressure, her physician, surgeon and apothecary all retracted their testimonies. In particular, the surgeon and apothecary admitted that they had wrongly trusted their patient's testimony, while the physician stated he had trusted in the testimony of the surgeon, the apothecary and his patient. De Berty characterized Massaron's medical practitioners as reckless, attributing their excessive trust in their patient's testimony to 'a blind zeal for the prodigies of today' (de Berty 1735: 59).

However, Marie Massaron's medical practitioners were not the only sources of information about her miraculous recovery. Slighted by de Berty's conclusions, Massaron published a letter to the archbishop that denounced her medical practitioners as dishonest. She also denied suffering from any menstrual irregularity, as de Berty had reported. She reminded readers that citing menstrual irregularity was a common (but illegitimate) method for disregarding women who claimed miraculous healings (Wilson 1993: 23–5). Massaron's case shows how boundaries of medical authority shifted during the Saint-Médard debates. Despite the disputed ability of patients (especially female ones) to accurately report the state of their bodies, patients and their familiars were becoming the default authority – boosted by the reluctance of medical practitioners to join debates over miracles. Supporters of reported miracles presented patients as the most reliable source of information about their health.

The Saint-Médard controversy faded after the cemetery closed in 1732, but it remained at the forefront of French debates over the supernatural. By mid-century, the miracles had become a favoured target of the French philosophes – many of whom had been personally influenced by the events at the cemetery, whether as eyewitnesses or as contemporaries. For d'Holbach, the convulsionaries revealed how piety and deceit might go together, with 'all of Paris run[ning] to see miracles, healings, *convulsions*, and to hear the predictions that were obvious frauds conjured up by "good souls", in order to support their party, which they qualified as the cause of God' (original emphasis; d'Holbach 1770: 337–8). In *Philosophical Thoughts* (1746), Diderot recounted his Saint-Médard experience:

> There the ashes of a predestinarian worked more wonders in a single day than Jesus Christ had in his entire life . . . I looked, and I saw a little lame boy who walked with the aid of three or four charitable people who marveled at him, repeating 'Miracle! Miracle!' Where then is this miracle, idiotic people? Do you not see that this swindler has simply changed crutches?

—113–15

Miracles had come to be associated with partisanship, deceit, superstition and ignorance, providing further motivation for medical practitioners to withhold their testimony.

Despite the political controversy and diatribes against the supernatural, there were many miracle reports in the second half of the eighteenth century. Although these reports were less overtly polemical than those of the 1730s, many miracles were publicized by Jansenist authors, who continued to seek vindication of their cause through an association with divine signs and to combat the rise of religious scepticism. Instead of appealing to formal medical judgement, authors took a two-pronged approach to proving the divine nature of the cures they reported. First, they stressed the extended period of the patient's ailments, which typically worsened despite, or because of, medical treatment. Earlier narratives had discussed medical ineffectiveness, but with the goal of showing that all earthly treatments had failed, leaving God's grace as the only possibility. Later accounts highlighted, by contrast, the inefficacy of medicine specifically, aiming to erode its practitioners' credibility. Second, later reports suggested that the testimony of common people on its own was sufficient to prove a miracle. The judgement of the untrained eye, they argued, was perhaps even superior to that of educated people, who might be misled by their own prejudices. With licensed medical practitioners unwilling to testify, defenders of miracles had little choice but to eliminate the need for medical judgements altogether; laypeople, particularly women, were instead considered better authorities to judge medical matters. As Anne Vila, Cathy McClive and others have shown, legal authorities and medical experts tended to distrust the judgement and testimony of women during this period on the grounds that women had a pathological sensibility and biological disposition to deception (Vila 1998; McClive 2008). The narratives' emphasis on the reliability of women's testimony is all the more significant, revealing a willingness to accept testimony that would ordinarily be considered questionable, for the sake of verifying miracles.

The relations of miracles were often unflattering to the medical profession. The author who publicized the miraculous recovery of Madame Gardet at a procession of the Eucharist on 6 September 1778 stressed that she had been 'abandoned by the men of the art' and 'prey to her sufferings, the end of which she saw no mortal could procure for her' (*Relation de la maladie de la Dame Gardet* 1778: 6). Many contested the miracle because of the lack of doctors' testimonies, but the author insisted that these were unnecessary. The character of the lay witnesses made their testimony sufficient, since they were 'honest people, who have their fixed dwelling ... who have a reputation of integrity amongst all those who know and employ them' and are 'penetrated with respect for religion' (41–2). The author acknowledged that doctors might add credibility to the account but said that they would 'never make that which is true and real not so. The truth is by itself. It is independent' (44–5). Stressing the reliability of lay witnesses, particularly those with faith and good reputations, the author placed the authority to judge medical matters into the hands of average people.

Similarly, the published narrative of a nun's miraculous recovery in 1790 included an extensive account of her ailments, showing that all the physicians' remedies had actually made her sicker (*Relation de la guérison de la sœur Ste. Geneviéve* 1790). After nine days of prayer to the Virgin Mary, her fellow sisters brought her a piece of the True Cross, by which she was reportedly healed on 17 August 1790. According to witnesses, her physician proclaimed, 'you are a marvel . . . It was not medicine that healed you because you had none . . . Do you realize that you are going to force doctors to believe in miracles?' (21–2). He nonetheless refused to provide written certification for the miracle. The narrative's author disregarded the significance of this certification; 'one does not need the testimony of medicine . . . it is only necessary to have eyes to assure oneself that a person reduced to the most extreme weakness by a sickness for many years passed all of a sudden to perfect health' (24). This author, like others of the time, portrayed medicine as ineffectual and the judgement of its practitioners unnecessary.

In the second half of the eighteenth century, a rift grew between those who prioritized the testimony of simple, pious lay witnesses and those who prioritized the judgement of sophisticated, scientifically minded medical experts. Some authors, such as Vauvilliers, professor of Greek at the Collège Royal and member of the Académie des Inscriptions et Belles-Lettres, argued that anyone was capable of judging the state of their own body and bemoaned the fact that piety and simplicity no longer sufficed to prove someone a reliable witness as it had in Biblical times. When a woman was healed after touching the robe of Jesus Christ, he noted, 'I do not believe that one supposes she carried with her the certificates of doctors' (Vauvilliers 1785: 37). Others, however, found the philosophes' view more compelling, seeing piety as a cloak for deception and simplicity as a breeding ground for ignorance. Although printed works threatened to undermine the authority and reputation of France's medical elite, these prestigious practitioners used print to their own ends. From mid-century on, elite medical practitioners in France launched a print campaign in which they represented themselves as the only legitimate medical authority in France, as their judgement was unquestionably reliable, while the judgement of the unlearned was disputable, even laughable.

MEDICAL MARVELS AND THE TESTIMONY OF WOMEN

As the example of miracles shows, the efficacy of medicine in the eighteenth century was ambiguous. The French medical elite sought alternative means to prove themselves the most reliable medical authority. One method was to investigate, debunk and publicize reported cases of extraordinary illnesses. While at one time church authorities in France had attributed such illnesses to divine or diabolical causes, these interpretations were rare by mid-century. Medical investigators ran little risk of being accused of unorthodoxy, leaving them with ample opportunities to display their scientific skill by debunking superstitions, hated by the Church and philosophes alike. When people across France reported medical marvels – ranging from women birthing animals to people living without food or drink for years – medical practitioners (especially elite Parisian physicians) investigated. Their reports drew on their experiences to prove that superstitious fools abounded; they alone, armed with scepticism and medical knowledge, could expose the ploys of deceitful patients. Elite practitioners used newspapers, pamphlets, journals and other publications (intended for medical practitioners and lay audiences alike) to emphasize their investigative skills. They stressed the importance of examining extraordinary illnesses by questioning the mental state and intentions of patients. In so doing, they attacked the reputation and judgement of patients, especially women, to reinforce their own authority over medical matters. Still, just as in the case of miracles, some authors defended those patients accused of ignorance or deceit and appealed to their readers to vindicate laypeople's ability to judge the state of their own bodies.

The hotly disputed case of Geneviève Martin displays this tension between the authority of patients and elite medical practitioners. In the 1750s, the bishop of Langres requested an official inquiry into a young woman in his diocese who reportedly expelled rocks in her vomit and urine. A member of the Faculty of Medicine in Paris, Jean-François-Clément Morand (1726–1784), was called to investigate. After a month-long investigation, he concluded that her illness, which some locals believed to be supernatural in origin, was a hoax. The Faculty of Medicine issued a statement confirming that the young woman did not suffer from lithiasis and placed Geneviève among the rank of other 'hysterical girls' who 'imagine different strategies to seduce credulous minds, to make a spectacle of themselves to attract some consideration or some alms' (Morand 1754b: 146). News of the hoax spread across France as the judgement was published in various popular periodicals of the time, including the *Mercure de France* and the *Journal œconomique*. After returning to Paris, Morand published a short, six-page account of his investigation (*Éclaircissement abrégé sur la maladie d'une fille de Saints-Geosmes*) in which he mocked the credulity of the locals who trusted a deceitful young woman.

In response, Jacques Hugony, a local surgeon with first-hand knowledge of Geneviève's ailment, defended her integrity. He insisted that it was absurd to believe that she had 'deceived her relatives, her friends, and some people who took care of her' and argued that Morand was 'persecuting an innocent' for the sake of an interesting story (Hugony 1754b: 4). He noted that local physicians, surgeons and priests were well acquainted with her 'Christian virtues' and that 'never did one see a young woman of her condition more upright, more naïve, more sincere, and more truthful' (Hugony 1754a: 4–5). Hugony claimed that 'one owes it to the progress of medicine . . . to discover the cause and remedy of the sickness in question', instead of simply disregarding the ailment as fraud (Hugony 1754a: 4). In a private letter to Morand, Hugony declared 'there are monsters in nature, Sir, and I would rather believe that the sickness of this girl is a miracle than to doubt . . . its reality' (Wellcome MS 3468: no. 9). Hugony trusted this woman's character and testimony to the point of believing that if the human body could not produce such rocks, then her illness must be supernatural.

Morand berated Hugony for respecting the character of Geneviève 'to the point of inspiring the idea of a *miracle*, and of converting a fable into an object of taciturn and respectful admiration, and not of philosophical contemplation' (original emphasis; Morand 1754b: 140). Following Hugony's attack on the Faculty's judgement, Morand published a second, more extensive work. He praised those who were convinced by his initial work, noting that it was 'this part of the public [that] always knows to yield to those who can be the only judges in all sorts of matters' (Morand 1754b: 27). He commended the bishop of Langres for calling on his expertise; under his auspices, 'medicine enjoyed the appropriate prerogative in this affair that is reserved for it to disabuse the public on such occasions' (Morand 1754b: 23). Morand asserted that through their knowledge of nature, physicians were in the best position to 'appropriately avoid the dangerous extremes of credulity and incredulity in regard to *miracles*. If popular credulity establishes only too often false ones, the lights of medicine do not at all refuse to recognize true ones' (original emphasis; Morand 1754b: 27). The debate between Hugony and Morand reveals the divide between those who defended the ability of laypeople to judge the state of their own bodies and those who insisted that elite practitioners knew best.

To defend the rightful position of elite urban physicians as arbiters in cases of miracles and medical marvels, Morand provided 150 pages of documentation to support his conclusions and the official judgement of the Paris Faculty. He also presented extensive evidence to prove that the stones Geneviève expelled were minerals produced in a quarry, not in a human body. However, a considerable portion of the evidence stemmed not from his medical training but from his interactions with Geneviève and other locals. Morand's manuscript notes from his visit and the publications that followed characterized Geneviève as cunning and emotionally unstable. In a letter to Bagard, president of the Royal College of Medicine in Nancy, Morand wrote that his commission was especially difficult because Geneviève, 'although a girl born in the countryside, is not an idiot'. Part of her plan to maintain her charade was to avoid contact with medical professionals by feigning behaviour that would suggest she was simple, pious and shy. He noted, for example, that she 'has a resolute aversion for all men that she takes indistinctly for physicians and surgeons' (Morand 1754b: 33). According to Morand, only the keen eye of a learned medical practitioner, being a man of science, could so easily discern deceit in medical matters.

Locals, by contrast, lacked the objectivity and experience necessary to see through her ruse. Morand characterized locals as 'naïve' and their testimony as 'amusing' (Morand 1754b: 39). Above all, he mocked them for trusting Geneviève's own account of events, simply 'because they knew the sick girl for a long time' (Morand 1754b: 36). True medical professionals needed to be better, Morand contended. He reminded his readers of the need for a 'wise distrust' and hoped that those who practised medicine 'without knowing all the traps sown under their feet' would learn from his experience. He used the surgeon Hugony to show that 'those who practice the art of medicine' had to be 'on guard against all extraordinary cases' and 'all that resembles a prodigy' in order 'to protect their reputation' (Morand 1754b: 26). Comparing Geneviève's feigned ailment with other impostures of his age, Morand conceded that at one time people trusted the testimony of simple people, while adding that 'good faith is no longer anything but weakness and silliness'. 'In this century', he claimed, 'the progress made in the sciences and medicine' left such stories only to 'the people and the vulgar' (Morand 1754b: 129). Morand's celebration of distrust represents one aspect of a larger tendency on the part of France's medical elite to push patients, perhaps especially women, out of diagnostics in cases of unusual illnesses.

Judging by the support Morand gained from the medical community, this sentiment was widely shared. A medical student wrote to Morand praising him for having debunked 'all that was marvelous and supernatural in this girl' and revealed for posterity that such an ailment could only be found amid 'afflictions of the mind and sicknesses of artifice' (*Journal de médicine*, hereafter JdM, 1759: 468). The Paris Faculty of Medicine praised his accomplishments, stating that 'Mr. Morand, our colleague, a judge enlightened by his knowledge of physics, anatomy, animal economy, medical practice, and even natural history, worked to open the eyes of an entire province, shocked by a so-called extraordinary sickness'. The story, they suggested, was valuable for both physicians and the general public. It was useful for physicians 'in showing them how it is necessary to challenge extraordinary things and how it is necessary to proceed to confirm a fact or unmask a lie'. It was useful for the public 'in showing them how it is necessary to keep guard against novelty and credulity, which follows ignorance' and that they must be suspicious of 'all events which appear to surpass the forces of nature' (Morand 1754b: ii). The tale was meant to teach both medical practitioners and the reading public to be sceptical of marvels and those who reported them, while trusting instead the judgement of France's most highly trained medical practitioners.

The case of Geneviève Martin was only one among many that emphasized the competence of elite medical practitioners, the deceit of patients and the ignorance of the untrained. The narratives that appeared in medical journals, particularly the *Journal de médecine*, in the second half of the century cautioned both lay readers and medical practitioners against having too much trust in the testimony of patients. The authors cautioned that there were tricksters, pious dupes and gullible healers around every corner. In 1761, the journal published a letter written by a priest from Leroux in the Auvergne who recounted the bizarre ailment of twenty-six-year-old Jeanne Charle, who claimed literally to have rocks in her head that gave her headaches and made unpleasant sounds. Unable to explain the cause of this ailment, a local 'charlatan, a peasant of good reputation' diagnosed her with a 'gravelous humor' and told her that upon smoking the powder he prescribed, she would begin to expel the stones. She then began to expel stones from her nostrils, some of which were the size of a pea (JdM 1761: 363). Combined, 'the bad faith of the charlatan', 'the criminal maneuver of the sick woman' and 'the credulity of the respectable person who reported this story' made this a teachable anecdote (374). Stressing 'the impossibility of the formation and expulsion of these mysterious stones', the editor observed that 'we have published this letter only to teach everyone to be on guard against these sorts of *prestiges*' (374). The journal's editors found themselves combatting not only the credulity of sick people desperate for a cure, but also the credulity of medical practitioners who were too quick to trust the testimony of their patients.

Nearly all of these stories published in the *Journal de médecine* illustrated the deceitful nature of young women, in particular. In 1757, the journal published an article about a pious girl who suffered from the appearance of needles, nails and pieces of chain link under her skin. The article's author, Boucher, a physician from Lille, asserted that '[t]he lights of our century do not permit us to pause for an instant on the question of whether or not this singular event is the product of an unknown cause' and diagnosed her with a 'sick brain' (JdM 1757: 167; 173). In 1783, the journal published a report by Jean-Baptiste Desgranges (1751–1832), a graduate surgeon in Lyon, in which he recounted the tale of Marie Didier, who was widely believed to have lived for seven years without eating. He noted that this was a teachable anecdote because it showed medical practitioners that they needed to be aware of 'the innumerable strategies one can use to mislead them' (JdM 1783: 425). These stories were meant to teach practitioners to be circumspect and sceptical of patients' assertions, and the extraordinary nature of the reported ailments made it easy to disregard their testimony. Because most of the patients were women, these tales also encouraged readers – most of whom were medical practitioners – to associate women with deception.

And yet, there was still a place in the medical debates of the Enlightenment for defending the testimony of patients, regardless of sex. Authors of miracle narratives highlighted the reliability of pious women and the unreliability of medicine. Local practitioners like Hugony took up their pens in defence of patients like Geneviève Martin, characterizing Parisian physicians as haughty and dishonest. These authors avowed that no one was in a better position to judge the state of the human body than the afflicted and those closest to them. As the members of the corporative medical community in France grew increasingly unwilling to entertain reports of any sickness or cure that seemed out of the ordinary, whether preternatural or supernatural, the testimony of the untrained eye became more important than ever for the authentication of these reports. Those who discredited miracles or medical marvels pointed to the unreliability of witnesses, while the printed works defending those same miracles and marvels countered with the reliability of witnesses and the inefficacy of medicine. There was a deep disagreement about where medical authority ought to rest and who was most capable of judging the nature of sicknesses and cures. It was this disagreement that was also at the heart of debates over mesmerism.

ON MESMERISM, OR TOWARDS A CONCLUSION

Perhaps no single controversy better exemplifies the competition between legally sanctioned and popularly acclaimed medical authority than that over mesmerism. On the eve of the French Revolution, the French reading public thirsted for both science and the supernatural; mesmerism seemed to deliver a bit of both. Although mesmerism appeared supernatural, its defenders declared it was scientific. Like the medical elite who published in the *Journal de médecine*, mesmerists professed authoritative knowledge of nature. And yet, rejected by that same medical elite and by the royal government, they turned to evidence more commonly used by defenders of miracles and medical marvels: the testimony of patients. In doing so, Mesmer's supporters took the authority to judge medical matters out of the hands of licensed professionals and placed it into the hands of laypeople. Mesmer's opponents struck back, arguing that witness testimony was inherently flawed, and that laypeople were not qualified to judge matters of health and healing, even when it pertained to their own bodies. The printed debates surrounding mesmerism in the 1780s reveal that despite all the efforts of France's elite practitioners to advertise their purportedly superior judgement, in the public sphere at least, their authority was at best shared, and at worst, rejected.

The theoretical framework that supported mesmerism sounded scientific enough. According to Franz Anton Mesmer (1734–1815), his healing technique manipulated animal magnetism, a universal force or 'fluid' that pervaded all matter. The idea of a universal, invisible force was not particularly objectionable. To many it appeared akin to gravity, the existence of which was widely accepted by the educated reading public of Enlightenment France. Mesmer's healing

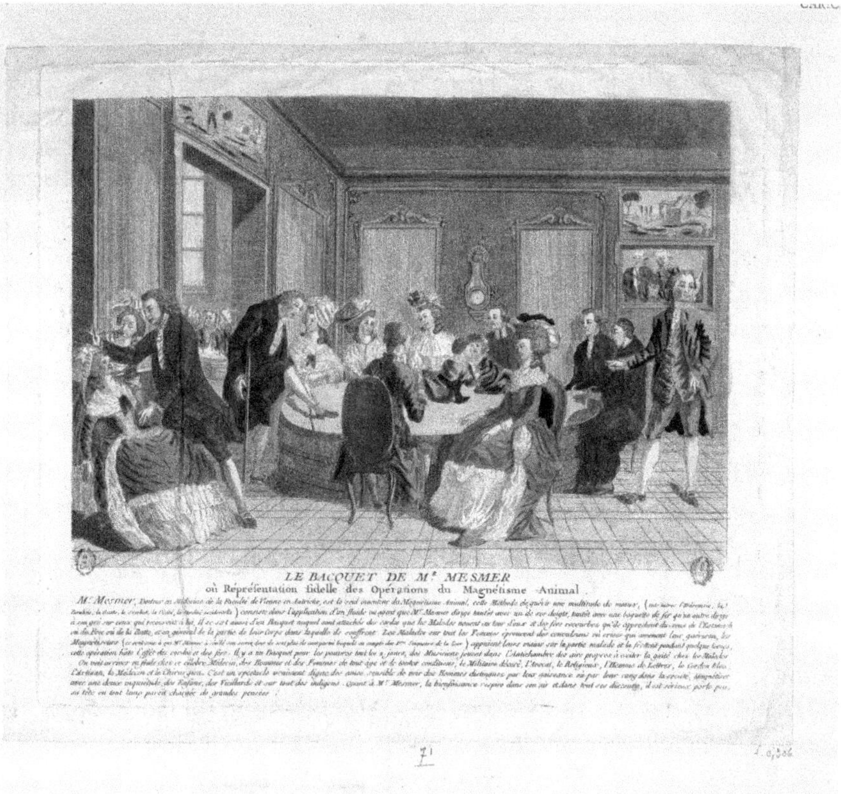

FIGURE 8.2: *The tub of Mr Mesmer, or the Faithful representation of the operation of animal magnetism. (Le bacquet de Mr. Mesmer ou Représentation fidelle des Opérations du Magnétisme Animal).* Credit: Bibliothèque Nationale de France, Paris.

methods, however, raised more than a few eyebrows. According to him, it was the obstruction of this universal fluid that caused disease. Health could be restored by 'magnetizing' the poles of the body to get the fluid flowing again. This was done in a variety of ways: massaging with 'magnetized' hands or metal rods, or in group sessions by gathering around tubs of iron filings (*baquets*). Those who practised this healing technique, called 'magnetizers', carefully regulated the environment with scientific instruments – including thermometers, barometers and hygrometers – as well as with music. Although those who championed this healing method declared that it was a scientific medical procedure developed through careful observation of natural laws, the theatrical characteristics gave many pause.

In 1784, the royal government created two commissions to investigate these cures, one drawn from the Royal Society of Medicine and the other from the Paris Faculty of Medicine and the Academy of Sciences. Like the commissions designed to investigate the Saint-Médard miracles, both reported unequivocally that the healings were a sham. Only those who were judged ignorant or impoverished felt any discernible change after the treatments, which suggested that the changes were imaginary. Above all, the commissioners could find no physical proof of the existence of a universal fluid. The commissioners from the Academy of Sciences printed upwards of 12,000 copies of their report in hopes of winning the hearts of the reading public and dealing a final, devastating blow to the mesmerist movement in France. Still, many remained convinced of Mesmer's theory and frustrated that the testimony of hundreds of cured people was not considered sufficient proof that his healing technique was valid.

Like authors of miracle narratives, supporters of animal magnetism attacked the formally trained where they were weakest. Marie-André-Joseph Bouvier defended animal magnetism, reminding detractors that sick people 'find so little help in ordinary medicine' that it would be absurd to disregard reports of cures by other means (Bouvier 1784: 26). Another of Mesmer's supporters reminded readers that 'if doctors have some rules for understanding sickness, they have almost none at all for knowing the remedy' (*Lettre de M. le marquis* 1783: 2) He suggested that he, armed only with 'reason and good faith', could judge better than 'an academician or a Member of the Faculty who has systems, conventional opinions, and above all a partisan spirit and personal interests' (1783: 1). Those who supported Mesmer's healing technique, and especially those who practised it, attacked the medical establishment in France as defunct, elitist, even aristocratic (Darnton 1968; Brockliss and Jones 1997). In their eyes, the authority that was legally placed in the hands of the elite medical institutions of France was undeserved. Furthermore, like defenders of miracles, defenders of cures by animal magnetism argued that the personal experience of patients held more evidentiary weight than the purportedly biased impressions of the Paris Faculty of Medicine.

The printed debate over mesmerism mirrored that over miracles in another way, in that opponents used a familiar tactic – attacking the judgement of lay witnesses and those who claimed to have been healed. The parallels between the cures of Saint-Médard and mesmerism were difficult to ignore, as the naturalist Charles Devillers (1724–1809) described: the sick had similar ailments (many fevers and nervous disorders), reacted similarly to their 'treatments' (often with convulsions) and had comparable long-term prognoses. For Devillers, the likeness was proof that 'the imagination had the greatest influence on the human body' (1784: 54). Jean-Baptiste Nougaret (1742–1823) also considered Mesmer's supporters to be the same as 'people who were simple enough, credulous enough, to have faith in convulsions and the miracles operated at the tomb of the deacon Pâris' (1787: 205). Even Condorcet averred that despite all the testimony in favour of animal magnetism, he remained unconvinced. After all, he reminded his readers, 'one is shocked by the names

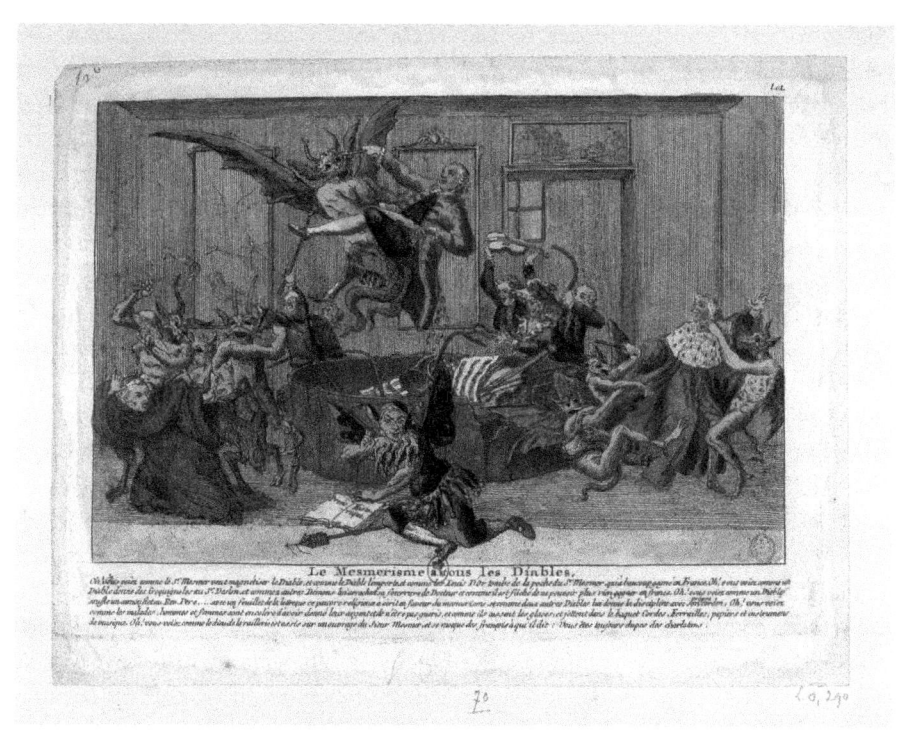

FIGURE 8.3: *Mesmerism has all the devils. (Le Mesmerisme a tous les diables)*. Credit: Bibliothèque Nationale de France, Paris.

that one encounters at the bottom of [certificates attesting to] some of the miracles of Saint-Médard' (Darnton 1968: 189). That mesmerist healings were widely attested proved nothing. After all, these other healings, here assumed to be obvious fakes, were at least as well attested. Patients, then, who were untrained in the art of medicine, could not be trusted to relay information about the state of their own bodies.

Likening their cures to those at Saint-Médard, which by the 1780s were widely (although not universally) derided, was a tactic meant to embarrass magnetizers and their proponents. In his *Research and Doubts on Animal Magnetism* (1784), the physician Michel-Augustin Thouret (1749–1810) stressed the absurdity of accepting mesmerist cures when they were so similar to other healings that had long been derided by intellectuals of the age. Writing about the miracles and convulsions at Saint-Médard, he wondered, 'were they not also numerous events, visible and adorned in the appearance of the greatest authenticity? Who would dare to adopt or defend them today?' (Thouret 1784: 221).

Thouret might have been surprised to learn that some were not, in fact, afraid to defend the reality of these historical events. Recognizing the inescapable parallel, some defenders actually co-opted miraculous healings of the historical record in order to suit them to Mesmer's system. Galart de Montjoie (1746–1816), a lawyer in the Parlement of Aix and professor of French law, defended the judgement of the untrained eye in medical matters, insisting that the testimony of those who claimed to have been cured both at the tomb of François de Pâris and at mesmerist séances was reliable. In his *Letter on Animal Magnetism* (1784), Montjoie argued that many extraordinary historical events had been poorly understood in their own time. 'One example will give my thought a useful extension', he wrote. 'No one dares to cite this example seriously, out of fear of ridicule. But I, who do not fear ridicule, will cite it.' Montjoie claimed that the cause of the Jansenist miracles and convulsions was never properly examined, 'first, because religion was mixed up in it, and then, because of the jokes of a sect that one has honored, I do not know why, with the name of *philosophes*'. Although he claimed the healings were not miracles, the detailed testimonies of the cured proved that they were nevertheless real. Saint-Médard was extraordinary only in the unlikely coincidence that the tomb of François de Pâris acted as a *baquet magnétique*, like those used in mesmerist séances. Although the 1730s was an 'unpleasant age', he claimed that 'today the causes are known', which explained how it could be that 'people of great clout' attested to these cures (Montjoie 1784: 9–11). While stressing the absurdity of a belief in miracles, Montjoie demanded a re-evaluation of the testimonial evidence in light of the recent discovery of animal magnetism.

Earlier debates over miracles had set a precedent for how the testimony of patients was valued and by whom. While discussions of controversial miracles worked their way into the debates over mesmerism, some publicized miracle reports of the 1780s similarly addressed the concurrent discussions of mesmerism. One anonymous author presented an extensive narrative of the recently reported miraculous cure of Louise Guélon. The narrative contained familiar elements: a long-suffering patient, useless doctors who refused to testify publicly, a miraculous healing following prayers to François de Pâris, and sceptical clerics who feared connections with Jansenism. After providing detailed testimonial evidence in favour of the miracle, the author emphasized that if the cures by animal magnetism were as well attested as those worked by Pâris, 'I protest that one would soon abandon all your systems of medicine as pure charlatanry, and all the drugs of chemists as poisons that one would allow to decay in the boutiques of apothecaries' (*Relation de la maladie de Mlle. Louis Guélon* n. d.: 48). While the author resented the attribution of the miracles of Saint-Médard to animal magnetism, he found even more disturbing those who contested both miracles and mesmerism on the grounds that the testimony of the cured was unreliable. He attacked Thouret, for example, whom he claimed was driven by a 'medical enthusiasm' and 'trembles at the sight of all that which could favor mesmerism' (*Relation de la maladie de Mlle. Louis Guélon* n. d.: 40). Thouret had had thus taken the 'dishonest, but very convenient' position of arguing that the witnesses of alleged healings by animal magnetism were just like those who attested to the miracles of François de Pâris – that is, unreliable (2). He reminded Thouret that the miracles of Saint-Médard had been 'attested and certified mostly by people in the learned class, recounted by the sick themselves, of which a certain number appeared to be from a higher social position' and that it was unreasonable 'to condemn multiple, irreproachable witnesses' (41–3). Although supporters of miracles and animal magnetism disagreed as to the origin of the healings, they did share a key sentiment: that laypeople were capable of judging medical matters and able to discern the state of their own health, irrespective of the preconceived notions of elite practitioners like Thouret.

Printed debates over miracles, medical marvels and mesmerism in eighteenth-century France suggest that there was little progress made towards the triumph of a medical profession that based its judgements solely on observational science. By contrast, the judgements of medical experts were also shaped by fear of reprimand or mockery, insecurity because of their lack of reliable remedies, and concerns over their reputation. In the early debates over miracles, medical judgement was so fluid that it could be used to support both sides of the debate. Even on the eve of the French Revolution, the remedies of the most prestigious medical practitioners were so ineffective that many authors suggested their judgement was useless. Elite physicians such as Morand and Thouret may have argued that their knowledge of the human body was superior to that of all others, but others argued that those educated in France's medical institutions were no more – and perhaps considerably less – capable of judging the nature of sicknesses and cures than those who were untrained.

That supernatural and preternatural phenomena were so hotly debated during the Enlightenment reinforces how useful they are for understanding medical authority during this period. Even as many within the medical community distanced themselves from 'non-natural' phenomena, the reading public remained fascinated with them, which meant that there was a potential audience to which supporters of miraculous and marvellous cures could appeal. These debates, which were hashed out across books, pamphlets, journals, newspapers and ephemera, reveal competing visions of medical authority. One of these visions, that of the medical elite themselves, aligns closely with earlier teleological histories of the rise of the rational male professional. However, these debates also reveal an alternative vision, one that challenged the authority of ineffective physicians and surgeons and resented the alienation of patients from discussions of their own illnesses, medical treatments and cures. Without a cultural historical approach, this alternative vision would be lost. The proponents of this vision lacked the power of their opponents. Jansenists lacked the support of church and state that their detractors enjoyed; the rural surgeon Hugony lacked the prestigious credentials and status of his competitor, the

Parisian physician Morand; and mesmerists lacked the institutional support enjoyed by their critics, many of whom were members of the Faculty of Medicine in Paris. And yet, medical authority was not established solely by means of power, much less legal power. Rather, as these debates show, medical authority was discursive, malleable and largely in the eyes of the beholder.

NOTE

1. Variations on portions of this chapter appear in my articles in *Social History of Medicine* and *The Journal for the Western Society for French History*.

REFERENCES

ARCHIVAL SOURCES

Archives nationales de France (Paris)

Magalhães, João Jacinto de, letter to Gabriel de Bory, "Extrait d'une lettre de Mr Magalhain a M.^r Le Chev.^{er} de Bory chef d'escadre, luë a l'accademie des Sciences. Procédé pour faire la Conserve de Carottes", f. 208, Dossier 5, Mar-D³

Poissonnier, Pierre-Isaac, letter to Antoine de Sartine 21 January 1772, dossier 5, pièce 76, Mar-G 179

Le Bègue de Presle, Achille-Guillaume, letter to Antoine de Sartine 22 February 1777, dossier 2, Mar-G 179

Bibliothèque nationale de France (Paris)

Rapports de police sur ce qui se passe chaque jour dans l'église et le cimetière de Saint Médard, Archives de la Bastille, MS 10196.

British Library (London)

Collectanea: or, a Collection of Advertisements and Paragraphs from the Newspapers Relating to Various Subjects, Printed at Strawberry-Hill by Thomas Kirgate, for the Collector, Daniel Lysons. Mic. C.20452/C 103.k11. Vol. 1, n. p., f. 96, v. – M. P. [Morning Post] Nov. 6 1787, 'A PARODY on a MODERN PUFF'.

Leiden University Special Collections (Leiden)

Tulbagh, Rijk, letter to Arnout Vosmaer 1766, BPL 246.

National Maritime Museum (London)

'Sick and Hurt Board, In-Letters and Orders', (1797–1798), ADM/E/46.

Natural History Museum Archives and Library (London)

Sloane, Hans (1687), Manuscript catalogues of Sir Hans Sloane's collections: 'Fossils', Volume 1, 'Coralls, Sponges, Crustaceae, Humana'.

The National Archives (London)

Instructions for the Royal Naval Hospital at Haslar & Plymouth (1808), London: Philanthropic Society, St. George's Fields, ADM 106/3091.
'Jamaica (Pay Lists)', (1742), ADM 102/461.
'Regulations respecting Nurses and Other Servants of the Royal Hospital', (1760) in 'Instructions and Precedents', ADM 98/105.

The Wellcome Library (London)

Fergusson, William (1811), 'Observations re Regimental Hospitals and Duties of the Brigade Surgeon', RAMC 210/3.
Fergusson, William, (1815–1816), 'In Barbados and Guadaloupe, including Reports on Disease among African Recruits, from Sierra Leone, and on Suitable Footwear for Africans', RAMC 210/2.
Martin, Geneviève (1716–1759), MS 3468, no. 9.

Yale University Library (New Haven, CT)

Fergusson, William, (n. d. [likely 1817], 'The Memorial of William Fergusson Inspector of Hospitals to His Royal Highness Field Marshall The Duke of York', William Fergusson Papers, MS 1287, Folder 10: 1815–1831, Yale University Library.

DIGITIZED PRIMARY SOURCES

Dictionnaires d'Autresfois Public Access Collection, https://artfl-project.uchicago.edu/content/dictionnaires-dautrefois (accessed 13 October 2020).
Hume, David ([1739]), *A Treatise of Human Nature*, Vol. 1, in Amyas Merivale and Peter Millican (eds), *Hume Texts Online*, https://davidhume.org (accessed 8 October 2020).
Pilloud, Séverine, Micheline Louis-Courvoisier and Vincent Barras, eds, *Fonds Tissot: Archives du corps et la santé au 18e siècle*, http://tissot.unil.ch/fmi/webd/Tissot (accessed 13 October 2020).
Seventeenth and Eighteenth Century Burney Newspapers Collection, www.gale.com/intl/c/17th-and-18th-century-burney-newspapers-collection (accessed 13 October 2020).
Shuttleton, David (n.d.), *The Cullen Project*, www.cullenproject.ac.uk (accessed 13 October 2020).
Smith, Lisa Wynne (2016), *The Sloane Letters Project*, www.sloaneletters.com (accessed 11 November 2020).

JOURNALS AND NEWSPAPERS

Avant-Coureur
Felix Farley's Bristol Journal
Gazette de Santé
Gazetteer and New Daily Advertiser
Gothaische gelehrte Zeitungen
Journal de médecine, chirurgie, pharmacie, etc. (1754–1793), 88 vols, Paris.

Morning Chronicle
Morning Herald
Public Advertiser
World

PRINTED PRIMARY SOURCES

Adams, Thomas (1616), *Diseases of the Soule: a Discourse Divine, Morall and Physical*, London: by George Purslowe for John Budge.
Allen, John (1749), *Synopsis Medecinae; or a Summary View of the Whole Practice of Physick*, 2 vols, London: W. Innys et al.
Arbuthnot, John (1731), *An Essay concerning the Nature of Aliments, and the Choice of Them, according to the Different Constitutions of Human Bodies*, London: J. Tonson.
Arbuthnot, John (2006), *The Correspondence of Dr. John Arbuthnot*, ed. Angus Ross, Paderborn: Fink.
Arthy, Elliot (1798), *The Seamen's Medical Advocate*, London: Richardson and Egerton.
Banier, A. (1732), *Les Métamorphoses d'Ovide*, 3 vols, Amsterdam: R. and J. Wetstein and G. Smith.
Blagrave, Jonathan (1693), *The Nature and Mischief of Envy: A Sermon*, London: John Southby.
Blane, Gilbert (1785), *Observations on the Diseases Incident to Seamen*, London: Joseph Cooper.
Blane, Gilbert (1822), *Select Dissertations on Several Subjects of Medical Science*, London: Thomas and George Underwood.
Boerhaave, Herman (1715), *Boerhaave's Institutions in Physick. By Which the Principles and Fundamentals of That Art Are Digested and Fully Explained*, London: Jonas Browne.
Boerhaave, Herman (1735), *Boerhaave's Aphorisms: Concerning the Knowledge and Cure of Diseases*, London: A. Bettesworth, et al.
Bond, William (1720), *The History of the Life and Adventures of Mr. Duncan Campbell*, London: E[dmund] Curll.
Bouvier, Marie-André-Joseph (1784), *Lettres sur le magnétism animal; où l'on discute l'Ouvrage de M. Thouret, intitulé Doutes & Recherches sur la découverte du Magnétisme animal, & le Rapport de MM. les Commissaires sur l'existence & l'efficacité de cette découverte*, Brussels : [s. n.].
Brooks, Thomas (1657), *The Unsearchable Riches of Christ*, London: John Hancock.
Buchan, William (1772), *Domestic Medicine: Or, a Treatise on the Prevention and Cure of Diseases by Regimen and Simple Medicines*, 2nd edn, London: W. Strahan and T. Cadell.
Buchan, William (1774), *Domestic Medicine; or, The Family Physician*, London: Joseph Cruikshank for R. Aitken.
Burton, John (1738), *A Treatise on the Non-Naturals, in Which the Great Influence They Have on the Bodies is Set Forth and Mechanically Accounted For*, York: A. Staples.
Camper, Petrus (1791), *Verhandeling Van Petrus Camper, over Het Natuurlijk Verschil der Wezenstrekken in Menschen van Onderscheiden Landaart en Ouderdom*, Utrecht: B. Wild and J. Altheer.

Caylus, Charles Daniel Gabriel de Thubières de (1735), *Instruction pastorale de Monseigneur l'évêque d'Auxerre au sujet de quelques Ecrits & Libelles répandus dans le public contre son mandement du 26.décembre 1733, à l'occasion du miracle opéré dans la ville de Seignelay, de ce diocese*, [s. l.; s. n.]

Cheyne, George (1724), *An Essay of Health and Long Life*, London: George Strahan.

Cheyne, George (1733), *The English Malady; or, a Treatise of Nervous Diseases of All Kinds*, London: G. Strahan.

Chomel, Jean-Baptiste (1712), *Abregé de l'histoire des plantes usuelles*, Paris: Charles Osmont.

Clark, James (1797), *A Treatise of the yellow fever, as it appeared in the island of Dominica, in the years 1793-4-5-6*, London: J. Murray and S. Highley.

Clossy, Samuel (1763), *Observations on Some of the Diseases of the Parts of the Human Body, chiefly taken from Dissections of Morbid Bodies*, London: G. Kearlsly.

Cocchi, Antonio (1743), *Del vitto Pitagorico per uso della medicina*, Firenze: Francesco Moücke.

Collins, Dr (1803), *Practical Rules for the Management and Medical Treatment of Negro Slaves, in the Sugar Colonies by a Professional Planter*, London: Venor and Hood.

Dancer, Thomas (1809), *The Medical Assistant, or Jamaica Practice of Physic Designed Chiefly for the Use of Families and Plantations*, 2nd edn, St Jago de la Vega: John Lunan.

De Berty, Nigon (1735), *Requête du Promoteur Général de l'Archevesché de Paris*, Paris.

De l'Épée, Charles-Michel (1759), *Relation de la Maladie et de la Guerison Miraculeuse, opérée le 14 juin 1759 à la suite d'une Neuvaine au Saint Sacrement, sur Marie Anne Pigalle, épouse du sieur Denis Mascrey, bourgeois de Paris, y demeurant rue de la Sourdiere, Paroisse S. Roch*, Paris: [s. n.].

Devillers, Charles (1784), *Le colosse aux pieds d'Argille*, [s. l.: s. n.].

D'Holbach, Paul-Henri Thiry Baron (1770), *Histoire critique de Jésus-Christ, ou, analyse raisonnée des Evangiles*, [s. l.: s. n.].

Dictionnaire de l'académie française (1762), 4th edn.

Diderot, Denis (1746), *Pensées Philosophiques*, The Hague: [s. n.].

Douglas, G. A. (1758), *The Nature and Causes of Impotence in Men, and Barrenness in Women*, London: P. Brett.

Duncan, Daniel (1705), *Avis salutaire a tout le monde, contre l'Abus des Choses Chaudes, et particulierement du Café, du Chocolat, et du Thé*, Rotterdam: Abraham Acher.

Falconer, William (1788), *A Dissertation on the Influence of the Passions upon Disorders of the Body*, London: C. Dilly.

The Family Magazine in Two Parts (1741), London: J. Osborn.

Fergusson, William (1846), *Notes and Reflections on a Professional Life*, London: Longman, et al.

Fordyce, William (1773), *A New Inquiry into the Causes, Symptoms, and Cure, of Putrid and Inflammatory Fevers*, London: T. Cadell, J. Murray, and W. Davenhill.

Forrester, James (1748), *Dialogues on the Passions, Habits and Affections Particular to Children*, London: R. Griffiths.

Forster, William (1745), *A Treatise on the Causes of Most Diseases Incident to Human Bodies, and the Cure of Them*, Leeds: James Lister.

Gottlieb, Salomon (1804), 'Neue Entdeckungen und Erfindungen', *Journal Fur Die Neueste Hollandische Medizinische und Naturwisseschaftliche Literatur*, 1 (4): 561–5.

Green, Francis (1783), *'Vox oculis subjecta': A Dissertation on the Most Curious and Important Act of Imparting Speech, and the Knowledge of Language, to the Naturally Deaf, and (Consequently) Dumb*, London: [s.n.].

The High-German Doctor (1720), London: Booksellers of London and Westminster.

Hodson, James (1791), *Nature's Assistant to the Restoration of Health*, London: E. Hodson.

Hugony, Jacques (1754a), *Défense de Geneviève Martin, fille de Saint Geômes, contre un écrit qui ne se trouve qu'à Paris, quoi-qu'imprimé à Langres, sous le nom de M. Morand*. Neufchâteau: Monnoyer.

Hugony, Jacques (1754b), *Lettres du sieur Jacques Hugony, maître en l'art et science de la chirurgie demeurant à Langres, à un de ses amis; ou justification de Geneviève Martin fille de St. Geômes près Langres, accusée dans le Receuil de M. Morand docteur en medecine &c. de s'être introduit les pierres qu'elle a rendues et qu'on lui a tirées grand nombre de fois, par l'operation*, Neufchâteau: [s. n.].

Hume, David (1739–40), *A Treatise of Human Nature*, London: John Noon.

Hunter, John (1788), *Observations on the Diseases of the Army in Jamaica; and on the Best Means of Preserving the Health of Europeans, in That Climate*, London: G. Nicol.

Instructions from the Army Medical Board of Ireland, to Regimental Surgeons Serving on That Establishment, for Regulating the Concerns of the Sick and the Hospital (1806), Dublin: [s.n.].

Instructions from the Army Medical Board of Ireland to Regimental Surgeons Serving on That Establishment (1813), Dublin: A. B. King.

Instructions to Regimental Surgeons, for regulating the Concerns of the Sick, and of the Hospital (1808), 3rd edn, London: Gilbert & Reed.

Jackson, Robert (1805), *A System of Arrangement and Discipline for the Medical Department of Armies*, London: J. Murray.

Jackson, Robert (1824), *A View of the Formation, Discipline and Economy of Armies; with an Appendix, containing Hints for Medical Arrangement in Actual War*, Stockton: William Robinson.

Johnson, Samuel (1755), *A Dictionary of the English Language: in which the Words Are Deduced from Their Originals, and Illustrated in Their Different Significations by Examples from the Best Writers*, 2 vols, London: W. Strahan et al.

Jones, Absalom (1794), *A Narrative of the Proceedings of the Black People during the Late Awful Calamity in Philadelphia in the Year 1793*, Philadelphia: William W. Woodward.

Kant, Immanuel (1784), 'Beantwortung der Frage: Was ist Aufklärung?' *Berlinische Monatsschrift*: 481–94.

The Ladies Dispensatory: or Every Woman Her Own Physician (1739), London: James Hodges.

Lambe, John (1695), *A Sermon Preached Before the King, at Kensington*, London: Walter Kettilby.

Le Clerc, C.-G. (1719), *La Medecine aisée*, new edn, Paris: Laurent d'Houry.

Lemnius, Levinus (1576), *The Touchstone of Complexions*, trans. Thomas Newton, London: Thomas Marsh.

Lempriere, William (1799), *Practical Observations on the Diseases of the Army in Jamaica, as They Occurred between the Years 1792 and 1797*, Vol. 2, London: T. N. Longman and O. Rees.

Lettre à un confesseur touchant le devoir des Medecins & Chirurgiens: Au sujet des Miracles, & des Convulsions (1733), [s. l.: s. n.].
Lettre de M. le marquis de *** à un médecin de province (1783), [s. l. : s. n.].
Lind, James (1778), *An Essay on the Most Effectual Means of Preserving the Health of Seamen in the Royal Navy*, London: J. Murray.
Lister, Martin and George Baglivi, eds (1742), *Sanctorii Sanctorii de Statica medicina aphorismorum Sectiones Septem*, Batavia: J. Manfrè.
Lloyd, G. E. R., John Chadwick and W. N. Mann, eds (1978), *Hippocratic Writings*, New York: Penguin.
Lobb, Theophilus (1739), *A Practical Treatise of Painful Distempers, with Some Effectual Methods of Curing Them*, London: James Buckland.
Locke, John (1694), *An Essay oncerning Human Understanding*, 2nd edn, London: Thomas Dring.
Locke, John (1745 [1693]), *Some Thoughts concerning Education*, London: A. Ward, S. Birt, et al.
Long, Edward (1774), *The History of Jamaica*, Vol. 2, London: T. Lowndes.
Louis XV of France (1732), *Ordonnance du Roy, qui ordonne que la porte du petit Cimetiere de la Paroisse de Saint Medard sera & demeurera fermée, &c.*, Paris: [s. n.].
Lynch, Bernard (1744), *A Guide to Health through the Various Stages of Life*, London: the author.
Lyser, Michael (1740), *The Art of Dissecting the Human Body, in a Plain, Easy, and Compendious Method*, trans. George Thomson, London: Joseph Davidson.
Lyser, Michael and Thomas Bartolin (1653), *Culter Anatomicus: Hoc Est Methodus Brevis Facilis Ac Perspicua Artificiosè [et] Compendiosè Humana Incidendi Cadavera: Cum Nonnulorum Instrumentorum Iconibus*, Copenhagen: Lamprecht.
MacKrill, Joseph (1796), *The History of the Yellow Fever, with the Most Successful Method of Treatment*, Baltimore: John Hayes.
Maddox, Isaac (1743), *The Duty and Advantages of Encouraging Public Infirmaries . . .*, London: H. Woodfall.
Malthus, T. R. (1798), *An Essay on the Principle of Population; or, a View of Its Past and Present Effects on Human Happiness*, London: J. Johnson.
Mendelssohn, Moses (1784), 'Ueber die Frage: was heißt aufklären?' *Berlinische Monatsschrift*: 193–200.
Mesmer, Franz Anton (1798–9), *Mémoire de F. A. Mesmer, docteur en médecine, sur ses découvertes*. Paris: [s. n.].
Monro, Donald (1780), *Observations on the Means of Preserving the Health of Soldiers; and of Conducting Military Hospitals*, vol. 1, 2nd edn, London: J. Murray and G. Robinson.
Montjoie, Galart de (1784), *Lettre sur le magnétisme animal, où on examine la conformité des Opinions des Peuples Anciens & Modernes, des Sçavans, & notamment de M. Bailly avec celles de M. Mesmer; & où l'on compare ces mêmes opinions au* Rapport des Commissaires chargés par le Roi de l'Examen du Magnétisme, Philadelphia: Chez Pierre – J. Duplain.
Morand, Jean-François-Clément (1754a), *Éclaircissement abregé sur la maladie d'une fille de St. Geosmes, à laquelle depuis 8 ans, on a fait 12 Extractions de Pierres de la Vessie, & qui en jette par la bouche, & par la voye des Urines*, Langres: Estinne Bonnin.

Morand, Jean-François-Clément (1754b), *Recueil pour servir d'Éclaircissement détailée sur la maladie de la Fille d'un tireur des Pierres du Village de S. Geomes, près Langres*, Paris: Chez Delaguette.

Morley, Henry (1859), *Memoirs of Bartholomew Fair*, London: Chapman and Hall.

[Muletier] (1784), *Réflexions sur le magnétisme animal, d'après lesquelles on cherche à étabir le degré de croyance que peut mériter jusqu'ici le sytème de M. Mesmer*, Brussels: [s. n.].

Noguez, Pierre (1725), *Sanctorii Sanctorii, de Statica medicina Aphorismorum sectionibus Septem distinctorum explanatio physico-medica. Cui Statica Medicina, tum Gallica Cl. Dodart; tum Britannica Cl. Keill Notis aucta*, Paris: Noël Pissot.

Nougaret, Pierre-Jean-Baptiste (1787), *Tableau mouvant de Paris, ou variétés amusantes, ouvrage enrichi de Notes historique & critiques, & mis au jour par M. Nougaret*, London: [s. n.].

Ovid ([E. J. Kenne] ed. 1986), 'The Envy of Aglauros', In *Metamorphoses*, trans. A. D. Melville, 46–49, Oxford: Oxford University Press.

Parmentier, Antoine A. (1781), *Recherches sur les végétaux nourrissans, qui, dans les temps de disette, peuvent remplacer les alimens ordinaires*, Paris: Imprimerie Royale.

Paxton, Peter (1701), *An Essay concerning the Body of Man, Wherein Its Changes or Diseases are Consider'd*, London: Rich. Wilkin.

Pepys, Samuel (n.d. [1666]), *The Diary of Samuel Pepys: Daily Entries from the 17th Century London Diary*, ed. Phil Gyford, available online: www.pepysdiary.com/diary/1666/11/09/#fn1-1666-11-09 (accessed 15 August 2020).

Pole, Thomas (1790), *The Anatomical Instructor; or an Illustration of the Modern and Most Approved Methods of Preparing and Preserving the Different Parts of the Human Body and of Quadrupeds by Injection, Corrosion, Maceration, Distention, Articulation, Modelling, &C.*, London: Couchman & Fry.

Pomme, Pierre (1767), *Traité des Affections vapoureuses des deux Sexes*, 3rd edn, Lyon: Benoît Duplain.

Poole, Joshua (1972 [1657]), *The English Parnassus 1657*, Menston: Scholar Press Limited.

Pringle, John (1752), *Observations on the Diseases of the Army, in Camp and Garrison*, London: A. Millar, D. Wilson, and T. Payne.

Pringle, John (1753), *Observations on the Diseases of the Army, in Camp and Garrison*, 2nd edn, London: A. Millar, D. Wilson, and T. Payne.

Procès Verbaux de plusieurs médecins et chirurgiens, dresses par ordre de Sa Majesté au sujet de quelques personness soi-disantes agitées de convulsions (1732), Paris: Chez la Veuve Mazières et Jean Baptiste Garnier.

Quincy, John (1721), *The Dispensatory of the Royal College of Physicians*, London.

Relation de la guérison de la sœur Ste. Geneviéve, Religieuse de chœur aux Hospitaliers de la Miséricorde de Jesus, Rue Mouffetard, fauxbourg Saint-Marcel, à Paris, Obtenue par l'application de la vraie Croix & l'intercession de la Sainte Vierge, le 17 Août 1790 (1790), Paris: Chez Le Clere.

Relation de la maladie de la Dame Gardet, demeurant à Paris, rue Phelippeaux, paroisse S. Nicolas-des-Champs. Et de sa guérison subite, opérée dans l'église du Temple, à la procession du Saint-Sacrement, le premier dimanche du mois, 6 septembre 1778 ([1778]), [s. l.: s. n.].

Relation de la maladie et de la guérison miraculeuse de Mlle. Louis Guélon, de Troyes [n. d.], [s. l.: s. n.].

Remarks on Dr. Cheyne's Essay on Health and Long Life ([1725?]), London: Aaron Ward.

Rollo, John (1801), *A Short Account of the Royal Artillery Hospital at Woolwich: With Some Observations on the Management of Artillery Soldiers, Respecting the Preservation of Health*, London: J. Mawman.

Rousseau, Jean-Jacques (1763), *Émile, or On Education*, English edn, London : J. Nourse and P. Vaillant.

Rowley, William (1779), *Seventy-Four Select Cases, with the Manner of Cure, and the Preparation of the Remedies, in the Following Diseases . . .*, London: F. Newbery.

Rumford, Count (Benjamin Thompson) (1796), *Essays Political, Economical, and Philosophical*, Vol. 1, London: T. Cadell Jr and W. Davies.

Ruysch, Frederik (1744), *Alle de Ontleed- Genees- En Heelkundige Werken*, 3 vols., Vol. 1, Amsterdam: Janssoons van Waesberge.

Shelley, Percy Bysshe (1813), *A Vindication of Natural Diet. Being One in a Series of Notes to Queen Mab, a Philosophical Poem*, London: [s.n.].

Sibscota, George (1670), *The Deaf and Dumb Man's Discourse*, London: H. Bruges for William Crook.

Sloane, Hans (1707–1725), *A Voyage to the Islands of Madera, Barbados, Nieves, S. Christophers and Jamaica, with the Natural History of the Herbs and Trees, Four-Footed Beasts, Fishes, Birds, Insects, Reptiles, &c.*, Vols 1 and 2, London, B. M.

Smellie, William (1876), *Smellie's Treatise on the Theory and Practice of Midwifery*, ed. Alfred H. McClintock, London: The New Sydenham Society.

Swieten, Gerard (1776), *Commentaries upon Boerhaave's Aphorisms concerning the Knowledge and Cure of Diseases*, Vol. 1, Edinburgh: Charles Elliot.

Sydenham, Thomas (1848), *The Works of Thomas Sydenham M. D.*, Vol. 1, ed. R. G. Latham, trans. Dr Greenhill, London: The Sydenham Society.

Thouret, Michel-Augustin (1784), *Recherches et doutes sur le magnétisme animal*, Paris: Chez Prault.

Tissot, Samuel Auguste (1765), *Advice to the People in General, with regard to Their Health*, trans. J. Kirkpatrick, London: T. Becket and P. A. de Hondt.

Triller, Daniel Wilhelm (1764), *Dispensatorium Pharmaceuticum Universale*, Frankfurt am Main.

Vauvilliers (1785), *Lettre de M. Vauvilliers, professeur de la langue grecque, au Collége Royal & de l'Académie des Inscriptions & Belles-Lettres, à Monseigneur l'Archevêque de Paris, sur le miracle opéré à Gonesse le 30 juin 1785*, [s. l.: s. n.].

Vintimille, Charles Galpard Guillaume de (1731), *Mandement de Monseigneur l'Archevêque de Paris, au sujet d'un écrit qui a pour titre: Dissertation sur les miracles, et en particulier sur ceux qui ont été opérez au tombeau de M. de Pâris*, Paris: [s. n.].

Wesley, John (1747), *Primitive Physick: or, an Easy and Natural Method of Curing Most Diseases*, London: Thomas Trye.

Willich, Anthony Florian Madinger (1799), *Lectures on Diet and Regimen: Being a Systematic Inquiry into the Most Rational Means of Preserving Health and Prolonging Life*, London: T. N. Longman and O. Rees.

Wollstonecraft, Mary (1792), *A Vindication of the Rights of Woman*, Vol. 1, 2nd edn, London: J. Johnson.

SECONDARY SOURCES

Abad, R. (2006), 'La Fraude dans le commerce et l'approvisionnement alimentaires de Paris au XVIIIe siècle', in G. Béaur, H. Bonin and C. Lemercier (eds), *Fraude, contrefaçon et contrebande, de l'Antiquité à nos jours*, 539–61, Geneva: Droz.

Abruzzo, Margaret (2011), *Polemical Pain: Slavery, Cruelty, and the Rise of Humanitarianism*, Baltimore: Johns Hopkins University Press.

Agamben, Giorgio (2002), *The Open: Man and Animal*, trans. Kevin Attell, Stanford: Stanford University Press.

Adamson, Glenn (2009), 'The Case of the Missing Footstool: Reading the Absent Object', in Karen Harvey (ed.), *History and Material Culture. A Student's Guide to Approaching Alternative Sources*, 192–207, London: Routledge.

Aitken, George A. (1892), *The Life and Works of John Arbuthnot, MD*, Oxford: Clarendon.

Albala, Ken (2002), *Eating Right in the Renaissance*, Berkeley: University of California Press.

Albala, Ken (2005), 'Weight Loss in the Age of Reason', in Christopher E. Forth and Ana Carden-Coyne (eds), *Cultures of the Abdomen: Diet, Digestion, and Fat in the Modern World*, 169–83, London: Palgrave Macmillan.

Albury, William R. (1998), 'Corvisart and Broussais: Human Individuality and Medical Dominance', in Caroline Hannaway and Ann LaBerge (eds), *Constructing Paris Medicine*, 221–50, Amsterdam: Rodopi.

Alpers, Svetlana (1983), *The Art of Describing: Dutch Art in the Seventeenth Century*, Chicago: University of Chicago Press.

Appadurai, Arjun, ed. (1986), *The Social Life of Things*, Cambridge: Cambridge University Press.

Arnold, Dana (2013), *The Spaces of the Hospital: Spatiality and Urban Change in London 1680–1820*, London: Routledge.

Armand, Guilhem (2018), 'Des esprits animaux aux esprits élémentaires: Phyisologie et poétique chez Tiphaigne de La Roche in Sylvie', in Sylvie Kleiman-Lafon and Micheline Louis-Courvoisier (eds), *Les esprits animaux: Littérature, Histoire, Philosophie*, 159–70 *Epistémocritique*, available online: http://epistemocritique.org/actes-du-colloque-les-esprits-animaux (accessed 3 October 2020).

Bacopoulos-Viau, Alexandra and Aude Fauvel (2016), 'The Patient's Turn: Roy Porter and Psychiatry's Tales, Thirty Years on', *Medical History*, 60 (1): 1–18.

Ball, Daniela U. (1991), 'Introduction', in Daniela U. Ball (ed), *Coffee in the Context of European Drinking Habits*, 17–21, Zürich: Johann Jacobs Museum.

Bardell, Eunice Bonow (1979), 'Primitive Physick: John Wesley's Receipts', *Pharmacy in History*, 21, (3): 111–21.

Barker-Benfield, G. J. (1992), *The Culture of Sensibility: Sex and Society in Eighteenth-Century Britain*, Chicago and London: University of Chicago Press.

Bartoš, Hynek (2015), *Philosophy and Dietetics in the Hippocratic On Regimen: A Delicate Balance of Health*, Leiden: Brill.

Basas, Carrie Griffin (2012), 'Private, Public, or Compassionate: Animal Rights and Disability Rights Laws', in Anthony J. Nocella II, Judy K. C. Bentley and Janet M. Duncan (eds), *Earth, Animal, and Disability Liberation: The Rise of the Eco-ability Movement*, 187–204, New York: Peter Lang.

Bashford, Alison and Joyce E. Chaplin (2016), *The New Worlds of Thomas Malthus: Re-reading the Principle of Population*, Princeton: Princeton University Press.

Bashford, Alison and Claire Hooker (2001), 'Introduction: Contagion, Modernity and Postmodernity', in Alison Bashford and Claire Hooker (eds), *Contagion: Historical and Cultural Studies*, 1–14, London and New York: Routledge.

Baudot, Laura (2012), 'An Air of History: Joseph Wright's and Robert Boyle's Air Pump Narratives', *Eighteenth-Century Studies*, 46 (1): 1–28.

Baxandall, Michael (1980), *The Limewood Sculptors of Renaissance Germany*, New Haven: Yale University Press.

Beatty, Heather (2012), *Nervous Disease in Late Eighteenth Century Britain: The Reality of a Fashionable Disorder*, London: Pickering & Chatto.

Bela, Zbigniew (2013), *O starożytnych antidotach, złotych pigułkach i innych sprawach związanych z historią farmacji*, Krakow: Medycyna Praktyczna.

Benedict, Barbara (2000), 'Making a Monster: Socializing Sexuality and the Monster of 1790', in Felicity Nussbaum and Helen Deutsch (eds), *'Defects': Engendering the Modern Body*, 127–53, Ann Arbor: University of Michigan Press.

Benedict, Barbara (2001), *Curiosity: A Cultural History of Early Modern Inquiry*, Chicago and London: University of Chicago Press.

Bennett, Rachel E. (2017), *Capital Punishment and the Criminal Corpse in Scotland, 1740–1834*, London: Palgrave Macmillan.

Berry, Helen (2014), 'The Pleasures of Austerity', *Journal for Eighteenth-Century Studies*, 37 (2): 261–77.

Boddice, Rob (2008), *A History of Attitudes and Behaviours towards Animals in Eighteenth- and Nineteenth-Century Britain: Anthropocentrism and the Emergence of Animals*, New York: Edwin Mellen Press.

Boddice, Rob (2018), *The History of Emotions*, Manchester: Manchester University Press.

Bolens, Guillmette (2014), 'Les simulations perceptives et l'analyse kinésique dans le dessin et dans l'image poétique', *Textimage. Revue d'étude du dialogue texte-image*, 4, available online: www.revue-textimage.com/09_varia_4/bolens1.html (accessed 3 October 2020).

Bolens, Guillemette (2018), 'Les esprits animaux et la châtaigne de Phutatorius: kinésie et agentivité dans *Tristram Shandy* de Laurence Sterne', in Sylvie Kleiman-Lafon and Micheline Louis-Courvoisier (eds), *Les esprits animaux: Littérature, Histoire, Philosophie*, 209–224, *Epistémocritique*, available online: http://epistemocritique.org/actes-du-colloque-les-esprits-animaux (accessed 3 October 2020).

Bolster, Jeffrey (1997), *Black Jacks: African American Seamen in the Age of Sail*, Cambridge, MA: Harvard University Press.

Bondeson, Jan (1999), *The Feejee Mermaid and Other Essays in Natural and Unnatural History*, Ithaca: Cornell University Press.

Bonnet, Jean-Claude (1979), 'Le système de la cuisine et du repas chez Rousseau', in Serge A. Thériault (ed), *Jean-Jacques Rousseau et la médecine naturelle*, Montréal : L'Aurore, 117–50.

Bonnet, Jean-Claude (1983), 'Les manuels de cuisine'. *Dix-huitième siècle*, 15 (1): 53–63.

Boon, Sonja (2016), *Telling the Flesh: Life Writing, Citizenship, and the Body in the Letters to Samuel August Tissot*, Montréal: McGill-Queen's University Press.

Bound Alberti, Fay, ed. (2006), *Medicine, Emotion and Disease, 1700–1950*, Basingstoke: Palgrave Macmillan.

Bound Alberti, Fay (2010), *Matters of the Heart: History, Medicine, and Emotion*, Oxford: Oxford University Press.

Bourke, Joanna (2003), 'Fear and Anxiety: Writing about Emotion in Modern History', *History Workshop Journal*, 55 (1): 111–33.

Bourke, Joanna (2014), *The Story of Pain: From Prayer to Painkillers*, Oxford: Oxford University Press.
Boury, Dominique (2008), 'Irritability and Sensibility: Key Concepts in Assessing the Medical Doctrines of Haller and Bordeu', *Science in Context*, 21 (4): 521–35.
Braisted, Todd (1999), 'The Black Pioneers and Others: The Military Role of Black Loyalists in the American War for Independence', in John Pullis (ed.), *Moving On: Black Loyalists in the Afro-Atlantic World*, 3–38, New York: Garland Publishing.
Branson, Jan and Don Miller (2002), *Damned for Their Difference: The Cultural Construction of Deaf People as Disabled*, Washington: Gallaudet University Press.
Brant, Clare (2004), 'Fume and Perfume: Some Eighteenth-Century Uses of Smell', *Journal of British Studies*, 43 (3): 444–63.
Breen, Benjamin (2019), *The Age of Intoxication: Origins of the Global Drug Trade*, Philadelphia: University of Pennsylvania Press.
Brennan, T. (1988), *Public Drinking and Popular Culture in Eighteenth-Century Paris*, Princeton: Princeton University Press.
Briesen, D. (2010), *Das gesunde Leben. Ernährung und Gesundheit seit dem 18. Jahrhundert*, Frankfurt and New York: Campus Verlag.
Brockliss, Laurence (1994), 'Consultation by Letter in Early Eighteenth-Century Paris: The Medical Practice of Etienne-François Geoffroy', in Ann La Berge and Mordechai Feingold (eds), *French Medical Culture in the Nineteenth Century*, 79–117, Amsterdam and Atlanta: Rodopi.
Brockliss, Laurence and Colin Jones (1997), *The Medical World of Early Modern France*, Oxford: Clarendon Press.
Brooks, Eric St John (1954), *Sir Hans Sloane: The Great Collector and His Circle*, London: Batchworth Press.
Broomhall, Susan (2004), *Women's Medical Work in Early Modern France*, Manchester: Manchester University Press.
Brown, Bill (2001), 'Thing Theory', *Critical Enquiry*, 28 (1): 1–22.
Brown, Kevin (2011), *Poxed and Scurvied: The Story of Sickness and Health at Sea*, Annapolis, MD: Naval Institute Press.
Brown, Michael (2008), 'From Foetid Air to Filth: The Cultural Transformation of British Epidemiological Thought, ca. 1780–1848', *Bulletin of the History of Medicine*, 82 (3): 515–44.
Brown, Michael (2017), 'Surgery and Emotion: The Era before Anaesthesia', in Thomas Schlich (ed.), *Handbook of the History of Surgery*, 327–48, London: Palgrave Macmillan.
Brown, Theodore (1993), 'Mental Diseases', in William F. Bynum and Roy Porter (eds), *Companion Encyclopedia of the History of Medicine*, 438–63, London: Routledge.
Buchenau, Stefanie and Roberto Lo Presti, eds (2019), *Human and Animal Cognition in Early Modern Philosophy and Medicine*, Pittsburgh: University of Pittsburgh Press.
Buckley, Cali (2014) 'The Art of Medicine', *Rubenstein Library Magazine*, 3 (1): 14–15.
Buckley, R. Norman (1979), *Slaves in Red Coats: The British West Indian Regiments, 1795–1815*, New Haven: Yale University Press.
Buckley, R. Norman (1998), *The British Army in the West Indies: Society and the Military in the Revolutionary Age*, Gainesville: University Press of Florida.
Burnard, Trevor (1999), '"The Countrie Continues Sicklie": White Mortality in Jamaica, 1655–1780', *Social History of Medicine*, 12 (1): 45–72.

Carlyle, Margaret (2018), 'Phantoms in the Classroom: Midwifery Training in Enlightenment Europe', *Know: A Journal on the Formation of Knowledge*, 2 (1): 111–36.
Carnicero de Castro, Clara (2014), 'Le fluide électrique chez Sade', *Revue 18e Siècle*, 46 (1): 561–77.
Carrera, Elena (2013), 'Anger and the Mind–Body Connection in Medieval and Early Modern Medicine', in Elena Carrera (ed.), *Emotions and Health 1200–1700*, 95–146, Leiden and Boston: Brill.
Carroll, Patrick E. (2002), 'Medical Police and the History of Public Health', *Medical History*, 46 (4): 461–94.
Cavallo, Sandra and Tessa Storey (2013), *Healthy Living in Late Renaissance Italy*, Oxford: Oxford University Press.
Cessford, Craig (2017), 'Throwing Away Everything but the Kitchen Sink? Large Assemblages, Depositional Practice and Post-Medieval Households in Cambridge', *Post-Medieval Archaeology*, 51, (1): 164–93.
Chakrabarti, Pratik (2010), *Materials and Medicine: Trade, Conquest, and Therapeutics in the Eighteenth Century*, Manchester and New York: Manchester University Press.
Chang, Ku-ming (2011), 'Alchemy as Studies of Life and Matter. Reconsidering the Place of Vitalism in Early Modern Chemistry', *Isis: International Review devoted to the History of Science and Its Civilisation*, 102 (2): 322–29.
Charters, Erica (2014), *Disease, War, and the Imperial State: The Welfare of the British Armed Forces during the Seven Years' War*, Chicago: University of Chicago Press.
Churchill, Wendy (2012a), 'Efficient, Efficacious and Human Responses to Non-European Bodies in British Military Medicine, 1780–1815', *The Journal of Imperial and Commonwealth History*, 40 (2): 137–158.
Churchill, Wendy (2012b), *Female Patients in Early Modern Britain: Gender, Diagnosis, and Treatment*, Farnham: Ashgate.
Clark, Peter (1988), 'The "Mother Gin" Controversy in the Early Eighteenth Century', *Transactions of the Royal Historical Society*, 5th series, 38: 63–84.
Clever, Iris and Willemijn Ruberg (2014), 'Beyond Cultural History? The Material Turn, Praxiography, and Body History', *Humanities*, 3: 546–66.
Cody, Lisa Forman (2005), *Birthing the Nation: Sex, Science, and the Conception of Eighteenth-Century Britons*, Oxford: Oxford University Press.
Coleman, William (1974), 'Health and Hygiene in the *Encyclopédie*: A Medical Doctrine for the Bourgeoisie', *Journal of the History of Medicine*, 29 (4): 399–421.
Cook, Harold (1986), *The Decline of the Old Medical Regime in Stuart London*, Ithaca: Cornell University Press, 1986.
Cook, Harold (1994), 'Good Advice and Little Medicine: The Professional Authority of Early Modern English Physicians', *The Journal of British Studies*, 33 (1): 1–31.
Cook, Harold (2000), 'Boerhaave and the Flight from Reason in Medicine', *Bulletin of History of Medicine*, 74 (2): 221–40.
Cook, Harold and Timothy Walker (2013), 'Circulation of Medicine in the Early Modern Atlantic World', *Social History of Medicine*, 26 (3): 337–51.
Cooper, Alix (2007), *Inventing the Indigenous: Local Knowledge and Natural History in Early Modern Europe*, Cambridge: Cambridge University Press.
Cooter, Roger and Claudia Stein (2013), *Writing History in the Age of Biomedicine*, New Haven: Yale University Press.
Coquillard, Isabelle (2018), 'Le marché des remèdes antivénériens et les docteurs régents de la Faculté de médecine de Paris au XVIIIe siècle', in Philip Reider and François Zanetti (eds), *Materia medica: Savoirs et usages des médicaments aux époques médiévales et modernes*, 161–88, Geneva: Librairie Droz.

Coste, Joël (2014), *Les écrits de la souffrance. La consultation médicale en France (1525–1825)*, Seysell: Champvallon.
Craton, Lillian E. (2009), *The Victorian Freak Show: The Significance of Disability and Physical Difference in 19th-Century Fiction*, Amherst: Cambria Press.
Crewe, Duncan (1993), *Yellow Jack and the Worm: British Naval Administration in the West Indies, 1739–1748*, Liverpool: Liverpool University Press.
Cronon, William. (1996), 'The Trouble with Wilderness: Or Getting Back to the Wrong Nature', in William Cronon (ed.), *Uncommon Ground: Rethinking the Human Place in Nature*, 69–90, New York: W. W. Norton.
Cullather, N. (2007), 'The Foreign Policy of the Calorie', *American Historical Review*, 112 (2): 337–64.
Cullen, L. M. (1992), 'Comparative Aspects of Irish Diet, 1550–1850', in H.-J. Teuteberg (ed.), *European Food History: A Research Review*, 45–55, Leicester, London and New York: Leicester University Press.
Cunningham, Andrew (2010), *The Anatomist Anatomis'd: An Experimental Discipline in Enlightenment Europe*, Farnham: Ashgate.
Cunningham, Andrew and Roger French, eds (1990), *The Medical Enlightenment of the Eighteenth Century*, Cambridge: Cambridge University Press.
Cunningham, Andrew and Ole Peter Grell, eds (2007), *Medicine and Religion in Enlightenment Europe*, Aldershot: Routledge.
Curran, Andrew (2011), *The Anatomy of Blackness: Science and Slavery in an Age of Enlightenment*, Baltimore: Johns Hopkins University Press.
Curth, Louise Hill (2004), 'Seventeenth-Century English Almanacs: Transmitters of Advice for Sick Animals', in Willem de Blécourt and Cornelie Usborne (eds), *Cultural Approaches to the History of Medicine: Mediating Medicine in Early Modern and Modern Europe*, 56–70, London: Palgrave Macmillan.
Curtin, Philip (1961), '"The White Man's Grave": Image and Reality, 1780–1850', *The Journal of British Studies*, 1 (1): 94–110.
Cusset, François (2008), *French Theory: How Foucault, Derrida, Deleuze, & Co. Transformed the Intellectual Life of the United States*, Minneapolis: University of Minnesota Press.
Dabhoiwala, Faramerz (2012), *The Origins of Sex: A History of the First Sexual Revolution*, Oxford: Oxford University Press.
Dacome, Lucia (2001), 'Living with the Chair: Private Excreta, Collective Health and Medical Authority in the Eighteenth Century', *History of Science*, 39 (4): 467–500.
Dacome, Lucia (2012), 'Balancing Acts: Picturing Perspiration in the Long Eighteenth Century', *Studies in History and Philosophy of Biological and Biomedical Sciences*, 43 (2): 379–91.
Darnton, Robert (1968), *Mesmerism and the End of the Enlightenment in France*, Cambridge: Harvard University Press.
Daston, Lorraine and Peter Galison (2007), *Objectivity*, New York: Zone Books.
Daston, Lorraine and Katherine Park (1998), *Wonders and the Order of Nature, 1150–1750*, New York: Zone Books.
Daston, Lorraine and Katherine Park (2001), *Wonders and the Order of Nature: 1150–1750*, revised edn, New York: Zone Books.
Davis, Lennard J. (1995), *Enforcing Normalcy: Disability, Deafness, and the Body*, London: Verso.
De Beer, Gavin (1953), *Sir Hans Sloane and the British Museum*, London: Published for the Trustees of the Museum by Oxford University Press.

De Renzi, Silvia (2004), 'Old and New Models of the Body', in Peter Palmer (ed.), *The Healing Arts: Health, Disease, and Society in Europe 1500–1800*, 166–92, Manchester: Manchester University Press.
De Zulueta, Paquita (2013), 'Compassion in Healthcare', *Clinical Ethics*, 8 (4): 87–90.
DeLacy, Margaret (1999), 'Nosology, Morality, and Disease Theory in the Eighteenth Century', *Journal of the History of Medicine*, 54 (2): 261–84.
Delbourgo, James (2012), 'Collecting Hans Sloane', in Alison Walker, Arthur MacGregor and Michael Hunter (eds), *From Books to Bezoars: Sir Hans Sloane and his Collections*, 9–23, London: The British Library.
Delbourgo, James (2017), *Collecting the World: The Life and Curiosity of Hans Sloane*, London: Allen Lane.
Den Hartog, A. P. (ed) (1995), *Food Technology, Science and Marketing: European Diet in the Twentieth Century*, East Linton: Tuckwell Press.
Desowitz, Robert S. (1997), *Who Gave Pinta to the Santa Maria? Torrid Diseases in a Temperate World*, New York: W. W. Norton.
Deutsch, Helen and Felicity Nussbaum, eds (2000), *Defects: Engendering the Modern Body*, Ann Arbor: University of Michigan Press.
Devlin, Hannah (2018), '"Irish Giant" May Finally Get Respectful Burial after 200 Years On Display', *The Guardian*, 22 June.
Digby, Anne (1994), *Making a Medical Living: Doctors and Patients in the English Market for Medicine, 1720–1911*, Cambridge: Cambridge University Press.
Dobson, Mary (1989), 'Mortality Gradients and Disease Exchanges: Comparisons from Old England and Colonial America', *Social History of Medicine*, 2 (3): 259–97.
Dobson, Mary (1997), *Contours of Death and Disease in Early Modern England*, Cambridge: Cambridge University Press.
Drey, Rudolf E. A. (1978), *Apothecary Jars: Pharmaceutical Pottery and Porcelain in Europe and the East 1150–1850*, London and Boston: Faber & Faber.
Duden, Barbara (1991), *The Woman Beneath the Skin: A Doctor's Patients in Eighteenth- Century Germany*, Cambridge, MA: Harvard University Press.
Duden, Barbara (1992), 'Medicine and the History of the Body', in Jens Lachmund and Gunnar Stollberg (eds), *The Social Construction of Illness*, 39–51, Stuttgart: Franz Steiner Verlag.
Duffin, Jacalyn (2009), *Medical Miracles: Doctors, Saints, and Healing in the Modern World*, Oxford: Oxford University Press.
Duncan, Janet M. (2012), 'Interdependence, Capability, and Competence as a Framework for Eco-Ability', in Anthony J. Nocella II, Judy K. C. Bentley and Janet M. Duncan (eds), *Earth, Animal, and Disability Liberation: The Rise of the Eco-Ability Movement*, 38–58, New York: Peter Lang.
Dyde, Sean (2015), 'George Combe and Common Sense', *British Journal for the History of Science*, 48 (2): 233–59.
Earle, Rebecca (2012), *The Body of the Conquistador: Food, Race and the Colonial Experience in Spanish America, 1492–1700*, Cambridge: Cambridge University Press.
Edelstein, Dan (2010), *The Enlightenment: A Genealogy*, Chicago and London: University of Chicago Press.
Eden, Trudy (2008), *The Early American Table: Food and Society in the New World*, Chicago: Northern Illinois University Press.
Eichberg, Stephanie (2009), 'Constituting the Human via the Animal in Eighteenth-Century Experimental Neurophysiology: Albrecht von Haller's Sensibility Trials', *Medizinhistorisches Journal*, 44 (3–4): 274–95.

Eisenman, Stephen F. (2013), *The Cry of Nature: Art and the Making of Animal Rights*, London: Reaktion Books.
Ellis, Markman (1996), *The Politics of Sensibility: Race, Gender and Commerce in the Sentimental Novel*, Cambridge: Cambridge University Press.
Emch-Dériaz, Antoinette (1992a), 'The Non-Naturals Made Easy', in Roy Porter (ed.), *The Popularization of Medicine 1650–1850*, 134–59, London and New York: Routledge.
Emch-Dériaz, Antoinette (1992b), *Tissot: Physician of the Enlightenment*, New York: Peter Lang.
Eustace, Nicole, Eugenia Lean, Julie Livingston, Jan Plamper, William M. Reddy and Barbara H. Rosenwein (2012), 'AHR Conversation: The Historical Study of Emotions', *The American Historical Review*, 117 (5): 1487–1531.
Fiering, Norman (1976), 'Irresistible Compassion: An Aspect of Eighteenth-Century Sympathy and Humanitarianism', *Journal of the History of Ideas*, 2(37): 195–218.
Fink, Beatrice (1990), 'The Metamorphic Potato: A Revolutionary Root', in *Oxford Symposium on Food and Cookery 1989. Staple Foods. Proceedings*, 107–11. London: Prospect Books.
Fischler, Claude (1993), *L'Homnivore. Le goût, la cuisine et le corps*, Paris: Éditions Odile Jacob.
Fissell, Mary (1991), *Patients, Power, and the Poor in Eighteenth-Century Bristol*, Cambridge and New York: Cambridge University Press.
Fissell, Mary (1995), 'The Disappearance of the Patient's Narrative in the Invention of Hospital Medicine', in Roger French and Andrew Wear (eds), *British Medicine in an Age of Reform*, 92–109, London and New York: Routledge.
Fissell, Mary E. (2004), 'Making Meaning from the Margins: The New Cultural History of Medicine', in Frank Huisman and John Harley Warner (eds), *Locating Medical History; The Stories and their Meanings*, 364–89, Baltimore and London: Johns Hopkins University Press.
Fleming, John (2013), *The Dark Side of the Enlightenment: Wizards, Alchemists, and Spiritual Seekers in the Age of Reason*, New York: W. W. Norton & Company.
Fleming, James Roger and Ann Johnson (2014), 'Introduction', in James Roger Fleming and Ann Johnson (eds), *Toxic Airs: Body, Place, Planet in Historical Perspective*, ix–xiv, Pittsburgh: University of Pittsburgh Press.
Flynn, Karen (2009), 'Beyond the Glass Wall: Black Canadian Nurses, 1940–1970', *Nursing History Review*, 17: 129–52.
Fogel, Robert William (2004), *The Escape from Hunger and Premature Death, 1700–2100*, Cambridge: Cambridge University Press.
Forbes, Robert Jacobus (1958), 'The Rise of Food Technology (1500–1900)', *Janus*, 47: 139–55.
Forster, Robert and Orest Ranum, eds (1980), *Medicine and Society in France: Selections from the Annales Economies, Sociétés, Civilisations*, Vol. 6, trans. Elborg Forster and Patricia M. Ranum, Baltimore: Johns Hopkins University Press.
Foucault, Michel (1973), *The Birth of the Clinic: An Archaeology of Medical Perception*, New York: Pantheon Books.
Foucault, Michel (1977), *Discipline and Punish: The Birth of the Prison*, London: Allen Lane.
Foucault, Michel (1991), 'What is Enlightenment?' in P. Rabinow (ed), *The Foucault Reader: An Introduction to Foucault's Thought*, 32–50, London: Penguin.

Foucault, Michel (2007), *Security, Territory, Population: Lectures at the Collège de France 1977–1978*, London: Palgrave Macmillan.
Foucault, Michel (2011), *Le beau danger. Entretien avec Claude Bonnefoy*, Paris: Edition EHESS.
Frazer, Michael (2010), *The Enlightenment of Sympathy: Justice and the Moral Sentiments in the Eighteenth Century and Today*, Oxford: Oxford University Press.
Frevert, Ute (2014), 'Defining Emotions: Concepts and Debates over Three Centuries', in Ute Frevert, Christian Bailey, Pascal Eitler, Benno Gammerl, Bettina Hitzer, Margrit Pernau, Monique Scheer, Anne Schmidt and Nina Verheyen (eds), *Emotional Lexicons: Continuity and Change in the Vocabulary of Feeling, 1700–2000*, 1–31, Oxford: Oxford University Press.
Frevert, Ute (2016), 'Empathy in the Theater of Horror, or Civilizing the Human Heart', in Aleida Assmann and Ines Detmers (eds), *Empathy and Its Limits*, 79–99, London: Palgrave Macmillan.
Fudge, Erica (2002), 'A Left-Handed Blow: Writing the History of Animals', in Nigel Rothfels (ed.), *Representing Animals*, 3–18, Bloomington: Indiana University Press.
Fudge, Erica (2006), 'The History of Animals', *H-Animal*, available online: https://networks.h-net.org/node/16560/pages/32226/history-animals-erica-fudge (accessed 21 June 2019).
Gabbard, D. (2008). 'From Idiot Beast to Idiot Sublime: Mental Disability in John Cleland's "Fanny Hill"', *PMLA*, 123 (2): 375–89.
Gabbard, D. (2011), 'Disability Studies and the British Long Eighteenth Century', *Literature Compass*, 8 (2): 80–94.
Gage, John (1993), *Colour and Culture: Practice and Meaning from Antiquity to Abstraction*, London: Thames and Hudson.
Gaukroger, Stephen (2010), *The Collapse of Mechanism and the Rise of Sensibility: Science and the Shaping of Modernity 1680–1760*, Oxford: Oxford University Press.
Gelfand, Toby (1980), *Professionalizing Modern Medicine: Paris Surgeons and Medical Science and Institutions in the 18th Century*, Santa Barbara: Greenwood Press.
Genette, Gerard (1987), *Paratexts: Thresholds of Interpretation*, trans. Jane E. Lewin, Cambridge: Cambridge University Press.
Gentilcore, David (1998), *Healers and Healing in Early Modern Italy*, Manchester and New York: Manchester University Press.
Gentilcore, David (2006), *Medical Charlatanism in Early Modern Italy*, Oxford: Oxford University Press.
Gentilcore, David (2015), *Food and Health in Early Modern Europe: Diet, Medicine and Society, 1450–1800*, London: Bloomsbury.
Geyer-Kordesch, Johanna (1995), 'Whose Enlightenment: Medicine, Witchcraft, Melancholia, and Pathology', in Roy Porter (ed.), *Medicine in the Enlightenment*, 113–27, Amsterdam: Rodopi.
Gil Sotres, Pedro (1998), 'The Regimens of Health', in Mirko D. Grmek (ed.), *Western Medical Thought from Antiquity to the Middle Ages*, 291–318, Cambridge, MA: Harvard University Press.
Gilligand, Donald (2017), 'Restoration Reveals Human Remains in Famous Carnegie Diorama', *Tribune Review*, 26 January.
Ginzburg, Carlo (2013), 'Nos mots et les leurs. Une réflexion sur le métier d'historien aujourd'hui', *Essais. Revue interdisciplinaire d'humanités*, Special Issue 1 (*L'estrangement. Retour sur un thème de Carlo Ginzburg*): 192–209.
Godineau, Dominique (2012), *S'abréger les jours. Le suicide en France au 18e siècle*. Paris: Armand Colin.

Gómez, Pablo (2013), 'The Circulation of Bodily Knowledge in the Seventeenth-Century Black Spanish Caribbean', *Social History of Medicine*, 26 (3): 383–402.
Goody, Jack (1997), 'Industrial Food: Towards the Development of a World Cuisine', in Carole Counihan and Penny Van Esterik (eds), *Food and Culture: A Reader*, 338–56, New York and London: Routledge.
Grassi, Marie-Claire (1998), *Lire l'épistolaire*, Paris: Dunod.
Grigson, Caroline (2016), *Menagerie: The History of Exotic Animals in England, 1100–1837*, Oxford: Oxford University Press.
Grosz, Elizabeth (1993), 'Intolerable Ambiguity: Freaks at/as the Limit', in Rosemarie Garland Thomson (ed), *Freakery: Cultural Spectacles of the Extraordinary Body*, 55–66, New York: New York University Press.
Guerrini, Anita (1986), 'The Tory Newtonians: Gregory, Pitcairne, and Their Circle', *Journal of British Studies*, 25 (3): 288–311.
Guerrini, A. (1999a), 'The Hungry Soul: George Cheyne and the Construction of Femininity', *Eighteenth-Century Studies*, 32, (3), 279–91.
Guerrini, Anita (1999b), 'A Diet for a Sensitive Soul: Vegetarianism in Eighteenth-Century Britain', *Eighteenth-Century Life*, 23 (2): 34–42.
Guerrini, Anita (2000), *Obesity and Depression in the Enlightenment: The Life and Times of George Cheyne*, Norman: University of Oklahoma Press.
Guerrini, Anita (2003), 'Duverney's Skeletons', *Isis: International Review devoted to the History of Science and Its Civilisation*, 94 (4): 577–603.
Guerrini, Anita (2006), 'Alexander Monro Primus and the Moral Theatre of Anatomy', *Eighteenth Century: Theory and Interpretation*, 47 (1): 1–18.
Guerrini, Anita (2010), 'Advertising Monstrosity: Broadsides and Human Exhibition in Early Eighteenth-Century London', in Patricia Fumerton and Anita Guerrini (eds), *Ballads and Broadsides in Britain, 1500–1800*, 109–30, Farnham: Ashgate.
Guerrini, Anita (2012a), 'Health, National Character and the English Diet in 1700', *Studies in History and Philosophy of Biological and Biomedical Sciences*, 43 (2): 349–56.
Guerrini, Anita (2012b), 'The Value of a Dead Body', in Helen Deutsch and Mary Terrall (eds), *Vital Matters: Eighteenth-Century Views of Conception, Life, and Death*, 246–64, Toronto: University of Toronto Press.
Guerrini, Anita (2016a), 'The Ghastly Kitchen', *History of Science*, 54 (1): 71–97.
Guerrini, Anita (2016b), 'The Material Turn in the History of Life Science', *Literature Compass*, 13 (7): 469–80.
Haas, Angela (2020), 'Medical Marvels and Professional Medicine: Establishing Scientific Authority in Enlightenment France', *Social History of Medicine*, 33 (3): 704–27.
Hacking, Ian (2002), *Historical Ontology*, Cambridge, MA: Harvard University Press.
Hallam, Elizabeth (2010), 'Articulating Bones: An Epilogue', *Journal of Material Culture*, 15 (4): 465–92.
Hallam, Elizabeth and J. Hockey (2001), *Death, Memory and Material Culture*, Oxford: Berg.
Hamlin, Charles (2014a), *More Than Hot: A Short History of Fever*, Baltimore: Johns Hopkins University Press.
Hamlin, Charles (2014b), 'Surgeon Reginald Orton and the Pathology of Deadly Air: The Contest for Context in Environmental Health', in James Roger Fleming and Ann Johnson (eds), *Toxic Airs: Body, Place, Planet in Historical Perspective*, 23–49, Pittsburgh: University of Pittsburgh Press.

Hanafi, Nahema (2017), *Le frisson et le baume. Expériences féminines du corps au siècle des Lumières*, Rennes: Presses Universitaires de Rennes.
Handley, Sasha (2016), *Sleep in Early Modern England*, New Haven: Yale University Press.
Hannan, Leonie and Sarah Longair (2017), *History through Material Culture*, Manchester: University of Manchester Press.
Haraway, Donna (2003), *Companion Species Manifesto: Dogs, People, and Significant Otherness*, Chicago: Prickly Paradigm Press.
Haraway, Donna (2019), 'Roundtable', in *Humanimalia*, 10 (1), available online: www.depauw.edu/humanimalia/issue%2019/index.html (accessed 10 August 2020).
Harris, Bernard (2004), 'Public Health, Nutrition, and the Decline of Mortality: The McKeown Thesis', *Social History of Medicine*, 17 (3): 379–407.
Harrison, Mark (2010), *Medicine in an Age of Commerce and Empire: Britain and Its Tropical Colonies 1660–1830*, Oxford: Oxford University Press.
Harrison, Mark (2013), 'Scurvy on Sea and Land: Political Economy and Natural History, c. 1780–c. 1850', *Journal for Maritime Research*, 15 (1): 7–25.
Harvey, Karen, ed. (2009), *History and Material Culture: A Student's Guide to Approaching Alternative Sources*, London: Routledge.
Heise, Ulla (1987), *Coffee and Coffee Houses*, West Chester: Schiffer Publishing.
Hendriksen, Marieke M. A. (2014) 'The Fabric of the Body: Textile in Anatomical Models and Preparations, ca. 1700–1900', *Histoire, médecine et santé*, 5: 21–32.
Hendriksen, Marieke M. A. (2015a), *Elegant Anatomy: The Eighteenth-Century Leiden Anatomical Collections*, Leiden and Boston: Brill.
Hendriksen, Marieke M. A. (2015b), 'Weapon Salve, Tooth Hangers and Other "Sympathetic" Cures', *The Medicine Chest*, 21 July, available online: https://mariekehendriksen.nl/2015/07/21/weapon-salve-tooth-hangers-and-other-sympathetic-cures (accessed 7 December 2017).
Hendriksen, Marieke M. A. (2017) '"Art and Technique Always Balance the Scale": German Philosophies of Sensory Perception, Taste, and Art Criticism, and the Rise of the Term Technik, ca. 1735 – ca. 1835," *History of Humanities*, 2 (1): 201–19.
Hendriksen, Marieke M. A. (2018a), 'The Disappearance of Lapidary Medicine: Skepticism about the Utility of Gemstones in 18th-Century Dutch Medicine and Pharmacy', in Michael Bycroft and Sven Dupré (eds), *Gems in the Early Modern World: Materials, Knowledge, and Global Trade, 1450–1800*, 197–220, Basingstoke: Palgrave.
Hendriksen, Marieke M. A. (2018b), 'Nosce te ipsum. Veränderte Funktionen und Räumlichkeiten des Leidener anatomischen Theaters im achtzehnten Jahrhundert', in Johanna Bleker, Petra Lennig and Thomas Schnalke (eds), *Tiefe Einblicke. Das Anatomische Theater im Zeitalter der Aufklärung*, 171–84, Berlin: Kulturverlag Kadmos.
Hendriksen, Marieke M. A. (2019), 'Animal Bodies between Wonder and Natural History: Taxidermy in the Cabinet and Menagerie of Stadholder Willem V (1748–1806)', *Journal of Social History*, 52 (4): 1110–31.
Hendriksen, Marieke M. A., Hieke Huistra and Rina Knoeff (2013), 'Recycling Anatomical Preparations', in Sam Alberti and Elizabeth Hallam (eds), *Medical Museums*, 74–87, London: Royal College of Surgeons of England.
Hennig, Boris (2010), 'Science, Conscience, Consciousness', *History of the Human Sciences*, 23 (3): 15–28.
Herman, Bernard L. (1992), 'Introduction: The Discourse of Objects', in *The Stolen House*, 3–14, Charlottesville: The University Press of Virginia.

Herrstein Smith, Barbara (2016), 'What Was Close Reading? A Century of Method in Literary Studies', *Minnesota Review*, 87: 57–75.
Hirschmann, Albert O. (1997), *The Passions and the Interests: Political Arguments for Capitalism before Its Triumph*, 20th anniversary edn, Princeton: Princeton University Press.
Hitchcock, Tim (2012), 'The Reformulation of Sexual Knowledge in Eighteenth-Century England', *Signs: Journal of Women in Culture and Society*, 37 (4): 823–31.
Hogarth, Rana (2017), *Medicalizing Blackness: Making Racial Difference in the Atlantic World, 1780–1840*, Chapel Hill: University of North Carolina Press.
Hollis, Karen (2001), 'Fasting Women: Bodily Claims and Narrative Crises in Eighteenth-Century Science', *Eighteenth-Century Studies*, 34 (4): 523–38.
Holmes, Frederic L. (1975), 'The Transformation of the Science of Nutrition', *Journal of the History of Biology*, 8 (1): 135–44.
Hufbauer, Karl (1982), *The Formation of the German Chymical Community, 1720–1795*, Berkeley: University of California Press.
Huisman, Tim (2009), *The Finger of God: Anatomical Practice in 17th Century Leiden*, Leiden: Primavera Press.
Huistra, Hieke (2019), *The Afterlife of the Leiden Anatomical Collections: Hands On, Hands Off*, London: Routledge.
Hunter, Lynette (2004), 'Cankers in *Romeo and Juliet:* Sixteenth-Century Medicine at a Figural/Literal Cusp', in Stephanie Moss and Kaara L. Peterson (eds), *Disease, Diagnosis and Cure on the Early Modern Stage*, 171–80, Aldershot: Ashgate.
ICOM Code of Ethics for Museums (2017), Paris: ICOM, available online: https://icom.museum/wp-content/uploads/2018/07/ICOM-code-En-web.pdf (accessed 5 October 2020).
Ishizuka, Hisao (2012), '"Fibre Body": The Concept of Fibre in Eighteenth Century Medicine, c. 1700–1740', *Medical History*, 56 (4): 562–84.
Ishizuka, Hisao (2016), *Fiber, Medicine, and Culture in the British Enlightenment*, New York: Palgrave Macmillan.
Israel, Jonathan I. (2006), *Enlightenment Contested. Philosophy, Modernity, and the Emancipation of Man 1670–1752*, Oxford: Oxford University Press.
Jackson, Stanley W. (1990), 'The Use of the Passions in Psychological Healing', *Journal for the History of Medicine and Allied Sciences*, 45 (2): 150–75.
Jacot Grapa, Caroline (2009), *Dans le vif du sujet. Diderot, corps et âme,* Paris: Classique Garnier.
Jankovic, Vladimir (2010), *Confronting the Climate: British Airs and the Making of Environmental Medicine*, New York: Palgrave Macmillan.
Jenner, Mark and Patrick Wallis, eds (2007), *Medicine and the Market in England and Its Colonies, c. 1450–c. 1850*, Basingstoke: Palgrave Macmillan.
Jewson, N. D. (1976), 'The Disappearance of the Sick-Man from Medical Cosmology, 1770–1870', *Sociology*, 10 (2): 225–44.
Johnston, James Andrew and Russel West-Pavlov (2015), 'Introduction. Performing the Politics of Passion: *Troilus and Criseyde* and *Troilus and Cressida* and the Literary Tradition of Love and History', in Andrew Johnston James, Russel West-Pavlov and Elisabeth Kempf (eds), *Love, History and Emotion in Chaucer and Shakespeare:* Troilus and Criseyde *and* Troilus and Cressida, 1–16, Manchester: Manchester University Press.
Jones, Colin (1996), 'The Great Chain of Buying: Medical Advertisement, the Bourgeois Public Sphere, and the Origins of the French Revolution', *The American Historical Review*, 101 (1): 13–40.

Jones, Ellis (1960), 'The Life and Works of Guilhelmus Fabricius Hildanus (1560–1634). Part I', *Medical History*, 4 (2): 112–34.
Jonsson, Fredrik Albritton (2005), 'The Physiology of Hypochondria in Eighteenth-Century Britain', in Christopher E. Forth and Ana Carden-Coyne (eds), *Cultures of the Abdomen: Diet, Digestion, and Fat in the Modern World*, 16–30, London: Palgrave Macmillan.
Jordanova, Ludmilla (1989), *Sexual Visions: Images of Gender in Science and Medicine between the Enlightenment and Twentieth Century*, London and New York: Harvester Wheatsheaf.
Jordanova, Ludmilla (2012), *The Look of the Past: Visual and Material Evidence in Historical Practice*, Cambridge: Cambridge University Press.
Jørgensen, Dolly and Sverker Sörlin (2013), 'Introduction: Making the Action Visible: Making Environments in Northern Landscapes', in Dolly Jørgensen and Sverker Sörlin (eds), *Northscapes: History, Technology, and the Making of Northern Environments*, 1–14, Vancouver: University of British Columbia Press.
Kafer, Alison (2012), 'Desire and Disgust: My Ambivalent Adventures in Devoteeism', in Robert McRuer and Anna Mollow (eds), *Sex and Disability*, 331–54, Durham, NC: Duke University Press.
Kamminga, Harmke and Andrew Cunningham, eds (1995), *The Science and Culture of Nutrition, 1840–1940*. Amsterdam and Atlanta: Rodopi.
Kaplan, S. L. (1996), *The Bakers of Paris and the Bread Question, 1700–1775*, Durham, NC, and London: Duke University Press.
Kennedy, Meegan (2014), '"Let Me Die in Your House": Cardiac Distress and Sympathy in Nineteenth-Century British Medicine', *Literature and Medicine*, 32 (1): 105–32.
Kiple, Kenneth (1984), *The Caribbean Slave: A Biological History*, Cambridge: Cambridge University Press.
Kirmayer, Laurence J. (1992), 'The Body's Insistence on Meaning: Metaphor as Presentation and Representation in Illness Experience', *Medical Anthropology Quarterly*, New Series, 6 (4): 323–46.
Kleiman-Lafon, Sylvie and Micheline Louis-Courvoisier (2018), 'Introduction' in Sylvie Kleiman-Lafon and Micheline Louis-Courvoisier (eds), *Les esprits animaux. Littérature, Histoire, Philosophie*, 1–12, available online: https://epistemocritique.org/actes-du-colloque-les-esprits-animaux (accessed 6 November 2020).
Klein, Herbert (1988), *African Slavery in Latin America and the Caribbean*, Oxford: Oxford University Press.
Klepp, Susan (1994), 'Seasoning and Society: Racial Differences in Mortality in Eighteenth-Century Philadelphia', *William and Mary Quarterly*, 51 (3): 473–506.
Knoeff, Rina (2007), 'Moral Lessons of Perfection: A Comparison of Mennonite and Calvinist Motives in the Anatomical Atlases of Bidloo and Albinus', in Ole Peter Grell and Andrew Cunningham (eds), *Medicine and Religion in Enlightenment Europe*, 121–43, Farnham: Ashgate.
Knoeff, Rina (2015), 'Touching Anatomy: On the Handling of Preparations in the Anatomical Cabinets of Frederik Ruysch (1638–1731)', *Studies in History and Philosophy of Biological and Biomedical Sciences*, 49: 32–44.
Knoeff, Rina and Robert Zwijnenberg, eds (2015), *The Fate of Anatomical Collections*, Farnham: Ashgate.
Koerner, Lisbet (1999), *Linnaeus: Nature and Nation*, Cambridge, MA: Harvard University Press.

Kosmin, Jennifer F (2020), *Authority, Gender, and Midwifery in Early Modern Italy*, London: Routledge.
Kracauer, Siegfried (2005), *L'histoire des avant-dernières choses*, Paris: Stock.
Kreiser, Robert B. (1978), *Miracles, Convulsions, and Ecclesiastical Politics in Eighteenth-Century Paris*, Princeton: Princeton University Press.
Laqueur, Thomas (1990), *Making Sex: Body and Gender from the Greeks to Freud*, Cambridge: Harvard University Press.
Laqueur, Thomas W. (2003), *Solitary Sex: A Cultural History of Masturbation*, New York: Zone Books.
Lane, Joan (1985), '"The Doctor Scolds Me": The Diaries and Correspondence of Patients in Eighteenth Century England', in Roy Porter (ed.), *Patients and Practitioners: Lay Perceptions of Medicine in Pre-Industrial Society*, 205–48, Cambridge: Cambridge University Press.
Langum, Virginia (2016), *Medicine and the Seven Deadly Sins in Late Medieval Literature Culture*, New York: Palgrave Macmillan.
Latour, Bruno (2005), *Reassembling the Social: An Introduction to Actor-Network-Theory*, Oxford: Oxford University Press.
Lawrence, Christopher (1996), 'Disciplining Disease: Scurvy, the Navy and Imperial Expansion, 1750–1825', in David Philip Miller and Peter Haans Reill (eds), *Visions of Empire: Voyages, Botany, and Representations of Nature*, 80–106, Cambridge: Cambridge University Press.
Lawrence, Christopher (2004), 'John Gregory', *Oxford Dictionary of National Biography*, Oxford: Oxford University Press.
Lebrun, François (1983), *Se soigner autrefois: Médecins, saints, et sorcières aux 17e et 18e siècles*, Paris: Messidor/Temps Actuels.
Leong, Elaine (2008), 'Making Medicines in the Early Modern Household', *Bulletin of the History of Medicine*, 82 (1): 145–68.
Leong, Elaine (2013), 'Collecting Knowledge for the Family: Recipes, Gender and Practical Knowledge in the Early Modern English Household', *Centaurus*, 55 (2): 81–103.
Lindemann, Mary (2010), *Medicine and Society in Early Modern Europe*, 2nd edn, Cambridge: Cambridge University Press.
Louis-Courvoisier, Micheline (2015), 'Rendre sensible une souffrance psychique. Lettres de mélancoliques au 18e siècle', *Dix-Huitième siècle*, 45: 87–101.
Louis-Courvoisier, Micheline (2017), 'L'univers physiopsychologique des malades au XVIIIe siècle: "Une pratique" du sensible', *Etudes Epistémè*, 31, https://doi.org/10.4000/episteme.1742 (accessed 13 October 2020).
Louis-Courvoisier, Micheline (2018a), 'La folie de Mme Fol (18e siècle). Une intranquillité de la chair', *Revue Epistémocritique*, 17, available online: https://epistemocritique.org/hors-dossier-la-folie-de-mme-fol-18e-siecle-une-intranquillite-de-la-chair (accessed 3 October 2020).
Louis-Courvoisier, Micheline (2018b) 'The Soul in the Entrails: The Experience of the Sick in the Eighteenth Century', in Rebecca Barr, Sylvie Kleiman-Lafon and Sophie Vasset (eds), *Bellies, Bowels and Entrails in the Eighteenth Century*, 80–97, Manchester: Manchester University Press.
Louis-Courvoisier, Micheline (2019), 'Inquiétude/Uneasiness: Between Mental Emotion and Bodily Sensation (18th–20th Centuries)', *Emotions: History, Culture, Society*, 3 (1): 94–115.
Louis-Courvoisier, Micheline and Alex Mauron (2002), '"He found me very well; for me I was still feeling sick": The Strange Worlds of Physicians and Patients in the

Eighteenth and 21st Centuries', *Journal of Medical Ethics: Medical Humanities*, 28 (1): 9–13.

Luyendijk-Elshout, Anthonie M. (1970) 'The Anatomical Illustrations in the London Edition (1741) of Part I of Herman Boerhaave's Institutiones Medicae', in G. A. Lindeboom (ed), *Boerhaave and His Time: Papers Read at the International Symposium in Commemoration of the Tercentenary of Boerhaave's Birth*, 83–92, Leiden: Brill.

Lyon-Caen, Judith (2016), 'Le "je" et le baromètre de l'âme', in Alain Corbin, Jean-Jacques Courtine and Georges Vigarello (eds), *Histoire des émotions*, Vol. 2, *Des Lumières à la fin du 19e siècle*, 168–88, Paris: Seuil.

Maerker, Anna (2011), *Model Experts: Wax Anatomies and Enlightenment in Florence and Vienna, 1775–1815*, Manchester and New York: Manchester University Press.

Maire, Catherine (1985), *Les Convulsionnaires de Saint-Médard: miracles, convulsions et prophéties à Paris au XVIIIe siècle*, Paris: Éditions Gallimard/Julliard.

Maire, Catherine (1998), *De la cause de Dieu à la cause de la Nation: Le jansénisme au XVIIIe siècle*, Paris: Éditions Gallimard.

Margócsy, Dániel (2011), 'A Museum of Wonders or a Cemetery of Corpses? The Commercial Exchange of Anatomical Collections in Early Modern Netherlands', in Sven Dupré and Christoph Lüthy (eds), *Silent Messengers: The Circulation of Material Objects of Knowledge in the Early Modern Low Countries*, 185–216, Berlin: LIT Verlag.

Marland, Hilary, ed. (1993), *The Art of Midwifery*, London and New York: Routledge.

Marr, Alexander (2016), 'Knowing Images', *Renaissance Quarterly*, 69 (3): 1000–13.

Mattfeld, Monica (2015), '"Genus Porcus Sophisticus": The Learned Pig and the Theatrics of National Identity in Late Eighteenth-Century London', in Jennifer Parker-Starbuck and Lourdes Orozco (eds), *Performing Animality: Animals in Performance Practices*, 57–76, New York: Palgrave Macmillan.

Mattfeld, Monica (2017), *Becoming Centaur: Eighteenth-Century Horsemanship and English Masculinity*, University Park: Pennsylvania State University Press.

McBride, William (1991), '"Normal" Medical Science and British Treatment of the Sea Scurvy, 1753–1775', *Journal of the History of Medicine and Allied Sciences*, 46 (2): 158–77.

McCants, Anne (2007), 'Exotic Goods, Popular Consumption, and the Standard of Living', *Journal of World History*, 18 (4): 433–62.

McClive, Cathy (2002), 'The Hidden Truths of the Belly: The Uncertainties of Pregnancy in Early Modern Europe', *Social History of Medicine*, 15 (2): 209–27.

McClive, Cathy (2008), 'Blood and Expertise: The Trials of the Female Medical Expert in the Ancien-Régime Courtroom', *Bulletin of the History of Medicine*, 82 (1): 86–108.

McClive, Cathy (2012), 'Witnessing of the Hands and Eyes: Surgeons as Medico-Legal Experts in the Claudine Rouge Affair, Lyon, 1767', *Journal for Eighteenth-Century Studies*, 35 (4): 489–503.

McCormick, Ian, ed. (1997), *Secret Sexualities: A Sourcebook of 17th and 18th Century Writing*, London: Routledge.

MacGregor, Arthur, ed. (1994), *Sir Hans Sloane: Collector, Scientist, Antiquary*, London: British Museum Press.

McKeown, Thomas (1979), *The Role of Medicine: Dream, Mirage, or Nemesis?* Princeton: Princeton University Press.

McNeill, John R. (2010), *Mosquito Empires: Ecology and War in the Greater Caribbean 1620–1914*, Cambridge: Cambridge University Press.

McRuer, Robert and Anna Mollow, eds (2012), *Sex and Disability*, Durham, NC: Duke University Press.

McTavish, Lianne (2005), *Childbirth and the Display of Authority in Early Modern France*, Aldershot: Ashgate.

Meli, Domenico Bertoloni (2013), 'Early Modern Experimentation on Live Animals', *Journal of the History of Biology*, 46 (2): 199–226.

Mennell, Stephen (1996), *All Manners of Food: Eating and Taste in England and France from the Middle Ages to the Present*, 2nd edn, Urbana and Chicago: University of Illinois Press.

Mennell, Stephen, Anne Murcott and Anneke H. van Otterloo (1992), *The Sociology of Food: Eating, Diet and Culture*, London: SAGE Publications.

Messbarger, Rebecca (2010), *The Lady Anatomist: The Life and Work of Anna Morandi Manzolini*, Chicago and London: University of Chicago Press.

Mikkeli, Heikki (1999), *Hygiene: In the Early Modern Medical Tradition*, Helsinki: Finnish Academy of Science and Letters.

Miller, Genevieve (1962), '"Airs, Waters, and Places" in History', *Journal of the History of Medicine and Allied Sciences*, 17 (1): 129–40.

Milles, Dietrich (1995), 'Working Capacity and Calorie Consumption: The History of Rational Physical Economy', in Harmke Kamminga and Andrew Cunningham (eds), *The Science and Culture of Nutrition, 1840–1940*, 75–96, Amsterdam and Atlanta: Rodopi.

Minou Lina (2017), 'Envy's Pathology: Historical Contexts [version 2; peer review: 2 approved]' *Wellcome Open Research* 2017, 2 (3), available online: https://doi.org/10.12688/wellcomeopenres.10415.2 (accessed 13 October 2020).

Mol, Annemarie (2002), *The Body Multiple: Ontology in Medical Practice*, Durham, NC, and London: Duke University Press.

Moody, Jane (2000), *Illegitimate Theatre in London, 1770–1840*, Cambridge: Cambridge University Press.

Morton, Timothy (1994), *Shelley and the Revolution in Taste: The Body and the Natural World*, Cambridge: Cambridge University Press.

Moscoso, Javier (2012), *Pain: A Cultural History*, Basingstoke: Palgrave Macmillan.

Muldrew, Craig (2011), *Food, Energy and the Creation of Industriousness: Work and Material Culture in Agrarian England, 1550–1780*, Cambridge: Cambridge University Press.

Müller, Rainer A. (1997), *Zeitalter des Absolutismus 1648–1789*, Stuttgart: Reclam.

Nahoum-Grappe, Véronique (1994), 'Le transport: Une émotion surranée', *Terrain. Anthropologie et sciences humaines*, 22: 69–78.

Neswald, Elizabeth, David Smith and Ulrike Thoms (2017), *Setting Nutritional Standards: Theory, Policies, Practices*, Rochester: University of Rochester Press.

Neveux, Julie (2013), *John Donne: Le sentiment dans la langue*, Paris: Editions Rue d'Ulm.

Newman, Lucille F., ed. (1995), *Hunger in History: Food Shortage, Poverty, and Deprivation*, Oxford and Cambridge, MA: Blackwell.

Newman, Simon (2013), *A New World of Labor: The Development of Plantation Slavery in the British Atlantic*, Philadelphia: University of Pennsylvania Press.

Newton, Hannah (2012), *The Sick Child in Early Modern England, 1580–1720*, Oxford: Oxford University Press.

Newton, Hannah (2015), '"Nature Concocts & Expels": The Agents and Processes of Recovery from Disease in Early Modern England', *Social History of Medicine*, 28 (3): 465–86.

Niebyl, Peter H. (1971), 'The Non-Naturals', *Bulletin of the History of Medicine*, 45 (5): 486–92.

Noble, Louise (2011), *Medicinal Cannibalism in Early Modern English Literature and Culture*, New York: Palgrave Macmillan.

Nocella II, Anthony J., Judy K. C. Bentley and Janet M. Duncan (2012), 'Introduction: The Rise of Eco-Ability', in Anthony J. Nocella II, Judy K. C. Bentley and Janet M. Duncan (eds), *Earth, Animal, and Disability Liberation: The Rise of the Eco-ability Movement*, xiii–xxii, New York: Peter Lang.

Nocella II, Anthony J., Amber E. George and J.L. Schatz, eds (2017), *The Intersectionality of Critical Animal, Disability, and Environmental Studies: Toward Eco-ability, Justice, and Liberation*, Lanham, MD: Lexington Books.

Nussbaum, Felicity A. (2003), *The Limits of the Human: Fictions of Anomaly, Race, and Gender in the Long Eighteenth Century*, Cambridge: Cambridge University Press.

Olivarius, Kathryn (2016), 'Necropolis: Yellow Fever, Immunity, and Capitalism in the Deep South, 1800–1860', PhD thesis, University of Oxford, Oxford.

O'Malley, Charles Donald (1964), *Andreas Vesalius of Brussels, 1514–1564*, Berkeley and Los Angeles: University of California Press.

Orland, Barbara (2010), 'Enlightened Milk: Reshaping a Bodily Substance into a Chymical Object', in Ursula Klein and E. C. Spary (eds), *Materials and Expertise in Early Modern Europe: Between Market and Laboratory*, 163–97, Chicago and London: University of Chicago Press.

Orland, Barbara (2014), 'Die Erfindung des Stoffwechsels – Wandel der Stoffwahrnehmung in der Experimentalkultur des 18. Jahrhunderts', in Kijan Espahangizi and Barbara Orland (eds), *Stoffe in Bewegung – Beiträge zur Wissensgeschichte der materiellen Welt*, 69–94, Zürich: Diaphanes.

Otter, Chris (2012), 'The British Nutrition Transition and Its Histories', *History Compass*, 10 (11): 812–25.

Outram, Dorinda (2013), *The Enlightenment*, 3rd edn, Cambridge: Cambridge University Press.

Owen, Harry (2016), *Simulation in Healthcare Education: An Extensive History*, Cham: Springer.

Palmer, Richard (1991), 'Health, Hygiene and Longevity in Medieval and Renaissance Europe', in Yosio Kawakita, Shizu Sakai and Yasuo Otsuka (eds), *History of Hygiene*, 75–98. Tokyo: Ishiyaku Euroamerica.

Paston-Williams, Sara (1993), *The Art of Dining: A History of Cooking and Eating*, London: The National Trust.

Paugh, Katherine (2017), *The Politics of Reproduction: Race, Medicine, and Fertility in the Age of Abolition*, Oxford: Oxford University Press.

Payne, Lynda (2007), *With Words and Knives: Learning Medical Dispassion in Early Modern England*, London: Ashgate.

Pelling, Margaret (1993), 'Contagion/Germ Theory/Specificity', in William F. Bynum and Roy Porter (eds), *Companion Encyclopedia of the History of Medicine*, Vol. 1, 30–3, London and New York: Routledge.

Pender, Stephen (2000), 'In the Bodyshop: Human Exhibition in Early Modern England', in Felicity Nussbaum and Helen Deutsch (eds), *'Defects': Engendering the Modern Body*, 95–126, Ann Arbor: University of Michigan Press.

Perkins, David (2003), *Romanticism and Animal Rights, 1790–1830*, Cambridge: Cambridge University Press.
Pigeaud, Jackie (1985), 'L'humeur des Anciens', *Nouvelle Revue de psychanalyse*, 32: 51–69.
Pilloud, Séverine (2013), *Les mots du corps. Expérience de la maladie dans les lettres de patients à un médecin du XVIIIe siècle: Samuel Auguste Tissot*, Lausanne: BHMS.
Pilloud, Séverine and Micheline Louis-Courvoisier (2003), 'The Intimate Experience of the Body in the Eighteenth Century: Between Interiority and Exteriority', *Medical History*, 47 (4): 451–72.
Plamper, Jan (2015), *The History of Emotions: An Introduction*, Oxford: Oxford University Press.
Plamper, Jan, William Reddy, Barbara Rosenwein and Peter Stearns (2010), 'The History of Emotions: An Interview with William Reddy, Barbara Rosenwein, and Peter Stearns', *History and Theory*, 49 (2): 237–65.
Polguère, Alain (2013), 'Les petits soucis ne poussent plus dans le champ lexical des sentiments', in Fabienne Baider and Georgeta Cislaru (eds), *Cartographie des émotions. Propositions linguistiques et sociolinguistiques*, 21–41, Paris: Presse de la Sorbonne.
Pollock, Linda (2004), 'Anger and the Negotiation of Relationships in Early Modern England', *The Historical Journal*, 47 (3): 567–90.
Pomata, Gianna (2016), 'The Devil's Advocate among the Physicians: What Prospero Lambertini Learned from Medical Sources' in Philip Gavitt, Christopher M. S. Johns and Rebecca Messbarger (eds), *Benedict XIV and the Enlightenment: Art, Science, and Spirituality*, 120–50, Toronto: University of Toronto Press.
Porter, Roy (1982), 'Was There a Medical Enlightenment in Eighteenth-Century England?', *Journal for Eighteenth-Century Studies*, 5 (1): 49–63.
Porter, Roy (1985), 'The Patient's View: Doing Medical History from Below', *Theory and Society*, 14 (2): 175–98.
Porter, Roy (1989), *Health for Sale: Quackery in England, 1660–1850*, Manchester: Manchester University Press.
Porter, Roy (1990) 'Foucault's Great Confinement', *History of the Human Sciences*, 3 (1): 13–26.
Porter, Roy (1993), 'Consumption: Disease of the Consumer Society?' in John Brewer and Roy Porter (eds), *Consumption and the World of Goods*, 58–84, London: Routledge.
Porter, Roy (1994), 'Gout: Framing and Fantasising Disease', *Bulletin of the History of Medicine*, 68 (1): 1–28.
Porter, Roy (2005), *Flesh in the Age of Reason*, London: Penguin.
Porter, Roy, ed. (1995), *Medicine in the Enlightenment*, Amsterdam: Rodopi.
Porter, Roy and Dorothy Porter (1989), *Doctors and Doctoring in Eighteenth-Century England*, Stanford: Stanford University Press.
Preece, Rod, ed. (2002), *Awe for the Tiger, Love for the Lamb: A Chronicle of Sensibility to Animals*, London: Routledge.
Preece, Rod (2005), *Brute Souls, Happy Beasts, and Evolution: The Historical Status of Animals*, Vancouver: UBC Press.
Principe, Lawrence, ed. (2007), *Chymists and Chymistry. Studies in the History of Alchemy and Early Modern Chemistry*, Sagamore Beach: Chymical Heritage Foundation and Science History Publications.
Prown, Jules David (1982), 'Mind in Matter: An Introduction to Material Culture Theory and Method', *Winterthur*, 17 (1): 1–19.

Puckrein, Gary (1979), 'Climate, Health and Black Labor in the English Americas', *Journal of American Studies*, 13 (2): 173–93.
Quinlan, Sean M. (2007), *The Great Nation in Decline: Sex, Modernity and Health Crises in Revolutionary France, c.1750–1850*, Aldershot: Ashgate.
Qureshi, Sadiah (2004), 'Displaying Sara Baartman, the "Hottentot Venus"', *History of Science*, 42 (136): 233–57.
Qureshi, Sadiah (2011), *Peoples on Parade: Exhibitions, Empire, and Anthropology in Nineteenth-Century Britain*, Chicago: University of Chicago Press.
Rabier, Christelle (2007), 'Defining a Profession: Surgery, Professional Conflicts and Legal Powers in Paris and London, 1760–1790', in Christelle Rabier (ed.), *Fields of Expertise: A Comparative History of Expert Procedures in Paris and London, 1600 to Present*, 85–114, Newcastle upon Tyne: Cambridge Scholars Publishing.
Ramsey, Matthew (1988), *Professional and Popular Medicine in France, 1770–1830: The Social World of Medical Practice*, Cambridge and New York: Cambridge University Press.
Reddy, William (2001), *The Navigation of Feeling: A Framework for the History of Emotions*. Cambridge: Cambridge University Press.
Reinhardt, Dirk, Uwe Spiekermann and Ulrike Thoms (eds) (1993), *Neue Wege zur Ernährungsgeschichte. Kochbücher, Haushaltsrechnungen, Konsumvereinsberichte und Autobiographien in der Diskussion*, Frankfurt am Main: Peter Lang.
Rennhak, Katharina (2011), 'Paratexts and the Construction of Author Identities: The Preface as Threshold and Thresholds in the Preface', in Isabel Karremann and Anja Müller (eds), *Mediating Identities in Eighteenth-Century England: Public Negotiations, Literary Discourses, Topography*, 57–70, Abingdon: Routledge.
Rey, Roselyne (2000), *Histoire de la douleur*, Paris: La Découverte.
Rheinberger, Hans-Jörg (2012) *On Historicizing Epistemology: An Essay*, Stanford: Stanford University Press.
Richardson, Ruth (2001), *Death, Dissection, and the Destitute*, Chicago: University of Chicago Press.
Rieder, Philip (2010), *La figure du patient au 18e siècle*, Geneva: Droz.
Rieder, Philip (2018), 'La figure de l'apothicaire (1500–1800): Artisan, entrepreneur et soignant' in Philip Rieder and François Zanetti (eds), *Materia medica: Savoirs et usages des médicaments aux époques médiévales et modernes*, 209–55, Geneva: Librairie Droz.
Rigoli, Juan (2001), *Lire le délire. Aliénisme, rhétorique et littérature en France au 19e siècle*, Paris: Fayard.
Risse, Guenter B. (1974), '"Doctor William Cullen, Physician Edinburgh": A Consultation Practice in the Eighteenth Century', *Bulletin of the History of Medicine*, 48 (3): 338–51.
Roosma, Maks (1969), 'The Glass Industry of Estonia in the Eighteenth and Nineteenth Century', *Journal of Glass Studies*, 11: 70–85.
Rosen, George (1953), 'Cameralism and the Concept of Medical Police', *Bulletin of the History of Medicine*, 27 (1): 21–42.
Rosen, George (1974), *From Medical Police to Social Medicine: Essays on the History of Health Care*, New York: Science History Publications.
Rosenwein, Barbara (2006), *Emotional Communities in the Early Middle Ages*, New York: Cornell University Press.
Rosenwein, Barbara, ed. (1998), *Anger's Past: The Social Uses of an Emotion in the Middle Ages*, Ithaca and London: Cornell University Press.

Rosner, Lisa (2010), *The Anatomy Murders: Being the True and Spectacular History of Edinburgh's Notorious Burke and Hare*, Philadelphia: University of Pennsylvania Press.

Ross, A. (2004), 'John Arbuthnot', in H. C. G. Matthew and B. Harrison (eds), *Oxford Dictionary of National Biography*, II, 325–9, London: Oxford University Press.

Rotberg, R. I. and Rabb, T. K., eds (1985), *Hunger and History: The Impact of Changing Food Production and Consumption Patterns on Society*, Cambridge: Cambridge University Press.

Roth, Udo (2015), '"Erlernung der Gesetze der Natur der Seele". Die Rezeption von Georg Friedrich Meiers Seelenlehre in der zeitgenössischen Medizin', in Frank Grunert and Gideon Stiening (eds), *Georg Friedrich Meier und die Philosophie als 'wahre Weltweisheit'*, 187–209, Berlin: Walter de Gruyter.

Rousseau, George S. (1976), 'Nerves, Spirits and Fibres', *Studies in the Eighteenth Century*, 3 (1): 137–57.

Rousseau, George S. (1993), '"A Strange Pathology": Hysteria in the Early Modern World, 1500–1800', in Sander L. Gilman, Helen King, Roy Porter, George S. Rousseau and Elaine Showalter, *Hysteria beyond Freud*, Berkeley and Los Angeles: University of California Press.

Rusnock, Andrea (2002), *Vital Accounts: Quantifying Health and Population in Eighteenth-Century England and France*, Cambridge: Cambridge University Press.

Rutman, Darrett B. and Anita H. Rutman (1976), 'Of Agues and Fevers: Malaria in the Early Chesapeake', *William and Mary Quarterly*, 33 (1): 31–60.

Saakwa-Mante, Norris (1999), 'Western Medicine and Racial Constitutions: Surgeon John Atkins' Theory of Polygenism and Sleepy Distemper in the 1730s', in Waltraund Ernst and Bernard Harris (eds), *Race, Science and Medicine, 1700–1960*, 29–57, London and New York: Routledge.

Santing, Catrien (2007), 'Tirami sù: Pope Benedict XIV and the Beautification of the Flying Saint Giuseppe da Copertino' in Andrew Cunningham and Ole Peter Grell (eds), *Medicine and Religion in Enlightenment Europe*, Aldershot: Routledge.

Santing, Catrien (2008), 'Andreas Vesalius's *De Fabrica corporis humana*, Depiction of the Human Model in Word And image', in Ann-Sophie Lehmann and Herman Roodenburg (eds), *Body and Embodiment in Netherlandish Art*, 59–85, Zwolle: Waanders Publishers.

Schiebinger, Londa (1986), 'Skeletons in the Closet: The First Illustrations of the Female Skeleton in Eighteenth-Century Anatomy', *Representations*, 14: 42–82.

Schiebinger, Londa (1993), *Nature's Body: Gender in the Making of Modern Science*, Boston: Beacon Press.

Schiebinger, Londa (2007), *Plants and Empire: Colonial Bioprospecting in the Atlantic World*, Cambridge, MA: Harvard University Press.

Schiebinger, Londa (2013), 'Medical Experimentation and Race in the Eighteenth-Century Atlantic World', *Social History of Medicine*, 26 (3): 364–82.

Schiebinger, Londa (2017), *Secret Cures of Slaves: People, Plants, and Medicine in the Eighteenth-Century Atlantic World*, Stanford: Stanford University Press.

Schillace, Brandy (2013), 'On the Trail of the Machine: William Smellie's "Celebrated Apparatus"', *Dittrick Medical History Centre Blog*, 3 April, available online: https://artsci.case.edu/dittrick/2013/04/04/on-the-trail-of-the-machine-william-smellies-celebrated-apparatus (accessed 5 October 2020).

Schmidt, James and Amelie Rorty (2009), *Kant's Idea for a Universal History with a Cosmopolitan Aim: A Critical Guide*, Cambridge: Cambridge University Press.

Scott, Joan W. (1991), 'The Evidence of Experience', *Critical Inquiry*, 17 (4): 773–97.
Sebastiani, Silvia (2013), *The Scottish Enlightenment: Race, Gender, and the Limits of Progress*, New York: Palgrave Macmillan.
Sechel, Daniela (2003), 'The Influence of Cameralism and Enlightenment upon the Sanitary Policy promoted by the Habsburgs in Transylvania (1740–1800)', *Revista Bistriței*, 17: 115–30.
Seela, Jacob (1974), 'The Early Finnish Glass Industry', *Journal of Glass Studies*, 16: 57–86.
Semonin, Paul (1996), 'Monsters in the Marketplace: The Exhibition of Human Oddities in Early Modern England', in Rosemarie Garland Thomson (ed.), *Freakery: Cultural Spectacles of the Extraordinary Body*, 69–81, New York: New York University Press.
Serjeantson, Richard (2001), 'The Passions and Animal Language, 1540–1700'. *Journal of the History of Ideas*, 62 (3): 425–44.
Seth, Suman (2018), *Difference and Disease: Medicine, Race, and the Eighteenth-Century British Empire*, Cambridge: Cambridge University Press.
Shapin, Steven (2010), *Never Pure: Historical Studies of Science as if it was produced by People with Bodies, Situated in Time, Space, Culture, and Society, and Struggling for Credibility and Authority*, Baltimore: Johns Hopkins University Press.
Shaw, Jane (2006), *Miracles in Enlightenment England*, New Haven: Yale University Press.
Shephard, Sue (2000), *Pickled, Potted and Canned: The Story of Food Preserving*, London: Headline.
Sheridan, Richard (1985), *Doctors and Slaves: A Medical and Demographic History of Slavery in the British West Indies, 1680–1834*, Cambridge: Cambridge University Press.
Sherman, Sandra (2001), *Imagining Poverty: Quantification and the Decline of Paternalism*, Columbus: Ohio State University Press.
Siegel, Rudolph (1968), *Galen's System of Physiology and Medicine: An Analysis of His Doctrines and Observations on Bloodflow, Respiration, Humors and Internal Diseases*, Basel: Karger.
Simmons, Dana (2015), *Vital Minimum: Need, Science and Politics in Modern France*, Chicago and London: University of Chicago Press.
Simms, Rupe (2001), 'Controlling Images and Gender Construction of Enslaved African Women', *Gender and History*, 15 (6): 879–97.
Singy, Patrick (2014), *L'usage du sexe au XVIIIe siècle. Lettres au Dr Tissot, auteur de L'Onanisme (1760)*, Lausanne: BHMS.
Skuse, Alanna (2015), *Constructions of Cancer in Early Modern England: Ravenous Natures*, Basingstoke: Palgrave Macmillan.
Smith, C. U. M., Eugenio Frixione, Stanley Finger and William Clower (2012), *The Animal Spirit Doctrine and the Origins of Neurophysiology*, Oxford: Oxford University Press.
Smith, Helen and Louise Wilson, eds (2011), *Renaissance Paratexts*, Cambridge: Cambridge University Press.
Smith, Justin E. H. (2017), 'Between Language, Music, and Sound: Birdsong as a Philosophical Problem from Aristotle to Kant', in Stefanie Buchenau and Roberto Lo Presti (eds), *Human and Animal Cognition in Early Modern Philosophy and Medicine*, 127–46, Pittsburgh: University of Pittsburgh Press.
Smith, Lisa Wynne (2003), 'Reassessing the Role of the Family: Women's Care in Eighteenth-Century England', *Social History of Medicine*, 16 (3): 327–42.

Smith, Lisa Wynne (2006), 'The Relative Duties of a Man: Domestic Medicine in England and France, *ca.* 1685–1740', *Journal of Family History*, 31 (3): 237–56.

Smith, Lisa Wynne (2008), '"An Account of an Unaccountable Distemper:" The Experience of Pain in Early Eighteenth-Century England and France', *Eighteenth-Century Studies*, 41 (4): 459–80.

Smith, Lisa Wynne (2011), 'The Body Embarrassed? Rethinking the Leaky Male Body in Eighteenth?Century England and France', *Gender and History*, 23 (1): 26–46.

Smith, Lisa Wynne (2013), 'Masturbation and the Dangerous Woman', in Holly Tucker (ed.), *Wonders and Marvels: A Community for Curious Minds Who Love History, Its Odd Stories, and Good Reads*, www.wondersandmarvels.com/2016/11/nursery-terrors.html (accessed 8 October 2020).

Smith, Lisa Wynne (2016), 'Nursery Terrors', in Holly Tucker (ed.), *Wonders and Marvels: A Community for Curious Minds Who Love History, Its Odd Stories, and Good Reads*, www.wondersandmarvels.com/2016/11/nursery-terrors.html (accessed 8 October 2020).

Smith, Lisa Wynne (2019), 'Remembering Dr Sloane: Masculinity and the Making of an Eighteenth-Century Physician', *Journal for Eighteenth-Century Studies*, 42 (4): 433–53.

Smith, Woodruff D. (2002), *Consumption and the Making of Respectability, 1600–1800*, New York and London: Routledge.

Spary, E. C. (2004), '"Peaches Which the Patriarchs Lacked": Natural History, Natural Resources, and the Natural Economy in Eighteenth-Century France', in Neil De Marchi and Margaret Schabas (eds), *History of Political Economy*, supplement to Vol. 35, 14–41, Durham, NC: Duke University Press.

Spary, E. C. (2009), 'Self Preservation: French Travels between *Cuisine* and *Industrie*', in James Delbourgo, Kapil Raj, Lissa Roberts and Simon Schaffer (eds), *The Brokered World*, 355–86, Canton, MA: Science History Publications.

Spary, E. C. (2011), 'Health and Medicine in the Enlightenment', in Mark Jackson (ed), *The Oxford Handbook of the History of Medicine*, 82–99, Oxford: Oxford University Press.

Spary, E. C. (2012), *Eating the Enlightenment: Food and the Sciences in Paris*, Chicago: University of Chicago Press.

Spary, E. C. (2014), *Feeding France: New Sciences of Food, 1760–1815*, Cambridge: Cambridge University Press.

Spencer, Colin (1993), *The Heretic's Feast. A History of Vegetarianism*, London: Fourth Estate.

Spierenburg, Peter (1984), *The Spectacle of Suffering: Executions and the Evolution of Repression, from a Preindustrial Metropolis to the European Experience*, Cambridge: Cambridge University Press.

Stahnisch, Frank (2004), 'Den Hunger standardisieren: François Magendies Fütterungsversuche zur Gelatinekost 1831–1841'. *Medizinhistorisches Journal*, 39: 103–34.

Starobinski, Jean (2012), 'L'invention d'une maladie', in *L'encre de la mélancolie*, Paris: Le Seuil.

Stead, Jennifer (1991), 'Necessities and Luxuries: Food Preservation from the Elizabethan to the Georgian Era', in C. Anne Wilson (ed), *'Waste Not, Want Not': Food Preservation from Early Times to the Present Day*, 66–103, Edinburgh: Edinburgh University Press.

Stein, Claudia (2021), 'Introduction', in Elaine Leong and Claudia Stein (eds), *A Cultural History of Medicine in the Renaissance*, London: Bloomsbury Press.
Stevenson, Christine (2000), *Medicine and Magnificence: British Hospital and Asylum Architecture, 1660–1815*, New Haven and London: Yale University Press.
Stevenson, Christine (2007), 'From Palace to Hut: The Architecture of Military and Naval Medicine, in Geoffrey Hudson (ed.), *British Military and Naval Medicine, 1600–1830*, 227–52, Amsterdam and New York: Rodopi.
Stewart, Mart A. (2002), *'What Nature Suffers to Growe': Life, Labor, and Landscape on the Georgia Coast 1680–1920*, Athens, GA: University of Georgia Press.
Stewart, Susan (1993), *On Longing: Narratives of the Miniature, the Gigantic, the Souvenir, the Collection*, Durham, NC: Duke University Press.
Stolberg, Michael (2000), 'An Unmanly Vice: Self-Pollution, Anxiety, and the Body in the Eighteenth Century', *Social History of Medicine*, 13 (1): 1–21.
Stolberg, Michael (2011), *Experiencing Illness and the Sick Body in Early Modern Europe*, Basingstoke: Palgrave Macmillan.
Stolberg, Michael (2012), '"Abhorreas pinguedinem": Fat and Obesity in Early Modern Medicine (c. 1500–1750)', *Studies in History and Philosophy of Biological and Biomedical Sciences*, 43 (2): 370–8.
Stolberg, Michael (2019), 'Emotions and the Body in Early Modern Medicine', *Emotion Review*, 11 (2): 113–22.
Strayer, Brian (2008), *Suffering Saints: Jansenists and Convulsionnaires in France, 1640–1799*, Brighton: Sussex Academic Press.
Stroup, Alice (1985), 'Some Assumptions behind Medicine for the Poor during the Reign of Louis XIV', in John David North and James Jeffrey Roche (eds), *The Light of Nature. Essays in the History and Philosophy of Science presented to A. C. Crombie*, 35–56, Dordrecht: Martinus Nijhoff.
Stuart, Tristram (2007), *The Bloodless Revolution: A Cultural History of Vegetarianism from 1600 to Modern Times*, New York and London: W. W. Norton & Company.
Sturm, Lars-Burkhardt (2007), 'Präparationstechniken und Ihre Anwendung in Den Meckelschen Sammlungen Zu Halle/Saale', in Rüdiger Schultka and Josef Neumann (eds), *Anatomie und Anatomische Sammlungen Im 18. Jahrhundert: Anlässlich Der 250. Wiederkehr Des Geburtstages von Philipp Friedrich Theodor Meckel (1755–1803)*, 377–88, Berlin: LIT Verlag.
Sugg, Richard (2013), *The Smoke of the Soul: Medicine, Physiology and Religion in Early Modern England*, New York: Palgrave Macmillan.
Sugg, Richard (2015), *Mummies, Cannibals and Vampires: The History of Corpse Medicine from the Renaissance to the Victorians*, London: Routledge.
Sutton, Robert (1998), *Philosophy and Memory Traces: Descartes to Connectionism*, Cambridge: Cambridge University Press.
Sysling, Fenneke (2010), 'Dead Bodies, Lively Debates: Human Remains in Dutch Museums', in Andrea Kieskamp (ed.), *Sense and Sensitivity: The Dutch and Delicate Heritage Issues*, 52–63, Rotterdam: ICOM Nederland.
Taylor, Barbara (2004), 'Feminists Versus Gallants: Manners and Morals in Enlightenment Britain', *Representations*, 87 (1): 125–48.
Taylor, Barbara (2005), 'Feminists versus Gallants: Manners and Morals in Enlightenment Britain', in Barbara Taylor and Sarah Knott (eds), *Women, Gender and Enlightenment*, 30–52, London: Palgrave.
Taylor, Sunaura (2011), 'Beasts of Burden: Disability Studies and Animal Rights', *Qui Parle: Critical Humanities and Social Sciences*, 19 (2): 191–222.

Teuteberg, Hans Jürgen (1995), 'History of Cooling and Freezing Techniques and Their Impact on Nutrition in Twentieth Century Germany', in A. P. den Hartog (ed), *Food Technology, Science and Marketing: European Diet in the Twentieth Century*, 51–65, East Linton: Tuckwell Press.
Teuteberg, Hans Jürgen (2007), 'Urbanization and Nutrition: Historical Research Reconsidered', in Peter J. Atkins, Peter Lummel and Derek J. Oddy (eds), *Food and the City in Europe since 1800*, 13–23. Aldershot and Burlington, VT: Ashgate.
Teuteberg, Hans Jürgen and Günther Wiegelmann (1972), *Der Wandel der Wahrungsgewohnheiten unter dem Einfluß der Industrialisierung*, Göttingen: Vandenhoeck & Ruprecht.
Teysseire, Daniel (1993), 'Le réseau européen des consultants d'un médecin des Lumières: Tissot (1728–1797)', in *Diffusion du savoir et affrontement des idées 1600–1770*, 263–97, Montbrison: Association du centre culturel de la ville de Montbrison.
Teysseire, Daniel (1995), *Obèse et impuissant, le dossier médical d'Elie de Beaumont, 1765–1776*, Grenoble: Jérôme Million.
Thatcher Ulrich, Laurel, Sarah Anne Carter, Ivan Gaskell, Sara Schechner and Samantha van Gerbig (2015), *Tangible Things: Making History through Objects*, New York: Oxford University Press.
Thirsk, Joan (2007), *Food in Early Modern England: Phases, Fads, Fashions 1500–1760*. London and New York: Hambledon Continuum.
Thomas, Keith (1983), *Man and the Natural World: Changing Attitudes in England 1500–1800*, London: Penguin.
Thomas, Keith (1991), *Man and the Natural World: Changing Attitudes in England 1500–1800*, London: Allen Lane.
Thompson, Catherine (2016), 'Questions of *Genre*: Picturing the Hermaphrodite in Eighteenth-Century France and England', *Eighteenth-Century Studies*, 49 (3): 391–413.
Thoms, Ulrike (2005), *Anstaltskost im Rationalisierungsprozeß. Die Ernährung in Krankenhäusern und Gefängnissen im 18. und 19. Jahrhundert*, Stuttgart: Franz Steiner Verlag.
Thomson, Rosemarie Garland (1996), 'Introduction: From Wonder to Error – A Genealogy of Freak Discourse in Modernity', in Rosemarie Garland Thomson (ed.), *Freakery: Cultural Spectacles of the Extraordinary Body*, 1–22, New York: New York University Press.
Thorne, Stuart (1986), *The History of Food Preservation*, Casterton Hall: Parthenon Publishing.
Todd, Dennis (1995), *Imagining Monsters: Miscreations of the Self in Eighteenth-Century England*, Chicago: University of Chicago Press.
Treitel, Corinna (2008), 'Max Rubner and the Biopolitics of Rational Nutrition', *Central European History*, 41 (1): 1–25.
Treitel, Corinna (2020), 'Nutritional Modernity: The German Case', *Osiris*, 35 (1): 183–203.
Tromp, Marlene (2008), *Victorian Freaks: The Social Context of Freakery in Britain*, Columbus: Ohio State University Press.
Turner, Brian S. (1982), 'The Government of the Body: Medical Regimens and the Rationalization of Diet', *British Journal of Sociology*, 33 (2): 254–69.
Turner, David M. (2012), *Disability in Eighteenth-Century England: Imagining Physical Impairment*, London: Routledge.

Van Calmthout, Martijn (2016), 'Ontdekking Museum Boerhaave: Oefenbaby blijkt echt skelet te bevatten', *De Volkskrant*, 25 November.
Van Wyhe, John (2002), 'The Authority of Human Nature: the Schädellehre of Franz Joseph Gall', *British Journal for the History of Science* 3 (1): 17–42.
Van Wyhe, John (2004), 'Was Phrenology a Reform Science? Towards a New Generalization for Phrenology', *History of Science*, 42 (3): 313–31.
Vasset, Sophie (2013), *Décrire, prescrire, guérir. Médecine et fiction dans la Grande Bretagne du 18e siècle*, Quebec City: Presses de l'Université de Laval.
Vermij, Rienk (2014), 'The Marginalization of Astrology among Dutch Astronomers in the First Half of the 17th Century', *History of Science: An Annual Review of Literature, Research and Teaching*, 52 (2): 153–77.
Vernon, James (2007), *Hunger: A Modern History*, Cambridge, MA, and London: The Belknap Press of Harvard University Press.
Veyne, Paul (1996), 'L'interprétation et l'interprète. A propos des choses de la religion', *Enquête*, 3: 2–19.
Vickery, Amanda (2009), *Behind Closed Doors: At Home in Georgian England*, New Haven and London: Yale University Press.
Vigarello, Georges (2014), Le sentiment de soi : Histoire de la perception du corps, Paris: Seuil.
Vila, Anne C. (1998), *Enlightenment and Pathology: Sensibility in the Literature and Medicine of Eighteenth-Century France*, Baltimore and London: Johns Hopkins University Press.
Vila, Anne C. (2014), 'Introduction: Powers, Pleasures, and Perils of the Senses in the Enlightenment Era', in Anne C. Vila (ed.), *A Cultural History of the Senses: In the Age of Enlightenment*, London: Bloomsbury.
Vila, Anne C. (2015) 'Medicine and the Body in the French Enlightenment', in Daniel Brewer (ed.), *The Cambridge Companion to the French Enlightenment*, 199–213, Cambridge: Cambridge University Press.
Voelz, Peter (1993), *Slave and Soldier: The Military Impact of Blacks in the Colonial Americas*, New York: Garland Publishing.
Von Engelhardt, Dietrich (1993), 'Hunger und Appetit. Essen und Trinken im System der Diätetik – Kulturhistorische Perspektiven', in A. Wierlacher, G. Neumann and H.-J. Teuteberg (eds), *Kulturthema Essen. Ansichten und Problemfelder*, 137–49, Berlin: Akademie Verlag.
Wagner, Corinna (2013), *Pathological Bodies: Medicine and Political Culture*, Berkeley, Los Angeles and London: University of California Press.
Wahrman, Dror (2004), *The Making of the Modern Self: Identity and Culture in Eighteenth-Century England*, New Haven and London: Yale University Press.
Wakefield, Andre (2009), *The Disordered Police State: German Cameralism as Science and Practice*, Chicago: University of Chicago Press.
Walker, Alison, Arthur MacGregor and Michael Hunter (eds), *From Books to Bezoars: Sir Hans Sloane and his Collections*, London: The British Library.
Wallace, Charles (2003), 'Eating and Drinking with John Wesley: The Logic of His Practice', *Bulletin of the John Rylands University Library of Manchester*, 85 (2–3): 137–55.
Wallace, Marina and Martin Kemp (2000), *Spectacular Bodies: The Art and Science of the Human Body from Leonardo to Now*, Berkeley: University of California Press.
Walsh, Sue (2015), 'The Recuperated Materiality of Disability and Animal Studies', in Karín Lesnik-Oberstein (ed.), *Rethinking Disability Theory and Practice*, 20–36, London: Palgrave Macmillan.

Walvin, James (1997), *Fruits of Empire: Exotic Produce and British Taste, 1660–1800*, Basingstoke and London: Macmillan.
Warren, Christian (1997), 'Northern Chills, Southern Fevers: Race-Specific Mortality in American Cities 1730–1900', *The Journal of Southern History*, 63 (1): 23–56.
Watts, Sydney (2011), 'Enlightened Fasting. Religious Conviction, Scientific Inquiry, and Medical Knowledge in Early Modern France', in Ken Albala and Trudy Eden (eds), *Food and Faith in Christian Culture*, 105–22, New York and Chichester: Columbia University Press.
Wear, Andrew (1989), 'Medical Practice in Late Seventeenth- and Early Eighteenth-Century England: Continuity and Union', in Roger French and Andrew Wear (eds), *The Medical Revolution of the Seventeenth Century*, 294–320, Cambridge: Cambridge University Press.
Wear, Andrew (2000), *Knowledge and Practice in English Medicine 1550–1680*, Cambridge: Cambridge University Press.
Wear, Andrew (2008), 'Place, Health, and Disease: The *Airs, Waters, Places* Tradition in Early Modern England and North America', *Journal of Medieval and Early Modern Studies*, 38 (3): 443–65.
Weisser, Olivia (2015), *Ill-Composed: Sickness, Gender, and Belief in Early Modern England*, New Haven: Yale University Press.
Wenger, Alexandre (2007), *La fibre littéraire. Discours médical sur la lecture au XVIIIe siècle*, Geneva: Droz.
Westerman, Frank (2004), *El Negro en ik*, Amsterdam: Atlas.
Weston, Robert (2013), *Medical Consulting by Letter in France, 1665–1789*, Farnham: Ashgate.
Wheeler, Roxanne (2000), *The Complexion of Race: Categories of Difference in Eighteenth Century British Culture*, Philadelphia: University of Pennsylvania Press.
White, Sara (2012), 'Crippling the Archives: Negotiating Notions of Disability in Appraisal and Arrangement and Description', *The American Archivist*, 75 (1): 109–24.
Whitterridge, Gweneth (1971), *William Harvey and the Circulation of the Blood*, London: Macdonald.
Wild, Wayne (2000) 'Doctor–Patient Correspondence in 18th Century Britain: A Change in Rhetoric and Relationship" in Erwin Mostfai (ed.), *Studies in the 18th Century Culture*, 47–64, Baltimore and London: John Hopkins University Press.
Wild, Wayne (2006), *Medicine-by-Post: The Changing Voice of Illness in XVIIIth century British Consultation Letters and Literature*, Amsterdam and New York: Rodopi.
Williams, Carolyn D. (2006), 'Bestiality in Eighteenth-Century English Literature: "The Dev'l himself is in that Mare"', *British Journal for Eighteenth-Century Studies*, 29 (2): 271–84.
Williams, Elizabeth (2012) 'Sciences of Appetite in the Enlightenment, 1750–1800', *Studies in History and Philosophy of Biological and Biomedical Sciences*, 43 (2): 392–404.
Wilson, Kathleen (2003), *The Island Race: Englishness, Empire and Gender in the Eighteenth Century*, New York: Routledge.
Wilson, Lindsay (1993), *Women and Medicine in the French Enlightenment: The Debate Over 'Maladies des Femmes'*, Baltimore and London: Johns Hopkins University Press.
Winston, Michael E. (2005), *From Perfectibility to Perversion: Meliorism in Eighteenth-Century France*, New York: Peter Lang.

Wise, M. Norton and Crosbie Smith (1990), 'Work and Waste: Political Economy and Natural Philosophy in Nineteenth-Century Britain (III)', *History of Science*, 28 (3): 221–61.

Withers, A. J. (2012), 'Disableism within Animal Advocacy and Environmentalism', in Anthony J. Nocella II, Judy K. C. Bentley and Janet M. Duncan (eds), *Earth, Animal, and Disability Liberation: The Rise of the Eco-ability Movement*, 111–25, New York: Peter Lang.

Withey, Alun (2011), *Physick and the Family: Health, Medicine and Care in Wales, 1600–1757*, Manchester: Manchester University Press.

Woods, Abigail, Michael Bresalier, Angela Cassidy and Rachel Mason Dentinger (2018), 'Introduction: Centring Animals Within Medical History', in Abigail Woods, Michael Bresalier, Angela Cassidy and Rachel Mason Dentinger (eds), *Animals and the Shaping of Modern Medicine: One Health and Its Histories*, 1–26, London: Palgrave Macmillan.

Wolfe, Charles T. (2017), 'Boundary Crossings: The Blurring of the Human/Animal Divide as Naturalization of the Soul in Early Modern Philosophy', in Stefanie Buchenau and Roberto Lo Presti (eds), *Human and Animal Cognition in Early Modern Philosophy and Medicine*, 147–72, Pittsburgh: University of Pittsburgh Press.

Wolloch, Nathaniel (2019), *The Enlightenment's Animals: Changing Conceptions of Animals in the Long Eighteenth Century*, Amsterdam: Amsterdam University Press.

Yancy, George (2008), 'Colonial Gazing: The Production of the Body as "Other"', *Western Journal of Black Studies*, 32 (1): 1–15.

Young, Robert Maxwell (1970), *Mind, Brain, and Adaptation in the Nineteenth Century: Cerebral Localization and Its Biological Context from Gall to Ferrier*, Oxford: Oxford University Press.

Young, Robert (1990), *Mind, Brain and Adaptation in the Nineteenth Century*, Oxford: Oxford University Press.

Zola, Irvin K. (1973), 'Pathways to the Doctor: From Person to Patient', *Social Sciences and Medicine*, 7 (9): 677–89.

Zuffi, Stefano (2012), *Color in Art*, New York: Abrahams.

CONTRIBUTORS

Roger Cooter is a cultural historian of science and medicine and the general editor of Bloomsbury's *A Cultural History of Medicine* series. He has authored and edited over twenty books on subjects ranging from phrenology to orthopaedics, war, childhood and historiography. His latest book, *The Man Who Ate His Cats*, is soon to be published. Now retired from University College London in the UK, he lives in Berlin.

Angela Haas is an associate professor of history at Missouri Western State University, USA. Her research focuses on the history of religion, print and medicine in eighteenth-century France. She has published on religious conflicts, miracles and medical marvels during the Enlightenment and French Revolution. She is currently working on a book titled *Miracles in the Press: Religious Authority and Intellectual Autonomy in Enlightenment France*.

Marieke M.A. Hendriksen is a researcher at the NL-Lab, part of the Humanities Cluster of the Royal Netherlands Academy of Arts and Sciences, the Netherlands. She is a historian of knowledge, whose main research interests are materiality and the senses, particularly taste, in eighteenth-century medicine and chemistry. Marieke is the author of *Elegant Anatomy* (2015), and she has published widely on the material and sensory culture of eighteenth-century arts and sciences.

Micheline Louis-Courvoisier is a historian and professor at the Faculty of Medicine and vice-rector of the University of Geneva, Switzerland. Her research focuses on epistolary consultations, the experience of suffering, and the articulation between the somatic and the psychological in the eighteenth century. She has published on melancholy and the physiopsychological universe of the sick. Her most recent article was on 'Inquiétude/Uneasiness: Between Mental Emotion and Bodily Sensation (18th–20th centuries)' (2019).

Monica Mattfeld is an assistant professor at the University of Northern British Columbia, Canada, in the Departments of English and History. Her research interests focus on animal studies, the history and literature of animal rights and disability, and gender in the English long eighteenth century. She has published on masculinity, performing animals and the early circus. Her most recent publication, *Horse Breeds and Human Society* (2019), is co-edited with Kristen Guest.

Lina Minou holds a research fellow post at University College London, UK, studying the experience of waiting for care. Her main research interests relate to health humanities and the ways insights from the history of medicine can help shape contemporary discussions about issues in healthcare. Part of her recently published work, which appeared in *Cultural History* (April 2019), focuses on suffering, emotion and compassionate language in eighteenth-century incarceration narratives.

Lisa Wynne Smith is a senior lecturer at the University of Essex, UK. She is writing a monograph on gender, health and the household in eighteenth-century England and France. She has published widely on domestic medical caregiving, pain, infertility and masculinity, and she is a founding co-editor of *The Recipes Project* collaborative blog (2012). Her recent publications look at Hans Sloane and masculinity, an Irish caesarean operation, and silence and family trauma.

E.C. Spary is a reader in the history of modern European knowledge at the University of Cambridge, UK, in the Faculty of History. Her books include *Feeding France: New Sciences of Food, 1760–1815* (2014), *Eating the Enlightenment: Food and the Sciences in Paris* (2012) and *Utopia's Garden: French Natural History from Old Regime to Revolution* (2000). She is currently at work on a study of drug-taking in the reign of Louis XIV.

Erin Spinney is a sessional lecturer at the University of Lethbridge and affiliated with the Department of History at Mount Allison University, Canada. Her research interests focus on nursing, labour and medical history in the long-eighteenth-century British Empire. She has published on eighteenth-century naval nursing and environmental history.

Claudia Stein is an associate professor at Warwick University, UK. The author of *Negotiating the French Pox in Early Modern Germany* (2009), she co-wrote several of the essays in Roger Cooter's *Writing History in the Age of Biomedicine* (2013). She is the co-editor, with Elaine Leong, of Volume 3 of Bloomsbury's *Cultural History of Medicine in the Renaissance* (2021). Her current work is on the cultural history of human nature.

INDEX

'A PARODY on a MODERN PUFF', 92–5, 98
abattement, 144–5, **145**
ableism, 79, 84, 95, 99
abolitionism, 95, 96
acclimatization, 23–4
Actor-Network-Theory, 104
Adams, Thomas, 58–9, 60, 62
aesthesis, 129–30, 131
Africanness, 11n1
Agamben, Giorgio, 75, 88
agency, patients, 7
Albinus, Bernard Siegfried, 119
alchemy, 110
allergies, 78
Alpers, Svetlana, 104
anatomical preparations, 117–9
anatomists, 110–6, 122
anatomy, study of, 110–6, **114**
anctorius, 39, **40**
anger, 55, 61, 65, **66**, 71
animal rationality, 81–5
animal research, 74
animal spirits theory, 126–7, 144, 154
animal studies, 76–8
animal turn, the, 76
animal welfare, 95, 96
animality
    and communication abilities, 80–5
    The Deaf and Dumb Man's Discourse, The (Sibscota), 80–5
    the deaf and mute, 79–87
    and disability, 73–102
    and human uniqueness, 100, 102
    and humanity, 90–1
    and monstrosity, 87–8, **89**, 90–102, **100, 101**
    objectifying gaze, 73
animalization, 84
animals, communication abilities, 80–5
anthropocentric absolutism, 74
anthropology, 156
apothecary handbooks, 109
apothecary jar, 103, 106–7, **107**, 122
Appadurai, Arjun, 104
appetite, 29
Arbuthnot, Dr John, 31, 35
Aristotle, 80, 81
army diseases, 18–9
Arthy, Elliot, 26
Augustine, St, 86
authority, 6

Bacon, Francis, 153
Banier, Antoine, 40–1
Banks, Sir Joseph, 2
Barker-Benfield, Graham, 68
Bashford, Alison, 16
Baxandall, Michael, 104
Beatty, Heather, 66, 68, 131
Bede, 86
Benedict, Barbara, 87

Benedict XIV, Pope, 174–5
Berty, Nigon de, 178–9
bestiality, 98
birthing models, 119–21, **120**
blackness, 11n1, 25–7
Blagrave, Jonathan, 59
Blane, Gilbert, 21, 25, 25–6
blood, circulation of, 61
bodily consistency, changes in, 144–5, **145**, 146
body, the, 11
   aberrant, 88
   alternative, 75
   assumptions about, 13
   concepts of, 61
   fibre, 64–5, 142
   historicity of, 133
   mechanical theories, 61–2
   and mind, 55, 143, 151
   and monstrosity, 87–8, **89**, 90–102, **100**, **101**
   racialized, 17
Boerhaave, Herman, 48, 61–2, 67–8
botany, 38
Bound Alberti, Fay, 52–3, 61, 72
Bourke, Joanna, 129–30, 131
Bouvier, Marie-André-Joseph, 188
Boyle, Robert, 37, 74
brain, the
   biologization, 166–8
   and mind distinction, 151–2
Branson, Jan, 80
British Museum, Enlightenment Gallery, 1, **2**, 3–5, 10
Brockliss, Lawrence, 172
Brooks, Thomas, 59
Broomhall, Susan, 171
Brown, Michael, 53, 72
Brown, Theodore, 51
Buchan, William, 18, 20, 21, 70
Buchenau, Stefanie, 74
Buc'hoz, Pierre, **36**
Buffon, Georges-Louis Leclerc Compte de, 102

Cadiz, yellow fever epidemic (1797), 25–6
Camper, Petrus, 116
cancer, 59
cardiac disease, 55
Carrera, Elena, 61

Cavallo, Sandra, 62, 64
cenesthesic chaos, 142
Chang, Ku-ming, 109–10
Charle, Jeanne, 185
cheerfulness, 64
Cheyne, Dr George, 35, 38–9, 42, 163
chocolate, 35
Chomel, Jean-Baptiste, 35
chymistry, 35, 37–8
class, 7, 14, 95, 121
   and disability, 88, 93
   and Enlightenment, 156–7
   and food, 29, 42, 45–7
   and letter-writing, 127. 146
   and nervous disorders, 131
   and self-regulation, 30, 31, 33
   and Sir Hans Sloane, 4
classical medicine 29, 31–3, 80–1, 162
classification
   sick, of the, 22
   nurses, of, 27
   food, of, 34
   animals, of, 75, 82–3, 91, 100
Clement XI, Pope, 175
Clever, Iris, 8
Clossy, Samuel, 69
Cocchi, Antonio, 41–2, 42
coffee, **33**, 35, 37, 46
cogito, ergo sum, 154
communication abilities, 80–5
comparative anatomy, 74, 162–3
compassion, 57, 70–1, 71, 140–1
compassionate care, 70
Condillac, Abbé de, 156
Congregation of Rites, 174
conjectural history, 160–1
consciousness, 154
consumption, 57–9, 62
contagion, 15–6, **16**, 18, 19
Cook, Harold, 171
Cook, Captain James, 43
Coquillard, Isabelle, 171
corpse medicine, 107, 109
Coudray, Angélique Marguerite du, 119–20
cranioscopie, 166
criminals, treatment, 74
Cullen, William, 131
cultural historians, 9
cultural meaning, 9

Cunningham, Andrew, 11
Curran, Andrew, 11n1
Curtin, Philip, 17

Daston, Lorraine, 173
Davis, Lennard J., 78, 79, 85, 87, 92
Deaf and Dumb Man's Discourse, The (Sibscota), 80–5
deaf and mute, the 79–87
  categorized as animal, 86
  communication abilities, 80–5
  education, 85–6
deformity
  and animality, 73–102
  animalization, 84
  and communication abilities, 80–5
  the deaf and mute, 79–87
  desire/disgust binary, 92–3, 98
  institutionalization, 86
  medicalization, 86
  and monstrosity, 87–8, **89**, 90–102, **100**, **101**
  objectifying gaze, 73
Descartes, René, 153–5, **153**
Desgranges, Jean-Baptiste, 185
Devillers, Charles, 188
d'Halgouet, Le Comte, 137, 139
Diderot, Denis, 179
diet. *see* food and diet
dietetic manuals, 32–4, **32**, **33**
dietetics, 31–2
disability
  and animal studies, 76–8
  and animality, 73–102
  animalization, 84
  and communication abilities, 80–5
  the deaf and mute, 79–87
  definition, 79
  desire/disgust binary, 92–3, 98
  discourses, 73–4
  institutionalization, 86
  language of, 79
  medicalization, 86
  and monstrosity, 87–8, **89**, 90–102, **100**, **101**
  objectifying gaze, 73
  and sexuality, 92–3
  visibility, 79
disability studies, 77–8
disciplinary spaces, 29, 42–3, 48

disease
  army, 18–9
  connection to emotion, 51–72
  definition, 61–2, 67–8
  holistic view of, 55
  humoral theory, 23–4 53–4, 57–60, **58**, 61, 113
  language of, 67–71
  nervous disorders, 64–6, 131, 163–4
  physiological understanding, 60–2, 64
  psychosomatic view, 66
  role of emotions, 52–3
dissection, 110
Dobson, Mary, 25
doctor–patient relationship, 125–6
Dodart, Denis, 39
Donne, John, 133
Douglas, G. A., 164
Duden, Barbara, 8, 133
Dunton, John, 86
dynamics, 61
dysentery, 27

East India Company, 22
economic bread, 42
Eichberg, Stephanie, 74
elephants, 82, **82**
embodiment, 8, 10
  internal movements, violence of, 142–4, 146
emotional communities, 52
emotional regime, 52
emotions, 8, **56**, **126**, 143
  anger, 55, 61, 65, **66**, 71–2
  beneficial, 65
  connection to disease, 51–72
  dangerousness, 59
  envy, 57–60, **58**, 60–1, 62, 71
  history of, 51–2, 55
  humoral theory, 53–4, 57–60, **58**, 61
  joy, 62, **63**, 64
  language of, 55, 67–71
  and mental disease, 51
  and nervous disorders, 64–6
  physiological understanding, 60–2, 64
  policing, 52
  political aspects of, 52
  role in surgery, 53
  role of, 52–3
Enlightenment ideals, 54

Enlightenment project, the, 5–6
environment, 13, 13–28, **14**
   definition, 14–7, **15**
   and health, 13–4
   hospitals, 15
   indoor, 13
   indoor/outdoor division, 15
   tropical regions, 17
envy, 57–60, **58**, 60–1, 62, 71
eyesight, 140

Falconer, William, 56, 62
femininity, 92, 94–5, 157–8, 160, 162, 178
Fergusson, William, 17, 19, 22, 24, 25, 27
fibre body, the, 64–5, 142
fibre medicine, 65, 141–2
fibrillar suffering, 141–2
Fiering, Norman, 70
Fissell, Mary, 52, 171
Fol, Madame, 125, 126, 140, 141, 143
food and diet, 29–50
   balance, 35
   dietetic manuals, 32–4, **32**, **33**
   fashionable, 35
   French cuisine, 36–7
   healthy, 29, 34
   and identity, 36
   and labour, 30
   low regimen, 38–9
   moral themes, 39–42
   nutrition transition, 35–6
   and political radicalism, 42
   politicization, 29
   precepts, 31–8
   and public health, 43–8
   reform, 38, 38–48, 48–9
   self-regulation, 29
   supply management, 46–7, 48
   vocabulary, 31
food chemistry, 29, 37–8
foodways, 35–8
Fordyce, William, 20
Forrester, James, 165
Forster, William, 65, 67
Foucault, Michel, 8–9, 29, 30, 170
Franc, Anne Le, 177
France, 11n1, 45–6
freak shows, 87–8
Frederick the Great, King of Prussia, 38, 46

French, Roger, 11
French cuisine, 36–7
Frevert, Ute, 68
Fudge, Erica, 76, 78
fumigation, 21

Galen, 111
Gall, Franz Joseph, 166–8, **167**
gender, 7, 10, 88, 95, 157, 168, 171
Genette, Gerard, 57, 67
Gentilcore, David, 171
Gil Sotres, Pedro, 61
Gillray, James, 99, **100**
Godineau, Dominique, 131
governance, 45
Greater Caribbean, 13–4, **14**, 17
Gregory, John, 162–3, 166
Grosz, Elizabeth, 87
Guélon, Louise, 190–1
Guerrini, Anita, 87, 112–3

Hacking, Ian, 106
Hallam, Elizabeth, 111
Haller, Albrecht von, 64, 68, 127, 156
Handley, Sasha, 7
Haraway, Donna, 76–7, 78
Harvey, William, 61, 170
Hay, William, 91–2
Hays, Mary, 161
health
   definition, 61–2
   and environment, 13–4
health authorities, 6
health data, collection of, 45
healthy eating, 29
heart, the, 61
Hérault, René, 178
Hill, Sir John, 163
historical materiality, 105
historiography, 5–10, 11
Hobbes, Thomas, 152
Hooker, Claire, 16
hospitals, 13, 15
   design, 17–22
   overcrowding, 19–20
   placement, 17–8, 28
   temperature regulation, 22–3
   ventilation, 19–22, 23, 28
   West Indies, 22–4
Hugony, Jacques, 182–3

human bone, 103–23
    child, 113
    commodification, 110, 116, 123
    display, 117–9, **118**, 122–3
    hidden, 119–22, **120**, 123
    historical context, 121–2, 123
    infant, 113, **114**
    preservation, 110–6, **114**, 122
    starting point, 106
    symbology, 117
    uses, 106–7, **107**, **108**, 109–10, 122
    whiteness, 112, 115
human exceptionalism, hierarchy of, 84
human uniqueness, 100, 102
humanitarian action, 70
humanity
    and animality, 90–1
    nature of, 75–6, 76–7
Hume, David, 155, 157, 160–1
humoral theory, 8, 31, 33–4, 53, 57–60, **58**, 61, 113, 126, 144
hunger, 29
Hunter, William, 112
hydrodynamic physiology, 61
hygiene, 31–2
hypochondria, 37, 70, 141, 163–4, 166
hysteria, 72, 163–4, 177, 182

identity, 36
illness, construction of, 7
imagination, 10, 141, 164–5, 168, 178, 188
Indigenous, 24, 121, 172
industrialization, 30, 48
infection, 15–6
inhumanity, 99
institutionalization, 86
Instructions for the Royal Naval Hospital at Haslar & Plymouth, 20
Instructions to Regimental Surgeons, 19
internationalism, 43
Irish Medical Board, 21
Ishizuka, Hisao, 11, 65, 142

Jackson, Robert, 17, 18
Jackson, Stanley, 64
Jamaica, 13–4, **14**, 22, **23**, 24, 26
Jankovic, Vladimir, 15
Jewson, Nicholas, 6–7
Johnston, Andrew, 134

Jones, Colin, 171, 172
Jordanova, Ludmilla, 105
Journal de médecine, 185, 186
joy, 62, **63**, 64

Kafer, Alison, 93
Kant, Immanuel, 38
Keill, James, 39
Kennedy, Meegan, 55
Kiple, Kenneth, 17
Kirmayer, Laurence, 133
kitchens, 34
Knoeff, Rina, 117–8
knowledge, source of, 154–6
Kracauer, Siegfried, 134

labour, and food and diet, 30
language, 79–80
    and animals, 80–5
    of disability, 79
    of disease, 67–71
    of emotions, 55, 67–71
    semantic ambiguity, 132–3
    of suffering, 125, 126, 127, 129, 131–3, 146
Latour, Bruno, 104, 106
Le Clerc, Charles-Gabriel, 39
Lebrun, François, 170
Leiden anatomical theatre, 117, 119, 120–1
Lelli, Ercole, **118**, 119
Lemnius, Levinus, 59, 60
Lempriere, William, 22–3
Lind, James, 21
Linnaeus, Carolus, 37, 75, 100
Lloyd, G. E. R., 13
Lo Presti, Roberto, 74
Locke, John, 152–6, 157, 164–5, 166
Louis-Courvoisier, Micheline, 8
Luyendijk-Elshout, Anthonie M., 62
Lynch, Bernard, 65
Lyser, Michael, 111–3, 116, 122, 123

McClive, Cathy, 8, 172, 180
McKeown, Thomas, 170
McNeill, J. R., 25
McTavish, Lianne, 171
Magalhães, João Jacinto de, 43
malaria, 25, 27
Malthus, Thomas, 46

Margócsy, Dániel, 119
Marland', Hilary, 171
marriage, 160–1
Marseille, plague of 1720, **15**
marshes, 17–8
Martin, Geneviève, 182–5, 186
masculinity, 88, 98–9, 164–5, 171–2
Massaron, Marie, 179
masturbation, 164
materia medica, 107, 110, 116
material turn, the, 8, 104–5
materiality, 8, 103–4, 106, 111, 121
mechanical physiology, 61
medical authority, 169–92
    alternative vision, 191–2
    debunking of medical marvels, 181–6
    defence of, 182–6, 191
    dispersal, 173
    frustration with, 169–70
    lay, 34, 132, 171, 182, 188
    legal, 172
    mesmerism debate, 186–92, **187**, **189**
    miracles debate, 174–81, **176**, 183
    nurses, 20, 27
    power dynamics, 172
    professionalization, 170
    rejection of, 186–92
    and reliability of testimony, 180–1, 181–6
    shared, 171
    social history approach, 170–1
    unreliability, 186
    women, 171–2, 180
medical bureaucracy, 48
medical interactions, 7
medical marketplace, the, 171
medical marvels, debunking of, 181–6
medical models, 117, 119–22, **120**
medical police, 46
medical revolution, 54–5
medullary oil, 112, 115, 123
Mendelssohn, Moses, 38
mental disease, 51, 88, 167
Mesmer, Franz Anton, 186–92, **187**
mesmerism, 186–92, **187**, **189**
miasma, 15–6
midwives, 171
military and naval medicine, 17, 18–9, 20–1, 28
    West Indies, 22–7

Miller, Don, 80
mind, 151–68
    biologization, 166–8
    and the body, 55, 143, 151
    and brain distinction, 151–2
    consciousness, 154
    educability of, 156
    Locke's conception of, 152–6
    and thinking, 151
    women, 156–65
miracles, 173–4, 174–81, **176**, 183, 188, 189–90, 191
    reliability of testimony, 180–1
    verification process, 176–7, 178, 178–9
modernity, 8
Mol, Annemarie, 8
monism, 133
monomania, 72
Monro, Alexander, 74
Monro, Donald, 21
monstrosity, 87–8, **89**, 90–102, **100**, **101**
    attractiveness, 91, 92
    charlatanism, 95–6
    desire/disgust binary, 92–3, 98
    eroticized, 92–8
    intellectual fascination, 90
    latent negative aspects, 91–2
    objectification, 93
Monstrous Craws, The, 88, **89**, 90–1, 93–9
Montjoie, Galart de, 190
moral geography, 9
moral themes, food and diet, 39–42
morality, 117–8, 152, 154–5
morality and gender, 158–61
morality and monstrosity, 87, 92, 94, 989
morality and nation, 37
Morand, Jean-François-Clément, 182–4, 191
Moreau, Edmond Thomas, 163
mortality, 38, 170
Moscoso, Javier, 130
mosquitos, 23
movement, excessive, 61
movements, **126**

natural, the, 157–8
natural rights, 159
naturalization, 173
Nazi Germany, 78
nerves, theory of, 127

nervous disorders, 64–6, 131, 163–4
nervous system, 64, 70, 127, **128**
neurophysiology, 61
Neveux, Julie, 133
Newman, Simon, 17
Newton, Hannah, 69
Newton, Sir Isaac, 1, 61
Noble, Louise, 107, 109
Nocella II, Anthony J., 77
non-naturals, doctrine of the, 55, 65
Nougaret, Jean-Baptiste, 188
nurses
    black, 25–7, 28
    ventilation duties, 20–2
nutrition science, 30
nutrition transition, 35–6, 48
    foreign foodways, 35–8

obesity, 39–40, **41**, 49
objects, as actors, 103–6
Orta, Garcia de, 82–3
osteogenesis, 113
Outram, Dorinda, 157–8, 161–2
Ovid, *Metamorphoses*, 40–1, 59

pain, 8, 67, 130, **136**, 137, **138**, 139, 142, **153**, 155
Pallison, William, 19–20
paratexts, 57, 67
Pâris, François de, 175–7, **176**, 190, 191
Park, Katherine, 173
Parmentier, Antoine-Augustin, 45–6
Pasley, Gilbert, 22
pathology, 59, 62, 65, 69, 72, 113
patients, agency, 7
Paulli, Simon, 112
Paxton, Peter, 69
Pelling, Margaret, 15–6
Pepys, Samuel, 83–4
pharmaceutics, human bone, 106–7, **107**, **108**, 109–10
pharmacopoeias, 35, 109
Philosophical Transactions (Royal Society), 2
phrenology, 166, **167**
physicians, position, 69
Pigalle, Marie-Anne, 169
Pigeaud, Jackie, 141
Pilloud, Séverine, 129
plague preventive costume, **16**
Pliny, 80

Plutarch, 80, 81
Pole, Thomas, 113–6, 122, 123
political radicalism, 42
politicization, food and diet, 29
Pollock, Linda, 130
Poole, Joshua, 59
poor management, 47–8
poor relief programmes, 46–7
Pope, Alexander, 10
popular belief, 5, 73, 152, 157, 164–5, 173–4, 177–8, 180, 182
Porter, Roy, 7, 9, 53, 171
postmodernism, 7, 9
poststructuralism, 7–8
Powell, Jacob, **41**
Power, 8, 30, 49
power dynamics, 53, 172
pregnancy, 8
preternatural, the, 173–4, 186, 191
preventative care, 62
Pringle, John, 18–9, 20–1
probability theory, 6
productivity, 6
professionalization, 54–5, 170
progress narrative, 5–10
public health, 6
    and food and diet, 43–8
Puckrein, Gary, 17
putrefaction, 19, 22

Quincy, John, 109
Qureshi, Sadiah, 91

race, 14, 17, 24–7, 98, 121
racialized medicine, 24–7
racism, 78
Ramsey, Matthew, 170
rationality, 8, 11, 81, 152
    animal, 81–5
Raw-head and Bloody-bones, 164–5
reason, 5–6, 8, 10, 74, 81–2, 84–6, 152–8, 163–5, 173, 188
reasoning, 153
Reddy, William, 52
regulation, lack of, 171
religion, 35, 81, 85–6, 90, 96, 151, 155, 175, 178, 179, 180
    Jansenism, 175–80, **176**, 190
    Roman Catholic Church, miracles debate, 174–81, **176**

Rieder, Philip, 132, 143, 171
Rijksmuseum Boerhaave, **118**, 120, **120**
Rosenwein, Barbara, 52
Rotalier. Le Chevalier de, 137
Rousseau, George, 163–4
Rousseau, Jean-Jacques, 42, 157, 159–60, 161, 162
Roussel, Pierre, 163
Rowlandson, Thomas, 99, **101**
Rowley, William, 69
Royal Society (London), 1–2, 80, 87, 153
Ruberg, Willemijn, 8
Rumford, Benjamin Thompson, Count, 43–5, **44**
Ruysch, Frederik, 112, 117–8

St Domingo expedition, 1815, 27
Saint-Médard controversy, 175–80, **176**, 188, 189, 191
Salomon, Gotllieb, 120–1
Schiebinger, Londa, 162
Scientific Revolution, 170
Scott, Joan, 131–2
scurvy, 19, 42–3
seasoning, 23–4, **23**
secular improvement, emphasis on, 38
secularism, 11
secularization, 173
self-regulation, 29, 31, 38, 46
Semonin, Paul, 87
senses, the, 125–6
    disturbances of, 140–1
sensibility, 11, 64, 66, 67, 68, 127
    culture of, 54, 71
sensual experiences, 155–6
sermons, 57, 70
Seth, Suman, 25
sex differences, 162–6
sexuality, 90, 92–3, 98
Shelley, Percy Bysshe, 42
Sibscota, George, 74, 75–6, 79
    The Deaf and Dumb Man's Discourse, 80–5
Skuse, Alanna, 52, 60
slavery and the slave trade, 4, 10, 24, 26–7
    abolitionism, 95, 96
    biological foundations of, 17
    enslaved people, 11 n.1, 24–7, 121, 156, 172

Sloane, Sir Hans, 1–4, **3**, 7, 11, 24, 109, 131, 163–4
    catalogue of fossils, **108**
    medical practice, 2–3
    removed from pedestal, 10
    trade card, **4**
smell, 17–8, 60
Smellie, William, 120
Smith, Lisa, 55, 67, 137, 168
social change, and medical intervention, 9
social status, 7, 14, 95, 121
    and disciplinary spaces, 30, 44, 47–8, 167
    and disease, 18
    and medical practitioners, 172
    and miracles, 177–8
    royalty, 93–5
Sondes, Lady Catherine, 163–4
soul, the, 154
Spary, E.C., 9
Spierenburg, Peter, 70
Spurzheim, Johann, 166, 168
Starobinski, Jean, 131
static medicine, 39–40
Stewart, Mart A., 17
stillrooms, 34
Stolberg, Michael, 54
Storey, Tessa, 62, 64
suffering, experience of, 125–47, **126**
    act of writing, 135–9, 146
    biases, 145–6
    changes in bodily consistency, 144–5, **145**, 146
    comparisons, 132, 140–1
    condensation, 145–6
    definition, 129–30
    disturbances of the senses, 140–1
    estrangement, 134
    fibrillar, 141–2
    importance of, 132
    importance of detail, 138–9
    intensification, 146
    language, 125, 126, 127, 129, 131–3, 146
    metaphors, 132
    narrative detail, 138–9
    narrative readings, 133–5
    narrative sources, 129–33
    operative machinery, 141
    pain, **136**, 137, **138**, 139

INDEX

sensations, 139–45
troubles of the flesh, 141–5
violence of internal movements, 142–4, 146
writing triggers, 136–8
Sugg, Richard, 107, 109, 133
supernatural, the, 164–5, 173–4, 179–80, 182–4, 186, 191
superstition, 5, 73, 152, 157, 164–5, 173–4, 177–8, 180, 182
surgery, role of emotions, 53
Sutton, John, 144
Sweden, 37
symbology, human bone, 117
sympathetic identification, 70–1
sympathetic medicine, 109–10
sympathy, 69, 70
taxidermy, 121, 123
Taylor, Sunaura, 73, 76, 78, 87
tea, 35
temperance, 45
temperature regulation, hospitals, 22–3
Thatcher Ulrich, Laurel, 104
thinking, 151, 152, 154
Thompson, Benjamin, 43–5, 44
Thomson, Rosemarie Garland, 88
Thouret, Michel-Augustin, 189, 190–1
Tissot, Samuel-Auguste-André-David, 46–7, 69, 125, 129, 131, 137–8, 139, 146
Todd, Dennis, 87, 91
Torrid Zone, the, 13–4, 14
tropical regions, environment, 17, 22
Turner, David, 79
typhus, 19
unnaturalness, 60
unwashed masses, the, 18
urbanization, 48
Vasset, Sophie, 132
vegetarianism, 38, 40–2
venereal diseases, 70
ventilation, 15, 19–22, 23, 28
ventilators, 19
Vermij, Rienk, 110
Verreaux, Jean Baptiste Édouard, 121, 123
Verreaux, Jules Pierre, 121, 123
Vesalius, Andreas, 111, 162, 170
Vigarello, Georges, 126
Vila, Anne, 11, 69–70, 127, 180
Vintimille, Charles Galpard Guillaume de, 177–8
vision-related disturbances, 140
vitalism, 109–10, 127
Vury de Remiremont, La Comtesse de, 137
Walsh, Sue, 77
Wear, Andrew, 55
Weisser, Olivia, 7
Wesley, John, 38, 42
West Indies, 22–7, 28
West-Pavlov, Russell, 134
White, William, 23
whiteness, 5–6, 10, 17, 27, 105, 156
Williams, Carolyn, 98–9
Willich, Anthony F. M., 60–1, 62, 64, 65
Willis, Thomas, 61
Wilson, Lindsay, 172, 174
Wollstonecraft, Mary, 157, 161
women, 6
 bodily experiences, 8
 brain size, 168
 conjectural history, 160–1
 control arrangements, 158
 deformity, 88, 90–3
 masturbation, 164
 medical evidence of difference, 162–6
 medical practices, 171–2
 mind, 156–65
 moral superiority, 161
 natures and natural place, 156–61, 159
 as the Other, 158, 160
 reliability of testimony, 180–1, 181–6
 role, 158–61
 sexual appetites, 164
 status, 157
Woods, Abigail, 76
workhouse reform, 44–5
yellow fever, 25–7